COLON AND RECTAL CANCER

Protocols in General Surgery

PROTOCOLS IN GENERAL SURGERY

SERIES EDITOR

JONATHAN M. SACKIER, M.D.

COLON AND RECTAL CANCER

VOLUME EDITOR

PETER S. EDELSTEIN, M.D.
Assistant Professor of Surgery
Stanford University School of Medicine
Stanford, CA, U.S.A.

WILEY-LISS

A JOHN WILEY & SONS, INC., PUBLICATION
New York • Chichester • Weinheim • Brisbane • Singapore • Toronto

This book is printed on acid-free paper. ♾

Published simultaneously in Canada.

For ordering and customer service, call 1-800-CALL WILEY.

Library of Congress Cataloging-in-Publication Data

Colon and rectal cancer / edited by Peter S. Edelstein.
p.; cm. - - (Protocols in general surgery)
Includes index.
ISBN 0-471-35145-8 (cloth: alk paper)
1. Colon (Anatomy) - - Cancer. 2. Rectum - - Cancer. I. Edelstein, Peter S. II. Series.
[DNLM: 1. Colonic Neoplasms. 2. Adenocarcinoma. 3. Rectal Neoplasms. WI 529 C7175 2001]
RC280.C6.C6335 2000
616.99′4347 - -dc21 99-462081

Printed in the United States of America.

10 9 8 7 6 5 4 3 2 1

To my teachers, from whom it has been a privilege to learn.
To my residents and students, to whom it is a privilege to teach.
To my wife, who is my greatest privilege.

CONTENTS

FOREWORD

I am one of those privileged to have been a teacher of Peter Edelstein. It was early in his medical career. He was but a junior medical student at the University of Chicago, assigned to do his surgical clerkship at Michael Reese Hospital. He was made a member of Team III and so we met.

I am happy to claim at least partial credit, or blame, for the fact that Peter ended up being a colon and rectal surgeon. I would like to think he still does some things the way we did them together back then—like being gentle and precise in his surgical technique and viewing the patient as a complete person who happens to have a cancer. That he does is reflected in his Preface to this book.

One of the most rewarding things that can happen to a teacher is to watch the future development of a pupil. Over the years, I have been delighted and more than a little bit proud of Peter. This book certainly adds to both these feelings. I am proud to have been his teacher. I am delighted to be his friend.

Integrity and a straightforward manner of writing are hallmarks of this book. The intent of the writing is not to impress with vaunted knowledge, but rather to truly educate, presenting data that is concise, readable, and imminently practical. The purpose of this book is to impart wisdom, not just provide information. The hope is that this wisdom will translate into critical patient care decisions that favorably impact the outcome for every colon and rectal cancer patient treated by the reader.

Ernestine Hambrick, M.D.
F.A.S.C.R.S., F.A.C.S., F.A.C.G

Founder and Chairman
STOP Colon/Rectal Cancer Foundation

PREFACE

One problem with the majority of texts discussing colorectal cancer is just that: they address colorectal cancer as if it were a single entity. But as we have learned more and more about the natural history and pathophysiology of large bowel cancers, it has become increasingly clear that maglignancies developing in the colon and those originating in the rectum must be viewed differently. Thus unique approaches are required when evaluating, treating, and following patients suffering from cancers arising in these two different sites. But two major advances have truly allowed for the development of distinct pathways in approaching colon and rectal tumors: first, the tremendous improvements that have occurred in endorectal ultrasonography, allowing for much more accurate staging of rectal tumors and surrounding lymph nodes; and second, the increasing variety in treatment options for rectal cancers of differing stages. Thus, although there have been few major advances to aid in the treatment of patients suffering from cancer of the colon, the evaluation and treatment options for patients suffering from rectal cancer continue to expand. No longer does a middle or distal rectal cancer always demand an abdominoperineal resection with a permanent colostomy. Nor do proctectomy patients who require irradiation need to undergo this adjuvant treatment after they have undergone resection, subsequently radiation damage to their neorectum with the associated worsening of bowel function and quality of life. With appropriate pretreatment staging, rectal cancer patients may now be accurately selected for one of a number of treatments aimed at curing their disease while generating the least morbidity and lowest risk of local and distant malignant recurrence.

Thus it is with these advances in mind that this work clearly separates colorectal cancer into two distinct entities. Patient presentation, evaluation, treatment, and follow-up in those haboring adenocarcinoma of the colon are addressed in chapters 7, 8, and 10, and similar topics are presented separately in relation to patients suffering from adenocarcinoma of the rectum (chapters 11 through 15). The first six chapters address issues applicable to both colon and rectal neoplasms, including a general introduction to genetics, polyps, preventative screening, and a variety of syndromes associated with an elevated risk of large bowel malignancy. Likewise, two later chapters discuss common issues, adjuvant therapy, and metastatic disease. Finally, chapter 17 presents current views regarding the role of laparoscopic surgery in cancer therapy, and chapter 18 addresses less common malignancies of the colon and rectum.

All chapters have been written with the practicing health care professional in mind. The focus of the work is clearly clinical, and every attempt has been made to keep the sections brief but clear. At the end of each chapter is a reference list for those readers wishing to delve more deeply into a specific topic. But the overriding theme of this book is to be of practical value and rapidly useful both to practitioners who only occasionally and to those who frequently encounter patients suffering from these all-to-common malignancies.

At times some of this work may seem cynical or even nihilistic, especially the sections discussing post-treatment patient follow-up. However, it is important to fully and objectively evalute the utility and value of all pretreatment and post-treatment studies, especially in this age of limited health are dollars. The testing techniques that fail to demonstrate any significant beneficial effect on our patients should be dropped from "routine" pre-treatment or post-treatment use. Such an approach, offering fewer medical tests, may be difficult, especially for health care providers who often desparately want to "do something" to help their cancer patients. Still, the best way to truly help our patients is to honestly scrutinize our current routines and to create clinical trials that allow us to responsibly evaluate staging, follow-up studies, and treatment modalities for those suffering from cancers of the colon and rectum.

I would like to thank all of the authors, the majority of whom are surgeons board certified in both general surgery and in colon and rectal surgery, others who are dedicated oncologists and gastroenterologists, and all of whom are experts in the field while at the same time being dedicated cancer physicians. Finally, I must thank my academic assistant, Nancy Riewerts, without whose tireless efforts this project would likely not have seen completion.

Peter S. Edelstein, M.D.

Contributors

John D.F. Allendorf, M.D.
Medical Student
Columbia Presbyterian School of Medicine
New York City, NY

Nasser Al-Sanea, M.D.
Surgical Resident
University of Minnesota
Minneapolis, MN

Paul E. Bernick, M.D.
Research Fellow
Memorial Sloan-Kettering Cancer Center
New York City, NY

David Blumberg, M.D.
Assistant Professor of Surgery
University of Pittsburgh Medical Center
Pittsburgh, PA

May C. Chen, M.D.
Postdoctoral Fellow
Stanford University Medical Center
Standford, CA

Bard C. Cosman, M.D.
Assistant Clinical Professor of Surgery
University of California, San Diego
San Diego, CA

ALVARO D. DAVILA, M.D.
Clinical Assistant Professor Medicine
Stanford University School of Medicine
Stanford, CA

MARTA A. DAVILA, M.D.
Assistant Professor of Medicine
Stanford University School of Medicine
Stanford, CA

WAYNE DE VOS, M.D., Ph.D.
Staff Surgeon
Reading Hospital and Medical Center
West Reading, PA

PETER S. EDELSTEIN, M.D.
Assistant Professor of Surgery
Stanford University School of Medicine
Standford, CA

CHARLES O. FINNE III, M.D.
Clinical Associate Professor of Surgery
University of Minnesota
Minneapolis, MN

JAMES M. FORD, M.D.
Assistant Professor of Medicine and Genetics
Stanford University School of Medicine
Standford, CA

JULIO A. GARCIA-AGUILLAR, M.D.
Clinical Associate Professor of Surgery
University of Minnesota Cancer Center
Minneapolis, MN

NEIL R. GLEASON, B.A.
Medical Student
Columbia Presbyterian School of Medicine
New York City, NY

HANNAH-NGOC HA, M.D.
Surgical Resident
University of California at San Diego
San Diego, CA

NIGEL R. HALL, M.D.
Surgical Resident
University of Minnesota
Minneapolis, MN

ALAN F. HORGAN, MBBCH
Surgical Fellow
Mayo Clinic
Rochester, MN

CLIFFORD KO, M.D.
Assistant Clinical Professor of Surgery
UCLA School of Medicine
Los Angeles, CA

EDWARD C. LEE, M.D.
Assistant Professor of Surgery
Albany Medical College
Albany, NY

HENRY T. LYNCH, M.D.
Professor and Chairman
Department of Preventative Medicine and Public Health
Creighton University Medical Center
Omaha, NE

JANE F. LYNCH, B.S.N.
Creighton University Medical Center
Omaha, NE

ROBERT D. MADOFF, M.D.
Clinical Associate Professor
University of Minnesota
Minneapolis, MN

KATHLEEN M. MANNING, M.D.
Surgical Resident
Stanford University School of Medicine
Stanford, CA

JAIME L. MAYORAL, M.D.
Assistant Professor of Surgery
The University of Texas Health Science Center at San Antonio
San Antonio, TX

FRANK G. OPELKA, M.D.
Staff Surgeon
Alton Ochsner Medical Foundation
New Orleans, LO

JOHN H. PEMBERTON, M.D.
Professor of Surgery
Mayo Clinic
Rochester, MN

PATRICIA L. ROBERTS, M.D.
Assistant Clinical Professor of Surgery
Tuffs School of Medicine
Lahey Clinic Medical Center
Burlington, MA

RAYMOND M. SHAHEEN, M.D.
Department of Surgery
Stanford University School of Medicine
Stanford, CA

ANDREW A. SHELTON, M.D.
Clinical Instructor of Surgery
University of Minnesota
Minneapolis, MN

TIMOTHY R. SHOPE, M.D.
Surgical Resident
Albany Medical College
Albany, NY

CHITTAMURU V. SURENDRANATH, M.D.
Staff Surgeon
The University of Texas Health Science Center at San Antonio
San Antonio, TX

RICHARD L. WHELAN, M.D.
Associate Professor of Surgery
Columbia Presbyterian School of Medicine
New York City, NY

W. DOUGLAS WONG, M.D.
Associate Attending Surgeon
Memorial Sloan-Kettering Cancer Center
New York City, NY

Colon and Rectal Cancer

Part

I

Common Issues in Colon and Rectal Cancer

CHAPTER

1

GENETICS AND THE POLYP-CANCER SEQUENCE

N. R. HALL, M.D., AND R. D. MADOFF, M.D.

CANCER IS A GENETIC DISEASE

At the cellular level, cancer is a genetic disease. Appreciation of this fact has revolutionized our understanding of what makes a malignancy. More important, it is the key to new methods of diagnosis, characterization of cancers, and ultimately, to new therapies. Colorectal cancer develops because of accumulation of alterations in certain important genes. These changes may come about as a result of spontaneous mutations or because of exposure to mutagenic agents (e.g., dietary, viral, or bile transported). They may arise in the context of a pre-existing hereditary susceptibility or on a background of chronic disease, such as ulcerative colitis. A degree of genetic instability also appears to be required for sufficient mutations to accumulate to allow progression of the carcinogenic process. This chapter outlines the current understanding of the genetics of the polyp-cancer sequence and its relevance to clinical practice. Although much is now known about the genetic pathways, there remains considerable uncertainty as to the triggers that initiate the process. Thus we can explain the genetic basis, at least in part, of *how*

Colon and Rectal Cancer, Edited by Peter S. Edelstein, M.D.
ISBN 0-471-35145-8

but not *why* cancers develop. For the latter, we must still look to epidemiologic and experimental studies.

GENES AND CANCER

Our genes control the cells that make up our bodies. They regulate growth, division, and death; control the response of the cell to the environment, to its neighbors, and to hormonal messages; and dictate the functional roles of the cell. Above all they are responsible for the maintenance of their own integrity for, without this, the cell loses its identity and becomes a liability to the organism. When a cell no longer responds to normal regulatory processes, starts to grow uncontrollably, and gains the ability to invade and metastasize, then it is malignant and threatens the life of the whole body.

The genetic events that must take place for the development of a cancer are now increasingly well characterized. Colorectal cancer is one of the best understood cancers in this regard, owing to the relatively slow process of transition from adenoma through to carcinoma and the relative ease of sampling polyps for analysis at various stages along that pathway. It has become clear that the phenotypic changes during the adenoma-carcinoma transition may come about through a variety of combinations of many possible genetic events. In broad terms, however, there appear to be only two principle genetic pathways for sporadic colorectal carcinogenesis to occur. These are referred to as the classical and microsatellite instability pathways.

HOW DO GENES WORK?

The DNA of cells is organized into 22 pairs of autosomal chromosomes and 1 pair of sex chromosomes (XX or XY). These contain the 100,000 or so genes that make up the genome. Each autosomal gene is represented by two copies, known as alleles, one inherited from the father and one from the mother. Although each allele of a gene lies at the same particular place (locus) on the maternal and paternal DNA strands, it does not have to be identical to its partner. Subtle differences from the wild-type allele at a locus may produce little or no discernable effect on the gene product and are termed polymorphisms. Other alterations, however, can radically change the way a gene works and lead to disease. Such changes are termed mutations. If one mutated copy is sufficient to cause a phenotypic change on its own then, according to Mendel's terminology, it is dominant. Huntington's disease, polycystic kidneys, and familial adenomatous polyposis are examples of dominant disorders. For recessive alleles to exert a phenotypic effect, both alleles must be mutated. The best known example of a recessive disorder is cystic fibrosis. With respect to carcinogenesis at the cellular level, oncogenes tend to act in a dominant fashion (a single mutated copy is sufficient for activation) whereas tumor-suppressor genes are recessive, requiring two inactivating steps (one on each allele) before function is lost.

Genes exert their influence through the proteins for which they encode. Such proteins may have direct actions (such as exported digestive enzymes or hormones) or function by altering the regulation of the cell's machinery. It is often these regulatory genes that become disordered in cancers. There are many ways in which gene function can change. A mutation of a single base nucleotide (A, C, T, or G) can lead to activation of the gene product. For example, a subtle change in the subsequent protein conformation can result in stronger binding at the active site. This is often the mechanism through which oncogene activation exerts its effects. Alternatively, complete or partial protein inactivation ensues if the genetic change results in a premature stop codon (Fig. 1.1). For many genes, inactivation of one allele still leaves the wild-type allele intact and active. To completely knock out the function of the gene, both alleles must be nonfunctional. When applied to carcinogenesis, genes such as these are termed tumor suppressors. This may happen in a variety

The DNA code consists of four nucleotides (A, C, T and G) arranged in three-letter codons which signal the order and type of amino-acids that make up the protein product. The genetic code can be likened to a sentence comprised of words. This illustration using a four letter codon demonstrates how small changes in the genetic code can have a profound effect on the encrypted message.

THIS DOOR MUST OPEN SOON

A change of a single letter (such as M to R) leads to a mis-sense mutation, with the change staying 'in frame':

THIS DOOR RUST OPEN SOON

A deletion of two letters (such as IS) leads both to a frame-shift (with loss of meaning) and a premature STOP codon:

THDO ORMU STOP

FIGURE 1.1. The genetic code and the effect of mutations.

of ways: through mutation, through deletion of the gene (or even part of the chromosome containing the gene), through abnormal separation of the chromosomes during mitosis (nondisjunction), through wild-type protein inactivation via direct interaction with the abnormal protein (dominant negative effect), or through somatic recombination. Genes implicated in colorectal cancer tumorigenesis are listed in Table 1.1.

Much of the DNA in the cell is not part of the coding regions (exons) of genes. Nevertheless, some of these regions are known to have important regulatory actions. Examples include the promoter regions upstream of the initiation codon, which control gene transcription, and the splice sites before and after each exon, which ensure that the exons are correctly joined during transcription. Alterations in these and other nonexon regions can explain in part why mutations are not always found even if the whole gene is sequenced.

The Polyp-Cancer Sequence

There is a considerable body of evidence to suggest that most if not all colorectal carcinomas develop from adenomatous polyps. This hypothesis serves as the basis for theories concerning the molecular genetics of colorectal carcinogenesis and current strategies for preventative screening. Broadly speaking, evidence for the adenoma-carcinoma sequence can be divided into histologic and epidemiologic.

Early investigators of familial adenomatous polyposis (FAP) could not help but suspect that, in some way, the development of cancer bore a relationship to the many thousands of adenomas that characterize the condition (1). Examination of colonic resections in FAP patients reveals a complete range from single crypt adenomas to invasive carcinomas. In sporadic cancer, about 15% of carcinomas are contiguous with adenomatous elements, suggesting that one might develop from the other. The prevalence of malignancy in polyps seems related to adenoma size, degree of villous content, and severity of dysplasia (2), consistent with the view that adenomas pass through stages of increasing size, villous architecture, and dysplasia during their transformation into malignancies.

Epidemiologic studies have revealed that the prevalence of adenomas (determined at autopsy) approximately mirrors that of colorectal cancer incidence in different populations (3,4). The cumulative incidence curve of adenomas has the same shape as that for cancer but precedes cancer development by at least 5 years (4). Also, the distribution of adenomas in the colon and rectum is similar to that of carcinomas (5). Furthermore, the presence of an adenoma is associated with an increased risk of colorectal cancer. For example, metachronous colorectal cancers are more common if a synchronous adenoma is found at the time of diagnosis of the first colorectal cancer, and the majority of patients with synchronous cancers also have adenomas (3).

The only major longitudinal study of the fate of untreated adenomas is that reported from the Mayo clinic (6). 226 patients with polyps at least 10 mm in diameter were followed for 12 to 229 months by sequential barium enema. A total of 37% of polyps enlarged and 21 lesions, on subsequent removal, were found to have developed cancer. A further 11 cancers developed at remote sites. The overall risk of cancer in the polyps was estimated to be 8% at 10 years and 24% at 20 years. More important, there is now

TABLE 1.1. GENES INVOLVED IN COLORECTAL CARCINOGENESIS

(a) Genes Also Implicated in Hereditary Colorectal Cancer Syndromes

Gene	Chromosomal Site	Syndrome	Protein Function
APC	5q21	FAP	Cell adhesion; apoptosis; repression of *c-myc*
hMSH2	2p16	HNPCC	DNA mismatch repair
hMLH1	3p21		
hPMS1	2q31		
hPMS2	7p22		
hMSH6	2p16		
PTEN	10q23	Familial juvenile polyposis	Tyrosine phosphorylase homology
SMAD4	18q21	Familial juvenile polyposis	Cytoplasmic mediator in TGF-β signaling pathway
LKB1	19p13	Peutz-Jeghers syndrome	Serine threonine kinase
(b) Genes Implicated in Tumorigenesis			
p53	17p13	Tumor suppressor	Cell cycle control, repair of DNA damage (especially from radiation), apoptosis

DCC	18q21	Tumor suppressor	Cell adhesion
MCC	5q21	Tumor suppressor	Unknown
K-*ras*	12p	Oncogenes	GTP binding proteins
N-*ras*	1p		Signal transduction
H-*ras*	11p		
c-*myc*	8q24	Oncogene	DNA synthesis, apoptosis
RII		Tumor suppressor	TGF-β2 receptor gene; intestinal cell growth inhibition; apoptosis
IGFIIR	6q26	Tumor suppressor	Binding to and activation of TGF-β (see above); degradation of IGF-2 (a growth stimulant)
BCL2		Tumor suppressor	Apoptosis
BAX		Tumor suppressor	Apoptosis (member of the *BCL2* gene family)
RB1	13q14	Tumor suppressor	Transcription factor
NM23	17q22	Tumor suppressor	NDP kinase activity

FAP, familial adenomatous polyposis; *HNPCC*, hereditary nonpolyposis colorectal cancer; *TGF*, transforming growth factor, *IGF*, insulin-like growth factor.

evidence that removal of polyps confers protection from colorectal cancer, presumably owing to the interruption of the adenoma-carcinoma pathway (7,8).

There are no valid alternative hypotheses to counter that of the adenoma-carcinoma sequence. Some authors have suggested that colorectal cancer may arise de novo (9). Even in such cases, the "flat adenoma" may be the precursor lesion (10), and thus the sequence of events would likely be similar, even if the clinical implications are more far-reaching (e.g., screening, might be less effective). Further confirmation of the adenoma-carcinoma pathway has come with a greater understanding of the molecular genetics of the carcinogenesis process.

LINKS BETWEEN HEREDITARY AND SPORADIC CANCER

Much of our current understanding of sporadic carcinogenesis has arisen from the study of the hereditary colorectal cancer syndromes. The proposition of a link between the two stems from Knudson's (11) analysis of retinoblastoma, a rare childhood tumor. Retinoblastoma can be divided into two forms: a sporadic form in which usually only one tumor develops and a second form in which the tumors are bilateral and multifocal and the age of onset is younger. In the second form there may be a family history in previous generations and/or evidence of dominant inheritance of susceptibility in subsequent generations. Knudson (11) hypothesized that two mutations, or "hits," in a single cell were required for a retinoblastoma to develop. In sporadic tumors both hits occur somatically, whereas in the hereditary form, one hit had already occurred in the germline and thus all cells in the eye (and throughout the body) already carried this mutation. The original two-hit hypothesis did not specify the nature of the two mutations. With further elaboration of the molecular and cytogenetics of retinoblastoma, it became clear that the two hits were likely to occur at the same locus, implying that each event is recessive (12). Typically, the first hit would be a mutation of the gene and the second would be a deletion. Such deletions were found to be characteristic of this kind of gene and can be demonstrated on DNA electrophoresis as the loss of one DNA band, termed loss of heterozygosity (Fig. 1.2). Knudson called these genes antioncogenes, but they are now known as tumor-suppressor genes; and many of the predicted mechanisms have been confirmed in a variety of tumors (13).

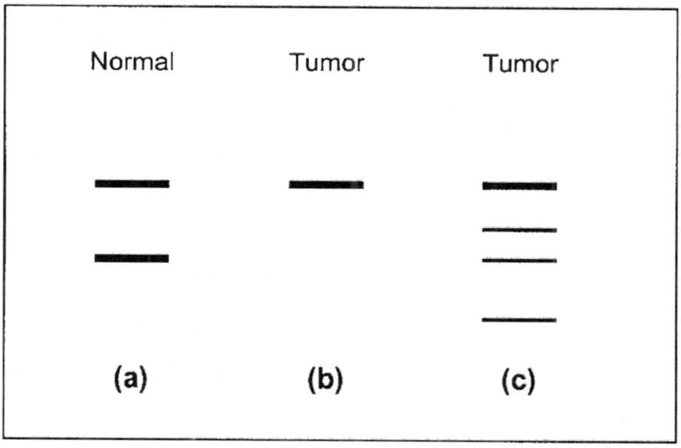

FIGURE 1.2. DNA electrophoresis of a microsatellite marker (**a**), demonstrating loss of heterozygosity (**b**) and microsatellite instability (**c**). At any particular locus, it is often possible to distinguish the parental alleles by looking for polymorphisms. Amplification of microsatellite markers is one of several methods used. When extracted DNA is electrophorised on a gel, smaller fragments travel faster than larger ones. For a given locus, alleles of different length will separate to form two bands on the gel. Electrophoresis of DNA from normal tissue in lane **a** shows heterozygosity at this locus. In the tumor tissue in lane **b**, the smaller fragment DNA band is absent: this is termed loss of heterozygosity (LOH) and indicates deletion of this fragment of the chromosome. This is a common mechanism for the second hit of tumor-suppressor gene inactivation. Thus finding of LOH is an indirect indicator of the presence of a tumor-suppressor gene. In lane **c** the main band for the smaller allele is less intense and there are two new bands seen. This indicates that in the tumor the DNA is not being faithfully replicated from one cell generation to the next. This is termed microsatellite instability and is the result of deficient DNA mismatch repair. For further details see text.

The genetic basis for the main hereditary colorectal cancer syndromes has now been identified (detailed in subsequent chapters) (14), and it is likely that most if not all of these genes are involved in sporadic carcinogenesis as well (Table 1.1).

THEORIES OF CARCINOGENESIS: THE MULTISTEP MODEL

Long before any of the genetic changes now known to be involved in colorectal carcinogenesis had been identified, epidemiologic studies in the 1950s predicted a multistep pathway. Nordling (15) recognized that in different populations, the mortality from most cancers increased with and rose proportional to the sixth power of age, indicating that cancer arose as a result of seven successive events. This kind of modeling based only on age-related mortality makes assumptions that necessarily are a crude representation of reality. For example, it assumes that the changes are independent of one another and occur in succession and that the exposure to risk is constant over time.

A more likely scenario for the development of cellular changes was proposed by Nowell (16). He was one of the first to advance the clonal theory of tumors (now well established) by proposing that each step of the carcinogenetic pathway resulted from selection of a subclone. Genetic damage caused by random mutation, chance events, or chemical or environmental carcinogens acting on a cell within a clone results in altered characteristics that might be deleterious or advantageous to growth. Alterations that are favorable to cellular proliferation lead to the establishment of a subclone that multiplies at the expense of its neighbors. By a process of natural selection occurring at the cellular level, further subclones of that subclone develop, and successive mutations accumulate within the mass of dividing cells. This process of genetic changes can lead to cancer (17). The clonal theory explains the common finding of areas of adenomatous tissue adjacent to a cancer. The malignancy is a malevolent subclone of the adenoma that outgrows the adenoma and determines the behavior of the entire neoplasm.

GENETIC INSTABILITY AND THE MUTATOR PHENOTYPE

Loeb (18) proposed that genetic instability leading to a "mutator phenotype" must underlie multistep carcinogenesis. Although it was initially thought that naturally occurring mutations would be sufficient to account for the malignant transformation process, Loeb argued that such rates were too slow to produce the numerous demonstrable mutations. The corollary of this idea is that in some way a mutator phenotype had to develop before the multistep pathway could be traveled. Loeb et al. (19) predicted that errors in DNA replication could be the basis of malignant change a full 20 years before this was confirmed by the discovery of the mismatch repair genes. Instability of the genome occurs in at least two different ways: instability affecting whole chromosomes and instability in short segments of repetitive DNA known as microsatellites. These differing mutator phenotypes underpin the two proposed pathways (referred to as the "classical" and "microsatellite instability" pathways) for sporadic colorectal carcinogenesis (Fig. 1.3; Table 1.2).

CHROMOSOMAL INSTABILITY

Many tumors of all types show a considerable degree of chromosomal aberration. Typical abnormalities include aneuploidy (an abnormal chromosome number) and loss of segments of chromosomes. This type of instability affects chromosomal segregation during cell division leading to losses or gains of whole chromosomes (20). The mechanisms controlling this instability are unclear, but it is likely that DNA hypomethylation is intimately involved (21,22), and there is one report suggesting that a mutated mitotic checkpoint gene

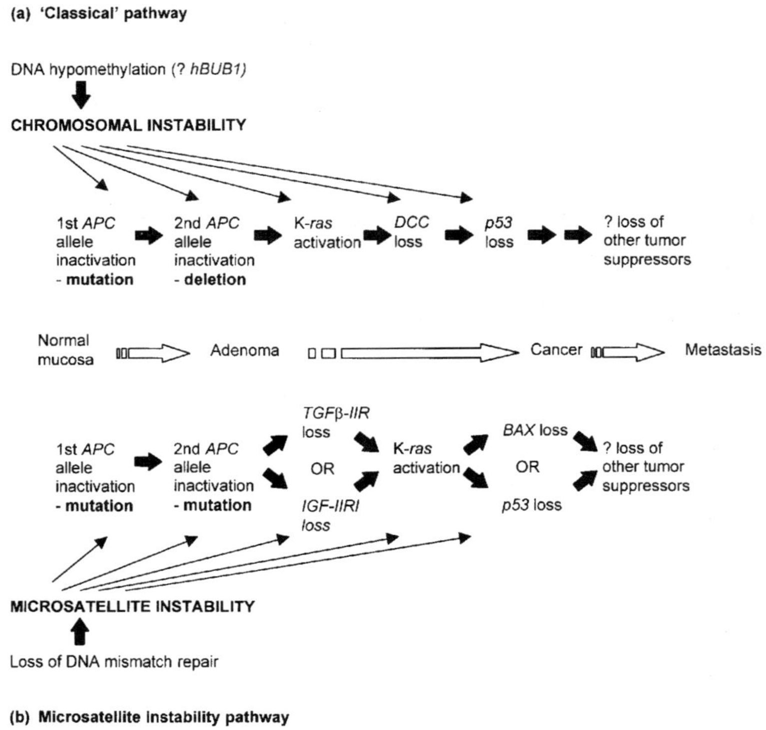

FIGURE 1.3. Possible multistep pathways of colorectal carcinogenesis.

called *hBUB1* may be responsible (23). Loss of whole or portions of chromosomes is probably the usual mechanism by which the second allele of tumor-suppressor genes is inactivated (24), and thus chromosomal disorders are likely to have a direct role in carcinogenesis.

MICROSATELLITE INSTABILITY

Microsatellites are repeated segments of DNA, commonly cytosine (C) and adenine (A) nucleotides, dinucleotides, or CA repeats, which are found scattered throughout the genome. Their function is not known, but they have been extremely useful to molecular geneticists owing to their ubiquity, their easy identification using polymerase chain reaction (PCR), and their high degree of polymorphism (the number of repeats at any one locus likely differs in the paternal and

TABLE 1.2. DIFFERENCES BETWEEN THE TWO PATHWAYS OF SPORADIC COLORECTAL CARCINOGENESIS

Feature	Classical Pathway	Microsatellite Instability Pathway
Frequency	85%	15%
Genomic instability	Chromosomal	Microsatellite
Ploidy	Aneuploid	Diploid
Loss of heterozygosity	Common	Rare
Mutations in genes	Point mutations, deletions, insertions	Insertions or deletions in repetitive sequences
Tumor location	66% left sided	80–90% right sided
Age	Older	Younger and perhaps very elderly
Prognosis	Poor	Good

the maternal chromosomes). They have been used to track segments of chromosomes through successive generations in families with hereditary disorders ("linkage") and to look for deletions of segments in tumors (loss of heterozygosity). Comparison of the allele sizes from paired samples of DNA from tumors and normal tissue in patients with hereditary nonpolyposis colorectal cancer (HNPCC) revealed instances in which, in the tumor DNA samples, a band representing one allele was diminished and additional bands had been formed (25) (Fig. 1.2). Under normal circumstances, the fidelity of replication of these repeat sequences is extremely high, and indeed, this is the basis on which CA repeat markers can be traced so accurately from one generation to the next in linkage studies. However, in the tumor samples the appearance of new alleles (always differing from the constitutional alleles by a multiple of two bases) indicated errors in DNA replication. This phenomenon was termed microsatellite instability (MSI) and is thought to result from slippage of DNA polymerase during normal replication. The abnormality in the tumor is not the slippage, but the failure of the cell to recognize and correct the mismatch. It was the serendipitous finding of MSI in HNPCC tumors that led to the original discovery of the DNA mismatch repair (MMR) genes.

MSI AND SPORADIC COLORECTAL CANCER

Defective DNA mismatch repair leading to MSI is thought to promote carcinogenesis through loss of a "caretaker" function (26). Accordingly, the resulting mutator phenotype allows the accumulation of DNA errors throughout the genome produced during mitotic replication. It is probably, therefore, by chance that mutations develop in important cancer-causing genes as well as in many other genes that have no bearing on tumorigenesis. Once such mutations have developed, they are selected for in successive generations of cells, resulting in increasing over-representation in cancer cells. Particularly susceptible to the loss of mismatch repair are stretches of DNA containing short repetitive sequences, and of course, this is why microsatellite instability is the hallmark of disordered DNA mismatch repair. The concept of disordered caretaker function as a permissive rather than directly causative mechanism for cancer development is new. Increasingly, other genes have been found to act in this way (27).

CAUSES OF MSI IN SPORADIC CANCER

MSI is a feature not only of HNPCC tumors but also of sporadic colorectal and extraintestinal malignancies (28). Many studies have shown that approximately 15% of apparently sporadic colorectal carcinomas display MSI (29). According to the tumor-suppressor hypothesis, such tumors could either be the result of an inherited MMR gene mutation with a second somatic hit (unsuspected HNPCC) or could show somatic mutations or deletions in both copies of an MMR gene. In fact, neither of these possibilities appears to be common, suggesting that other pathways for MSI may exist.

Analysis of constitutional DNA from patients who have developed MSI+ tumors without a family history has shown a very low incidence of germline MMR gene mutations (30,31), implying that the majority of such cases are indeed "sporadic." Perhaps more surprising is the apparent absence of somatic mutations in the MMR genes in tumors showing MSI (31). Nevertheless, there is convincing evidence that MMR genes are involved in the MSI phenotype in these cases, because a high proportion show absence of either the hMSH2 or hMLH1 protein (both MMR gene products), suggesting loss of the tumor-suppressor gene (32–34). A number of theories have been postulated to reconcile these apparent inconsistencies. First, other MMR genes may be involved, possibly genes not yet discovered. Second, there may be some dominantly acting germline mutations (a naturally occurring mutation of MMR gene *hPMS2* has been shown to inactivate its fellow wild type allele in a dominant negative manner without a second mutation occurring (35)). Third, differential methylation of the promoter region of MMR genes may prevent gene expression in an epigenetic manner (36,37).

MULTISTEP COLORECTAL CARCINOGENESIS: THE CLASSICAL PATHWAY

Colorectal cancer has become a paradigm for multistep carcinogenesis owing to the ability to analyze polyps at different stages along the pathway. The first real insight into the genetic steps involved came only 10 years ago when Vogelstein and co-workers (38) reasoned that, given the knowledge that a number of different genes were mutated or deleted somatically in colorectal cancers, the pattern and number of such changes might be reflected in the different stages of development from adenoma to carcinoma. They examined the frequency of occurrence of K-*ras* mutations and deletions of chromosomes 5q (site of *APC*), 17p (site of *p53*), and 18q (site of *DCC* and the newly discovered *SMAD4*) in adenomas and carcinomas. *APC* deletions were detected in approximately 30% of sporadic adenomas (now shown to be much more frequent) but not greatly more abundant in carcinomas, whereas 17p and 18q deletions were uncommon in small adenomas but displayed increasing frequency in adenomas with in situ carcinoma and even more frequently in invasive carcinomas. Frequency of K-*ras* mutations rose with increasing dysplasia and size of adenoma but increased no further in invasive carcinomas. These findings suggest that each of these genes may play roles in different parts of the process. For example, 5q loss may be required for adenoma formation, K-*ras* mutation for progression, and 17p and 18q loss for development of invasion. By examining the same tumors for all four alterations, it appeared that in early adenomas the number of genetic changes was small, but that in the carcinomas almost all tumors had two or more mutations. These findings led to the proposal of the, now "classical" model of carcinogenesis involving a stepwise accumulation of a number of genetic alterations (39,40). They stated that the number of acquired alterations in tumor-suppressor genes or oncogenes (usually four to six) is more important than the order in which they arise (Fig. 1.3).

Fearon and Vogelstein's classical model of cancer development as a stepwise accumulation of activated oncogenes and inactivated tumor-suppressor genes within a single cell has become widely accepted and acts as a framework on which to hang some more recent refinements, discussed below.

THE CRITICAL ROLE OF *APC* AS GATEKEEPER

The *APC* gene is now thought to play a fundamental role in the initiation of adenomas in both the classical and MSI pathways. Its importance in FAP is obvious in that germline mutations result in the carpet of polyps that characterizes the condition. For the majority of sporadic neoplasias, it is likely that both copies of *APC* must be inactivated before an adenoma can be initiated (41). In this respect *APC* can be thought of as a "gatekeeper" that prevents the neoplastic process from starting (42). Once the *APC* gene's function has been lost, a polyp forms, and the potential for malignant transformation is present (26). Although *APC* acts as a gatekeeper in the colon and rectum, it is not a universal gatekeeper. Its organ specificity is probably limited to the tissues in which there is an excess cancer risk as seen in FAP, the colorectum, the duodenum, and possibly the brain.

DOES THE MULTISTEP PATHWAY HOLD IN TUMORS WITH MSI?

Although for convenience we have chosen to describe the classical and MSI pathways as distinct carcinogenic mechanisms, there is considerable overlap between the two both conceptually and biologically (Fig. 1.3). Many of the same genes that contribute to the classical pathway of colorectal carcinogenesis, such as *APC*, K-*ras*, and *p53*, are also involved in MSI+ tumors. There are some important differences, however, and several additional tumor-suppressor genes have also been implicated (43).

INITIAL STEPS

Once again *APC* plays a crucial early role in adenoma formation. The mutations seen in the *APC* gene differ from those seen in MSI − tumors in that there is an excess of frameshift mutations in repetitive sequences (especially polyadenine tracts), exactly those expected where there is deficient MMR (44). This implies that the mutator phenotype must develop before *APC* mutation. Thus it is likely that the first step in the pathway is inactivation of the caretaker MMR, followed by mutation of the gatekeeper *APC* gene (42).

ONCOGENES AND TUMOR SUPPRESSORS

Mutations of K-*ras*, *APC*, and *p53* are seen less frequently in MSI + tumors than in those arising along the classical pathway (29,45), and significantly, there is a much lower frequency of loss of heterozygosity at sites of tumor-suppressor genes (29,45) in MSI + lesions. In other words, these genes are being hit less often and through a different mechanism.

ROLE OF OTHER TUMOR SUPPRESSORS

Further analysis of MSI + tumors has implicated certain other genes in the carcinogenesis pathway, owing first to the types of mutations seen and second to their over-representation in these tumors. The most important of these appears to be the *RII* gene, which codes for the transforming growth factor $\beta 2$ (TGF-$\beta 2$) receptor. This gene is interesting because it is a potent inhibitor of cell growth in the gut and is involved in induction of apoptosis. It also contains a tract of $(A)_{10}$ within its coding region, which renders it susceptible to mutation in MMR-deficient cells. In tumors with MSI, 80 to 90% have a mutated *RII* poly(A) tract with a frameshift, resulting in a premature stop codon (46,47). Another gene, the insulin-like growth factor II receptor (IGF-2r), is mutated in a similar manner although less frequently, but not usually in tumors in which a *RII* mutation is present (48). Thus one or another of these growth-controlling genes may be required for MSI carcinogenesis. A further gene, *BAX*, containing a $(G)_8$ tract, is mutated in approximately 50% of MSI + tumors (49). *BAX* interacts with *p53* and promotes apoptosis in normal cells, and thus mutations in MSI + tumors might be the counterpart to *p53* deletions in MSI − cancers.

Clinical Correlations of Genetic Changes

Cancers arising from each of the two main genetic pathways can be distinguished in a number of ways and also appear to behave differently in their growth and prognosis. These differences may have potential clinical applications.

Histopathologic Analysis

Tumors with MSI are often larger and have a more exophytic growth pattern than their MSI − counterparts (50). Moreover, they are often poorly differentiated or have a significant mucinous component (51). There is an increased presence of tumor and peritumoral infiltrating lymphocytes resembling a Crohn's-like lymphoid reaction. Such features are reliable enough to predict MSI status from the histopathologic features with a high degree of accuracy (51).

Patient Characteristics

The distribution of sporadic MSI + cancers shows a predominance of right-sided lesions with approximately 90% of tumors located proximal to the splenic flexure (29,50,51). This is an even higher proportion than that found in HNPCC, where only about two-thirds of the cancers (which are nearly all MSI +) are proximally located. In MSI − sporadic cancers, approximately two-thirds of tumors are distally situated. Taking all sporadic cancers as a group, however, only a 25 to 35% of right sided cancers show MSI (29,52). No studies have reported any gender-related differences.

Microsatellite instability appears to be more prevalent in younger patients with colorectal cancer (53), but is also seen at very old ages (52). It is more common in patients with multiple primaries both in the colon and in related sites (54). Such features lead one to hypothesize that MSI in apparently sporadic cancers may be the result of an unsuspected hereditary susceptibility, but the incidence of positive family history or detectable germline MMR gene mutations is low (30,52).

DIAGNOSIS

The high sensitivity of DNA-based tests has led to a large-scale pursuit for a molecular test to detect colorectal cancers. The K-*ras* gene lends itself to this approach because only a limited number of mutations are seen, and therefore, tests can be designed to recognize these few alterations. In one study, K-*ras* mutations were accurately detected in exfoliated cells present in the stool of colorectal cancer patients (55). Another analysis used similar techniques and found mutant K-*ras* DNA in the serum of patients with colorectal cancers (56). Unfortunately, K-*ras* is only mutated in approximately 40% of all colorectal cancers, limiting its general applicability as a diagnostic tool. Using the knowledge that cancer cells are frequently aneuploid and contain excess amounts of DNA, an assay of DNA density in stool (the stool DNA index) has been developed that appears to accurately discriminate between patients with and without cancers (57). Such molecular tests all show promise for colorectal cancer screening and diagnosis.

TUMOR BEHAVIOR

There are increasing data to suggest that the genetic changes present within a tumor correlate with its behavior and thus affect factors such as responsiveness to therapy and prognosis. This is not surprising because, ultimately, the character of a cancer must be dictated by its genetic makeup.

PROGNOSIS

The prognosis of a cancer depends on a variety of factors including tumor stage (itself governed both by the length of time the tumor has been growing and its ability to grow and invade), the surgery performed, the use of chemotherapy and radiotherapy, the patient's ability to mount an immune response to identify and eradicate tumor cells, and the tumor's ability to metastasize. DNA technology based on knowledge of the genetics of colorectal carcinogenesis is already finding uses in clinical practice. For example, certain genetic changes in the primary tumor have been shown to correlate with prognosis (58). Deletions of the gene *DCC*, overexpression of p53 (a measure of mutations in *p53*), and K-*ras* mutations have each been implicated as a poor prognostic indicator, although not all studies show a significant correlation. In contrast, the presence of MI within a tumor is associated with a significantly better prognosis (29). This is somewhat paradoxical given that some of the histologic features of MSI + tumors, such as poor differentiation or mucin secretion, usually indicate a poor prognosis.

Novel techniques have been used to identify micrometastases in lymph nodes of patients with stage II (node-negative) cancers based on conventional histopathology. For example, one group used PCR-based detection of identical mutations of *p53* and K-*ras* in nodes to those seen in the primary tumors as an indication of nodal metastases (59). When such metastases were found, the prognosis was worse. Similarly, detection of the messenger RNA for carcinoembryonic antigen as an indicator of lymph node micrometastases has also been shown to carry a poorer prognosis (60).

RESPONSE TO RADIOTHERAPY AND CHEMOTHERAPY

The *p53* gene has long been known to be intimately involved in control of DNA repair or cell death (apoptosis) after exposure to radiation. Some studies have demonstrated that tumors with mutated *p53* are more likely to be resistant to radiotherapy (61). Tumors with wild-type (nonmutated) K-*ras* and *p53* are more likely to benefit from adjuvant chemotherapy with 5-fluorouracil and levamisole than those with mutations (62). Theoretically at least, tumors with MSI will be resistant to alkylating agents because tolerance to such agents in cell lines has been shown to result from loss of mismatch repair function (63). Thus it is almost inevitable that future assessments of colorectal cancers will include genetic analysis to predict tumor responsiveness to adjuvant and neo-adjuvant therapies.

CONCLUSION

We now have an increasingly well understood model of the genetic basis of sporadic colorectal carcinogenesis. Although the advent of successful gene therapies may be many years away, we are close to the time when the pathology report we receive after biopsy or resection of a cancer will include a full genetic evaluation of the tumor. This will provide extremely valuable information that will aid in patient management. First, we should be able to select patients who are likely to have metastatic or recurrent disease and to whom further treatments should be directed. Furthermore, many patients with good prognoses will be spared unnecessary adjuvant therapy, representing a vast improvement over the rather crude histologic staging that is our current arbiter for further treatment. Second, we will be able to predict which tumors will respond to which forms of treatment, whether radiotherapy, different forms of chemotherapy. or possibly, newer treatments also based on genetic technology.

REFERENCES

1. Lockhart-Mummery P. Cancer and heredity. Lancet 1925;1:427–429.
2. Muto T, Bussey HJR, Morson BC. The evolution of cancer of the colon and rectum. Cancer 1975;36:2251–2270.
3. Morson BC, Bussey HJR, Day DW, Hill MJ. Adenomas of large bowel. Cancer Surv 1983;2:451–477.
4. Eide TJ. Natural history of adenomas. World J Surg 1991;15:3–6.
5. Morson BC. The evolution of colorectal carcinoma. Clin Radiol 1984;35:425–431.
6. Stryker SJ, Wolff BG, Culp CE, et al. Natural history of untreated colonic polyps. Gastroenterology 1987;93:1009–1013.
7. Winawer SJ, Zauber AG, Ho MH, et al. Prevention of colorectal cancer by colonoscopic polypectomy. N Engl J Med 1993;329:1977–1981.
8. Atkin WS, Morson BC, Cuzick J. Long-term risk of colorectal cancer after excision of rectosigmoid adenomas. N Engl J Med 1992;326:658–662.
9. Shimoda T, Ikegami M, Fujisaki J, et al. Early colorectal carcinoma with special reference to its development *de novo*. Cancer 1989;64:1138–1146.
10. Muto T, Kamiya J, Sawada T, et al. Small "flat adenoma" of the large bowel with special reference to its clinicopathologic features. Dis Colon Rectum 1985;28:847–851.
11. Knudson Jr AG. Mutation and cancer: statistical study of retinoblastoma. Proc Natl Acad Sci U S A 1971;68:820–823.
12. Knudson Jr AG. Hereditary cancer, oncogenes, and antioncogenes. Cancer Res 1985;45:1437–1443.
13. Stanbridge EJ. Functional evidence for human tumour suppressor genes: chromosome and molecular genetic studies. Cancer Surv 1992;12:5–24.
14. Hall NR. Hereditary colorectal cancer syndromes. Semin Colon Rectal Surg 1998;9:2–11.
15. Nordling CO. A new theory on the cancer-inducing mechanism. Br J Cancer 1953;7:68–72.
16. Nowell PC. The clonal evolution of tumor cell populations: acquired genetic lability permits stepwise selection of variant sublines and underlies tumor progression. Science 1976;194:23–28.

17. Bodmer W, Bishop T, Karran P. Genetic steps in colorectal cancer. Nature Genet 1994;6:217–219.
18. Loeb LA. Mutator phenotype may be required for multistage carcinogenesis. Cancer Res 1991;51:3075–3079.
19. Loeb LA, Springgate CF, Battula N. Errors in DNA replication as a basis of malignant change. Cancer Res 1974;34:2311–2321.
20. Lengauer C, Kinzler KW, Vogelstein B. Genetic instability in colorectal cancers. Nature 1997;386:623–627.
21. Chen RZ, Pettersson U, Beard C, et al. DNA hypomethylation leads to elevated mutation rates. Nature 1998;395:89–93.
22. Lengauer C, Kinzler KW, Vogelstein B. DNA methylation and genetic instability in colorectal cancer cells. Proc Natl Acad Sci USA 1997;94:2545–2550.
23. Cahill DP, Lengauer C, Yu J, et al. Mutations of mitotic checkpoint genes in human cancers [see comments]. Nature 1998;392:300–303.
24. Vogelstein B, Fearon ER, Kern SE, et al. Allelotype of colorectal carcinomas. Science 1989;244:207–211.
25. Aaltonen LA, Peltomäki P, Leach FS, et al. Clues to the pathogenesis of familial colorectal cancer. Science 1993;260:812–816.
26. Kinzler KW, Vogelstein B. Lessons from hereditary colorectal cancer. Cell 1996;87:159–170.
27. Kinzler KW, Vogelstein B. Landscaping the cancer terrain. Science 1998;280:1036–1037.
28. Ionov Y, Peinado MA, Malkhosyan S, et al. Ubiquitous somatic mutations in simple repeated sequences reveal a new mechanism for colonic carcinogenesis. Nature 1993;363:558–561.
29. Thibodeau SN, Bren G, Schaid D. Microsatellite instability in cancer of the proximal colon. Science 1993;260:816–819.
30. Liu B, Nicolaides NC, Markowitz S, et al. Mismatch repair gene defects in sporadic colorectal cancers with microsatellite instability. Nature Genet 1995;9:48–55.
31. Senba S, Konishi F, Okamoto T, et al. Clinicopathologic and genetic features of nonfamilial colorectal carcinomas with DNA replication errors. Cancer 1998;82:279–285.
32. Thibodeau SN, French AJ, Roche PC, et al. Altered expression of hMSH2 and hMLH1 in tumors with microsatellite instability and

genetic alterations in mismatch repair genes. Cancer Res 1996;56:4836–4840.

33. Dietmaier W, Wallinger S, Bocker T, et al. Diagnostic microsatellite instability: definition and correlation with mismatch repair protein expression. Cancer Res 1997;57:4749–4756.
34. Thibodeau SN, French AJ, Cunningham JM, et al. Microsatellite instability in colorectal cancer: different mutator phenotypes and the principal involvement of *hMLH1*. Cancer Res 1998;58:1713–1718.
35. Nicolaides NC, Littman SJ, Modrich P, et al. A naturally occurring hPMS2 mutation can confer a dominant negative mutator phenotype. Mol Cell Biol 1998;18:1635–1641.
36. Herman JG, Umar A, Polyak K, et al. Incidence and functional consequences of hMLH1 promoter hypermethylation in colorectal carcinoma. Proc Natl Acad Sci U S A 1998;95:6870–6875.
37. Veigl ML, Kasturi L, Olechnowicz J, et al. Biallelic inactivation of *hMLH1* by epigenetic gene silencing, a novel mechanism causing human MSI cancers. Proc Natl Acad Sci U S A 1998;95:8698–8702.
38. Vogelstein B, Fearon ER, Hamilton SR, et al. Genetic alterations during colorectal-tumor development. N Engl J Med 1988;319:525–532.
39. Madoff RD, Wong KS. The multistep model of colorectal carcinogenesis. Semin Colon Rectal Surg 1998;9:30–37.
40. Fearon ER, Vogelstein B. A genetic model for colorectal tumorigenesis. Cell 1990; 61:759–767.
41. Powell SM, Zilz N, Beazer-Barclay Y, et al. *APC* mutations occur early during colorectal tumorigenesis. Nature 1992;359:235–237.
42. Kinzler KW, Vogelstein B. Gatekeepers and caretakers. Nature 1997;386:761–763.
43. Cunningham JM, Boardman LA, Burgart LJ, Thibodeau SN. Molecular abnormalities in colorectal cancer: microsatellite instability pathway. Semin Colon Rectal Surg 1998;9:38–48.
44. Huang J, Papadopoulos N, McKinley AJ, et al. *APC* mutations in colorectal tumors with mismatch repair deficiency. Proc Natl Acad Sci U S A 1996;93:9049–9054.
45. Konishi M, Kikuchi-Yanoshita R, Tanaka K, et al. Molecular nature of colon tumors in hereditary nonpolyposis colon cancer, familial polyposis, and sporadic colon cancer. Gastroenterology 1996;111:307–317.
46. Markowitz S, Wang J, Myeroff L, et al. Inactivation of the type II TGF-β

receptor in colon cancer cells with microsatellite instability. Science 1995;268:1336–1338.

47. Parsons R, Myeroff L, Liu B, et al. Microsatellite instability and mutations of the transforming growth factors β type II recpetor gene in colorectal cancer. Cancer Res 1995;55:5548–5550.
48. Souza RF, Appel R, Yin J, et al. Microsatellite instability in the insulin-like growth factor II receptor in gastrointestinal tumours. Nature Genet 1996;14:255–257.
49. Rampino N, Yamamoto H, Ionov Y, et al. Somatic frameshift mutations in the BAX gene in colon cancers of the microsatellite mutator phenotype. Science 1997;275:967–969.
50. Kim K, Jen J, Vogelstein B, Hamilton SR. Clinical and pathological characteristics of sporadic colorectal carcinomas with DNA replication errors in microsatellite sequences. Am J Pathol 1994;145:148–156.
51. Jass JR, Do K-A, Simms LA, et al. Morphology of sporadic colorectal cancer with DNA replication errors. Gut 1998;42:673–679.
52. Samowitz WS, Slattery ML, Kerber RA. Microsatellite instability in human colonic cancer is not a useful clinical indicator of familial colorectal cancer. Gastroenterology 1995;109:1765—1771.
53. Liu B, Farrington SM, Petersen GM, et al. Genetic instability occurs in the majority of young patients with colorectal cancer. Nature Med 1995;1:348–352.
54. Brown SR, Finan PJ, Hall NR, Bishop DT. Incidence of DNA replication errors in patients with multiple primary cancers. Dis Colon Rectum 1998;41:765–769.
55. Sidransky D, Tokino T, Hamilton SR, et al. Identification of ras oncogene mutations in the stools of patients with curable colorectal tumors. Science 1992;256:102–105.
56. Kopreski MS, Benko FA, Leitzel KE, et al. Detection of mutant K-*ras* in plasma or serum of patients with colorectal cancer. Br J Cancer 1998;76:1293–1299.
57. Loktionov A, O'Neill IK, Silvester KR, et al. Quantitation of DNA from exfoliated colonocytes isolated from human stool surface as a novel noninvasive screening test for colorectal cancer. Clin Cancer Res 1998;4:337–342.
58. Chung DC. Molecular prognostic markers and colorectal cancer: the search goes on. Gastroenterology 1998;114:1330–1338.
59. Hayashi N, Ito I, Yanagisawa A, et al. Genetic diagnosis of lymph-node metastasis in colorectal cancer. Lancet 1995;345:1257–1259.

60. Liefers G-J, Cleton-Jansen A-M, van de Velde CJH, et al. Micrometastases and survival in stage II colorectal cancer. N Engl J Med 1998;339:223–228.

61. Fu C-G, Tominaga O, Nagawa H, et al. Role of *p53* and *p21/WAF1* detection in patient selection for proeoperative radiotherapy in rectal cancer patients. Dis Colon Rectum 1998;41:68–74.

62. Ahnen DJ, Feigl P, Quan G, et al. *Ki-ras* mutation and *p53* overexpression predict the clinical behavior of colorectal cancer: a Southwest Oncology Group study. Cancer Res 1998;58:1149–1158.

63. Karran P, Hampson R. Genomic instability and tolerance to alkylating agents. Cancer Surv 1996;28:69–85.

CHAPTER

2

COLON AND RECTAL POLYPS

T. R. SHOPE, M.D., AND E. C. LEE, M.D.

Although they are relatively common entities, polyps of the colon and rectum present a management dilemma to the clinician. The advent of fiberoptic endoscopy for the investigation of occult or overt lower gastrointestinal bleeding and for screening at-risk populations has allowed for the easier and more frequent identification of these lesions (1). However, even after histologic examination of a polypectomy or biopsy specimen, many clinicians are still uncertain of the implications for future patient management. The goal of this chapter is to fully describe these mucosal protrusions by presenting their natural history, risk for malignant transformation, metastatic potential, histologic characteristics, operative versus nonoperative management, and clinical outcomes. By describing the polyps of the colon and rectum in this manner, we will clarify the clinical dilemmas and outline appropriate management of patients with these lesions.

Colon and Rectal Cancer, Edited by Peter S. Edelstein, M.D.
ISBN 0-471-35145-8

NON-NEOPLASTIC COLON AND RECTAL POLYPS

The non-neoplastic colon and rectal polyps are a group of mucosal eruptions that vary in histologic appearance. Although they may appear grossly similar to their neoplastic counterparts, they have significantly less, and often no, malignant potential (Table 2.1) (2,3). In this section, we describe these lesions.

HYPERPLASTIC POLYPS

Hyperplastic polyps are characteristically small lesions of the distal colon and rectum, usually 5 to 10 mm in diameter (2–4). Although they become more prevalent with advancing patient age, they are generally asymptomatic and are usually incidental findings at endoscopy. As their name implies, they are a benign overgrowth of mucosal cells that protrude into the colonic lumen. Although they have no malignant potential, these polyps are grossly indistinguishable from adenomatous polyps and, therefore, demand biopsy (3,4). Histologic examination reveals the characteristic serrated appearance of benign glands and supporting tissue (3,5). The serrated appearance is created by elongation and infolding of the mucosal epithelium. Management of hyperplastic polyps, after tissue diagnosis, is expectant. Surgical intervention is not warranted, and there are no clinical sequelae (3).

TABLE 2.1. NON-NEOPLASTIC POLYPS OF THE COLON AND RECTUM

Hyperplastic
Inflammatory
Hamartomas
Juvenile polyps
Peutz-Jeghers syndrome
Hamartomatous polyposis
Submucosal lesions presenting as polyps

INFLAMMATORY POLYPS

Inflammatory polyps arise in the face of surrounding inflammation and mucosal ulceration (3,4). For this reason, they are found with relative frequency in patients with inflammatory bowel disease and chronic infectious colitis. At least one study reports the presence of these polyps in 12.5% of ulcerative colitis patients (6). These lesions are slightly larger than hyperplastic polyps, up to 15 mm, and may cause symptoms of bleeding, abdominal pain and obstruction (3,4). Note that these symptoms are not uncommon in conditions that predispose the patient to the development of inflammatory polyps. For this reason, inflammatory polyps are often found at endoscopy performed for the pre-existing condition

Inflammatory polyps lack malignant potential; however, they are associated with ulcerative colitis, a known premalignant process. Therefore, inflammatory polyps may be seen in patients with colorectal cancer. Histologic examination of the inflammatory polyp reveals an often severe mucosal inflammatory infiltrate along with granulation tissue (5). Management of these polyps should be directed at the underlying inflammatory process, once appropriate pathologic examination confirms the benign condition. There are no clinical sequelae of inflammatory polyps, and prognosis depends on the underlying disease process (3,6).

HAMARTOMATOUS POLYPS

JUVENILE POLYPS Juvenile polyps, also referred to as retention polyps, are found in as many as 1 to 2% of children (7). These polyps acquired their name from the fact that 75% of them occur in children under the age of 10 years (5). They are frequently solitary, pedunculated, cherry red lesions seen at endoscopy performed to evaluate gastrointestinal bleeding. The polyps are highly vascular and may bleed spontaneously. Their stalks lack a muscularis mucosa layer, and they may easily autoamputate. Other presentations include rectal prolapse in the case of a distal polyp and symptoms consistent with obstruction caused by intussusception precipitated by a more proximal lesion (5). There has been one report in the literature of an adenocarcinoma arising within a solitary juvenile polyp in a 9-year-old patient, but for the overwhelming majority of patients, isolated juvenile polyps are considered to have no malignant potential (4,5,8).

Unlike solitary juvenile polyps, the phenotype of juvenile polyposis coli (JPC) typically involves multiple hamartomas of the distal colon and rectum. Most frequently occuring in children in the preteen to mid-teen years, the syndrome classically presents with bright red rectal bleeding and rectal prolapse. A more impressive variant, called diffuse juvenile polyposis (DJP), involves harmartomatous lesions throughout the gastrointestinal tract, most frequently in the stomach, distal colon, and rectum. DJP is usually found in young children, also with rectal bleeding, intussusception, and even protein-losing enteropathy.

Histologic examination of juvenile polyps (in all syndrome variants) reveals large, cystic, mucus-filled glands with ample lamina propria, an absence of muscularis mucosa, and an inflammatory infiltrate (5). In a large review of patients suffering from JPC or DJP, Coburn et al. (9) found that colorectal adenocarcinomas developed in 17% of cases and noted that the risk of malignancy was increased with increased polyposis. These cancers were believed to be extremely aggressive, frequently harboring poor prognostic pathology (poor differentiation, signet ring formation), and were often well advanced at the time of diagnosis. In addition, the study found 31 cases in 218 patients in which adenomatous changes were identified within the juvenile polyps; dysplasia was identified in 7 lesions. Coburn and co-workers' (9) analysis supported a number of other reports suggesting that juvenile polyps in both JPC and DJP are indeed premalignant and actually progress through a polyp-adenoma-carcinoma sequence. (10–13). Published estimates of a 10% risk of adenomatous transformation within JPC and DJP polyps translates into a risk of cancer formation in 1 out of every 1000 juvenile polyps, if one accepts a 10% risk of malignant transformation in adenomatous lesions (based on estimates for sporadic adenomas in adults). Coburn et al. (9) go as far as suggesting a possible role for prophylactic total abdominal colectomy in selected JPC and DPJ patients with lesions involving the entire colon. Even if a less aggressive posture is taken, it is clear that patients suffering from JPC and DJP require close endoscopic monitoring, with surveillance colonoscopy and biopsy of any suspicious or symptomatic polyps performed routinely. If surgical resection is required for symptomatic treatment, such as for persistent bleeding or intussusception, it may be reasonable to consider total colectomy for patients with extensive polyposis, followed by surveillance proctoscopy.

PEUTZ-JEGHERS SYNDROME Peutz-Jeghers syndrome, a rare but well-described clinical syndrome, includes a characteristic pigmentation of the skin and oral mucosa as well as multiple gastrointestinal polyps (3–5). The syndrome follows autosomal dominant Mendelian genetics. The skin and oral pigmentation often lead to a presumptive diagnosis of Peutz-Jeghers syndrome in any patient in whom colon and rectal polyps are discovered. Presenting symptoms are frequently those of intestinal obstruction, usually secondary to intussusception. Hemorrhage may also occur (3–5).

The colon and rectal polyps associated with Peutz-Jeghers syndrome have no malignant potential; however, patients are at increased risk for small and large intestinal cancers as well as breast, pancreatic, and gonadal tumors (3–5). The clinician should be aware of these associations and have an appropriately low threshold for further evaluation. Grossly, the polyps found in patients suffering from Peutz-Jeghers syndrome are large and often multilobulated. Histologic examination reveals arborizing bands of smooth muscle associated with an overlying benign epithelium (5).

Management of these patients should be directed at their presenting symptoms. Polyps evident at endoscopy should be removed to prevent clinical sequelae. Surgery should be reserved for polyps that cannot be removed endoscopically and are causing intussusception or obstructive symptoms (symptomatic polyps are usually located in the small bowel) (3–5). Surveillance for the related neoplasms is recommended, and surgery may be indicated for the related pathology (4).

HAMARTOMATOUS POLYPOSIS Hamartomatous polyposis is a category of several rare, clinical, non-neoplastic polyp syndromes. These syndromes are described for completeness; however, the colorectal polyps associated with these syndromes lack malignant potential and require no specific surgical therapy once their identity has been established.

Canada-Cronkhite syndrome is an acquired syndrome characterized by gastrointestinal polyposis, onycholysis, alopecia, cutaneous hyperpigmentation, and severe chronic diarrhea with protein losing enteropathy. The polyps of Canada-Cronkhite syndrome are histologically similar to juvenile polyps. (4,5).

Ruvalcaba-Myrhe-Smith syndrome is the rare clinical presentation of macrocephaly, delayed psychomotor development, pigmented macules of the penis, and hamartomatous gastrointestinal polyps (4). Devon Family syndrome is an isolated description of three successive generations of females who presented with recurrent inflammatory polyps of the terminal ileum and right colon (4). Muir-Torre syndrome is the association of sebaceous neoplasms with adenocarcinomas of multiple sites. Polyps of the colon and rectum are frequently found (4).

Cowden syndrome is the presence of hamartomatous polyps of the gastrointestinal tract with multiple and varied facial lesions. The facial lesions arise from follicular epithelium and are histologically trichilemmomas. Patients with these lesions should be evaluated for gastrointestinal polyps to confirm the syndrome. The syndrome must be identified because of the associated risk for the development of breast and thyroid cancer (4,5).

Mucosal neurofibromatosis and neuromas are present as part of von Recklinghausens disease and multiple endocrine neoplasia type 2B (MEN-2B). Patients with these disorders may have neurofibromas of the gastrointestinal tract that are seen as mucosal protrusions (4). Management of patients with these syndromes should be directed at the more serious associated clinical problems.

SUBMUCOSAL LESIONS

Submucosal masses of the colon and rectum may create the appearance of a polyp at endoscopy by causing a protrusion of the overlying mucosa into the intestinal lumen (2–5). These lesions are often not diagnosed at biopsy secondary to limitations of the biopsy forceps, but they include lipomas, leiomyomas, lymphoid hyperplasia, and rare conditions such as pneumatosis cystoides intestinalis, colitis cystica profunda, and carcinoid tumors (2–5). Detailed discussion of these conditions is beyond the scope of this chapter.

SUMMARY

This section described the non-neoplastic polyps of the colon and rectum and discussed their presentation, natural history, histology, management, and outcomes. The majority of these lesions have in common the absence of malignant potential and are, therefore, generally managed nonoperatively. However, it is vital to appreciate the malignant potential, albeit limited compared to that of the neoplastic polyps, of the juvenile polyposis syndromes, and the increased risk of malignancy, including gastrointestinal, in patients diagnosed with Peutz-Jeghers syndrome. In virtually all cases in which non-neoplastic polyps are suspected, index polypectomy is required for diagnosis and confirmation of benign status. The next section describes colon and rectal polyps with the greatest malignant potential, the neoplastic polyps.

NEOPLASTIC POLYPS OF THE COLON AND RECTUM

The neoplastic polyps of the colon and rectum are somewhat simpler to classify than their non-neoplastic counterparts; i.e., they are either premalignant or malignant. However, because these polyps possess malignant potential, the consequences of our actions are greatly increased and the patient management planning process is vastly more complex. The molecular and genetic basis for the progression of premalignant polyps to malignant polyps is described elsewhere in this text, as is the sporadic versus hereditary nature of these polyps. Here, we discuss the histology, malignant potential, metastatic potential, management options, and clinical outcomes of neoplastic polyps. Specific attention will be drawn to the Haggitt system of classification as the histologic guide for the above considerations in the management of malignant polyps.

PREMALIGNANT POLYPS (ADENOMAS)

Adenomatous polyps make up >70% of endoscopically removed colon and rectal polyps (2,5). Adenomas are highly prevalent in demographic regions with high rates of colorectal adenocarcinomas. Autopsy studies reveal an overall prevalence of adenomas in up to 50% of individuals, increasing with age to 65% at age 70 years (3,5). Endoscopic studies suggest an adenomal prevalence of 20 to 40% overall. Age-associated prevalence rates indicate that adenomas appear 5 to 10 years before colorectal adenocarcinomas. Asymptomatic adenomas have a uniform distribution throughout the colon, but larger and symptomatic premalignant polyps tend to be located distal to the splenic flexure (5). Adenmatous polyps are categorized based on their histologic appearance as tubular, tubulovillous, or villous (2–5,14). Tubular adenomas contain branching tubules lined by tightly packed cells with <25% villous component. Villous adenomas contain elongated papillae that create fingerlike projections >75% of the polyp. Tubulovillous adenomas contain both types of histology with a villous component between 25 and 75% (2,3,5,14). Further categorization of adenomas is based on size and degree of dysplasia. All polyps may be considered as sessile, i.e., arising directly from the colonic wall or pedunculated, when the polyp protrudes into the intestinal lumen on a fibrous, highly vascularized stalk.

The cumulative risk for progression of an adenomatous polyp to a carcinoma is 2.5 to 8% over 10 years (3,5). The malignant potential directly correlates with an adenoma size >2 cm, increasing villous component, and increasing severity of dysplasia (Table 2.2) (2,3,5,15). Advancing patient age is a risk factor for the presence of polyps and for higher grade dysplasia, but aging is not itself an independent risk factor for the progression to carcinoma (2,3,5). Because carcinomas are more frequently found in the distal colon and rectum, location may also be a risk factor for malignant potential. The adenoma to carcinoma sequence is well described elsewhere, but note that, although colorectal polyps are relatively prevalent, the progression to carcinoma is slow and infrequent (3,5). Adenomas by definition have not progressed to carcinoma and, therefore, have no metastatic potential.

When a polyp is identified at colonoscopy, index polypectomy, preferably by the snare method with electrocautery, is indicated (1,3,5). Lesions that are large or sessile may be difficult to snare. Larger lesions have an increased malignant potential, as do villous adenomas, which tend to be sessile (15). Such lesions may be removed in piecemeal fashion. If the lesion is too large, it may be

TABLE 2.2. RISK FACTORS FOR MALIGNANCY IN NEOPLASTIC COLORECTAL POLYPS

Risk factors
Size >2 cm
Increasing villous component
Increasing degree of dysplasia

unsafe to remove all of the plyp at one time, as high and prolonged currents increase the potential for significant injury to the bowel wall. Therefore, repeat endoscopies may be necessary to remove residual tissue. If the lesion is not thought to be endoscopically resectable owing to its size or sessile morphology, surgical resection should be considered. Resection can be performed conventionally or laparoscopically. Other possible management includes laparoscopic-assisted polypectomy. This approach uses standard laparoscopic techniques to mobilize the colon and allow for an easier and safer endoscopic approach to areas of the colon that are technically difficult to visualize through the endoscope alone.

Because up to 50% of patients with one adenoma will harbor another synchronous lesion, the entire colon must be visualized endoscopically (3,5). Between 30 and 40% of patients with an index adenoma will have a metachronous lesion 3 years after the initial polypectomy (3,5). Most of these metachronous lesions are small tubular adenomas, and index polypectomy and 3-year surveillance colonoscopy have resulted in a 76 to 90% reduction in colorectal cancers (5). Currently, there is some debate regarding the need for 3-year follow-up, particularly in older individuals and in patients with small tubular index adenomas. Such patients have a very low incidence of malignant metachronous lesions (2,3,5).

MALIGNANT POLYPS (ADENOCARCINOMAS)

Polyps that have already undergone malignant transformation may be either invasive carcinomas or carcinomas in situ. Lesions in which the malignancy is superficially confined to the muscularis mucosa are defined as carcinoma in situ. Invasive carcinoma is defined as any lesion in which the malignancy has violated the muscularis mucosa (1–5,14,16). Malignant polyps may appear grossly similar to their premalignant counterparts. Thus histologic examination is critical both for the determination of malignancy and for the depth of invasion.

Haggitt et al. (16) described the prognosis of colorectal carcinomas arising in adenomas based on their level of invasiveness (Fig. 2.1). Haggitt level 0 indicates an absence of invasion of the muscularis mucosa (carcinoma in situ). Because there is no lymphatic drainage of the colonic lamina propria (the mucosal tissue superficial to the muscularis mucosa), these malignant lesions have no metastatic potential (3,6,16). The incidence of lymph node metastasis for Haggitt level 1 polyps, defined as invasion into the head of a pedunculated polyp, is 0 to 3% (17–19). For Haggitt levels 2 and 3, defined as invasion into the neck and into the stalk of a pedunculated polyp, respectively, the incidence of lymph node metastasis is 0 to 20% (A Mayo Clinic study (17) found a 0% incidence of lymph node metastases in Haggitt level 1, 2, and 3 polyps). Haggitt level 4 lesions, polyps with invasion into the bowel wall submucosa, are advanced growths with significant metastatic potential. Furthermore, histologic examination of a polypectomy specimen can determine several additional risk factors suggesting a greater risk for the presence of residual malignancy in the bowel wall or lymphatics. Risk factors include a poor degree of differentiation, invasion of lymphatics or veins, involved margins or margins of resection < 2 mm, and submucosal invasion. The presence of one or more of these risk factors increases the incidence of residual malignancy after polypectomy to approximately 25% (3).

Haggitt level 0 lesions may be safely excised endoscopically (3,6) Polypectomy should be considered curative for these lesions. Polyps at Haggitt level 1, 2, and 3 that are highly differentiated may be safely followed nonoperatively, provided that they have been completely excised endoscopically. Analysis of multiple studies reveals an incidence of recurrence of disease, presence of residual disease, or evidence of metastatic disease on follow-up examination in 0.7% of patients with Haggitt level 1 lesions (1). Increasing depth of invasion to Haggitt levels 2, 3, and 4 increases the incidence of these adverse outcomes to 5, 12.9, and 15 to 25%, respectively (1,3,16). In addition, the presence of severe dysplasia or vascular

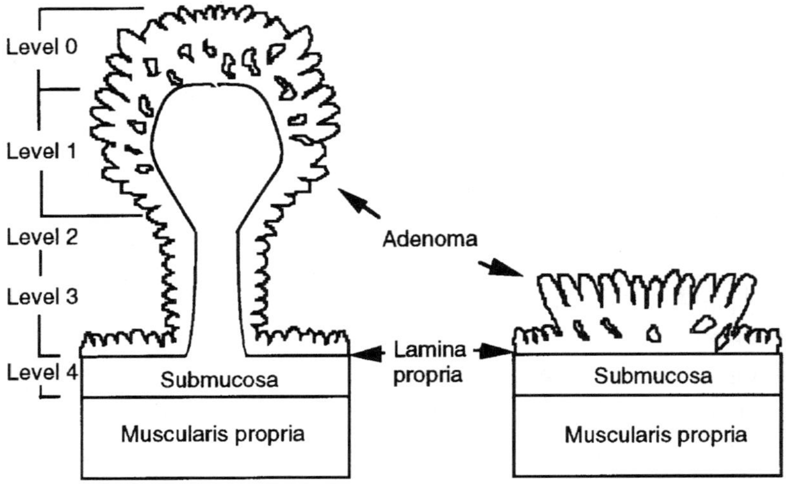

FIGURE 2.1. Pedunculated polyps versus sessile polyps in the Haggitt classification.

or lymphatic invasion by malignancy within a polyp carries an incidence of recurrent, residual, or metastatic disease of 37.5% (1). Excised polyps with clear margins have only a 6.6% incidence of such adverse outcomes versus 41.7% for those with involved or nearly involved margins (1). Therefore, Haggitt level 4 polyps have highly undifferentiated histology; are incompletely excised; or are large, sessile villous lesions demand formal oncologic colon resection and lymphatic examination (1,3–5).

As with any surgical procedure, the operative morbidity and mortality and potential benefits must be carefully weighed. The presence of risk factors suggesting a poorer prognosis should heavily influence the operative planning process. For each individual patient, the risk of future cancer-related morbidity and mortality from an incompletely excised malignant polyp needs to be carefully balanced against the risks of surgical resection (20).

Patients whose malignant polyps are adequately excised endoscopically require follow-up similar to patients who harbor purely premalignant lesions (21). The incidence of metachronous polyps is similar in patients with premaligant polyps and in those whose polyps are malignant. Completely excised, maligant, sessile polyps require more frequent colonoscopic follow-up (at 2 to 6 months) than do their pedunculated counterparts (20). Assuming local control by index polypectomy or colonic resection, prognosis for these patients is excellent.

SUMMARY This section described the neoplastic polyps of the colon and rectum. Specific attention was drawn to the Haggitt levels and histology as the basis for patient management. Recommendations for surgery and for colonoscopic follow-up were made.

DIMINUTIVE POLYPS

Diminutive polyps, as their name implies, are small lesions (< 5 mm). They are frequently encountered during endoscopy but lack clinical significance. Although studies have shown that up to 50% of diminutive polyps are adenomatous (neoplastic), < 1% are either villous or contain severe dysplasia and only rarely do they contain carcinoma. Diminutive polyps may be safely thermoablated without biopsy for histologic identification, because the risk of future malignancy is no greater than that found in the general population (2,3,5,22). Although they essentially have no malignant potential, diminutive polyps are discussed here because as many as half have been found to be neoplastic. They represent an interesting clinical finding with no clinical relevance.

CONCLUSION

This chapter described the polyps of the colon and rectum. The non-neoplastic polyps are varied and have multiple presentations and histology, but most lack malignant potential. It must be emphasized, however, that there is indeed a limited malignant potential in the lesions of juvenile polyposis patients and an increased risk of malignant tumor formation, including within the gastrointestinal tract, in patients suffering from Peutz-Jeghers syndrome. The neoplastic polyps were described with particular attention to their histology and Haggitt levels as the basis for patient management and follow-up. Finally, diminutive polyps were mentioned. The descriptions clarified the management dilemma proposed by the finding of colon and rectal polyps. The clinician, surgeon, and pathologist working in concert can provide acceptable and appropriate care for patients afflicted with these common lesions.

REFERENCES

1. Stein B, Coller J. Management of malignant colorectal polyps. Surg Clin North Am 1993;73:47–66.
2. Kim E, Lance P. Colorectal polyps and their relationship to cancer. Gastroenterol Clin North Am 1997;26:1–17.
3. Itzkowitz S, Kim Y. Colonic polyps and polyposis syndromes. In: Sleisinger M, Fordtran J, eds. Gastrointestinal disease: pathophysiology/diagnosis/management. 6th ed. Philadelphia: Saunders, 1997: 1905.
4. Watne A. Colon polyps. J Surg Oncol 1997;66:207–214.
5. Chang A. Colorectal cancer. In: Greenfield L, Mulholland M, Oldham K, et al., eds. Surgery: scientific principles and practice. 2nd ed. Philadelphia: Lippincott-Raven, 1997: 1128–1146.
6. DeDombal F, Watts J, xxxxx, et al. Local complications of ulcerative colitis: stricture, pseudopolyposis, and carcinoma of the colon and rectum. Br Med J 1966;1:1442–1447.
7. Jarvinen H. Juvenile gastrointestinal polyposis. Probl Gen Surg 1993;10:749–755.
8. Lie TH, Chen MC, Tseng HC. Malignant change of juvenile polyp of colon. A case report. Chin Med J 1978;4:434–439.
9. Coburn MC, Pricolo VE, DeLuca FG, Bland KI. Malignant potential in intestinal juvenile polyposis syndromes. Ann Surg Oncol 1995;2:386–391.
10. Lipper S, Kahn LB, Sandler RS, Varma V. Multiple juvenile polyposis: a study of the pathogenesis of juvenile polyps and their relationship to colonic adenomas. Hum Pathol 1981;12:804–813.

11. Sandler RS, Lipper S. Multiple adenomas in juvenile polyposis. Am J Gastroenterol 1981;75:361–366.

12. Rozen P, Baratz M. Familial juvenile colonic polyposis with associated colon cancer. Cancer 1982;49:1500–1503.

13. Mills SE, Fechner RE. Unusual adenomatous polyps in juvenile polyposis coli. Am J Surg Pathol 1982;6:177–183.

14. Konishi F, Morson B. Pathology of colorectal adenomas: a colonoscopic survey. J Clin Pathol 1982;35:830–841.

15. Muto T, Bussey H, Morson B. The evolution of cancer of the colon and rectum. Cancer 1975;36:2251–2270.

16. Haggitt R, Glotzbach R, Soffer E, et al. Prognostic factors in colorectal carcinomas arising in adenomas: implications for lesions removed by endoscopic polypectomy. Gastroenterology 1985;89:328–336.

17. Nivatvongs S, Rojanasakul A, Reiman H, et al. The risk of lymph node metastasis in colorectal polyps with invasive adenocarcinoma. Dis Colon Rectum 1991;34:323–338.

18. Coverlizza S, Risio M, Ferrari A, et al. Colorectal adenomas containing invasive carcinoma: pathologic assessment of lymph node metastatic potential. Cancer 1989;64:1937–1947.

19. Pollard C, Nivatvongs S, Rojanasakul A, et al. The fate of patients following polypectomy alone for polyps containing invasive carcinoma. Dis Colon Rectum 1992;35:933–937.

20. Wilcox G, Beck J. Early invasive cancer in adenomatous colonic polyps ("malignant polyps"): evaluation of the therapeutic options by decision analysis. Gastroenterology 1987;92:1159–1168.

21. Eckardt V, Fuchs M, Kanzler G, et al. Follow-up of patients with colonic polyps containing severe atypia and invasive carcinoma: compliance, recurrence, and survival. Cancer 1988;61:2552–2557.

22. Weston A, Campbell D. Diminutive polyps: histopathology, spatial distribution, concomitant significant lesions, and treatment complications. Am J Gastroenterol 1995;90:24–28.

CHAPTER

3

Screening for Colon and Rectal Cancer

M. L. Davila, M.D., and A. D. Davila, M.D.

Introduction

Colorectal cancer (CRC) is the second leading cause of cancer death in the United States. It is the third most common cancer both in men and in women. The lifetime incidence of colorectal cancer in the general population is 5 to 6%.

Risk factors for the development of colorectal cancer include advancing age, a personal history of CRC or adenomatous polyps, a family history of CRC or adenomatous polyps, inherited disorders such as familial adenomatous polyposis (FAP) and hereditary nonpolyposis colorectal cancer (HNPCC), inflammatory bowel disease, a diet high in fat and low in fiber, obesity, diabetes mellitus, and a sedentary lifestyle.

This chapter focuses on reviewing environmental risk factors for CRC and on screening for people at average and increased risk (i.e., first-degree relative diagnosed with colorectal cancer). Patients with inflammatory bowel disease and hereditary polyposis syndromes, those with a personal history of colorectal cancer, and those with

Colon and Rectal Cancer, Edited by Peter S. Edelstein, M.D.
ISBN 0-471-35145-8

signs or symptoms of colorectal cancer require individualized management and are addressed elsewhere in this book.

RISK FACTORS

Age is an important risk factor in the development of sporadic colorectal carcinoma. The incidence of malignancy begins to rise between the ages of 40 and 50. Age-specific incidence rates increase significantly in each subsequent decade thereafter (1).

Family history is also an important risk factor in sporadic disease. In a case-controlled study conducted in Australia involving relatives of 523 colorectal cancer patients and matched controls, 16% of the case patients and 7.5% of the control patients had one or more first-degree relatives with CRC (odds ratio 2.1; CI 1.4 to 3.0; $P < 0.001$) (2). The odds for CRC increased with the number of affected first-degree relatives, having two affected relatives was associated with an odds ratio of 5.7 (CI 1.7 to 19.3, $P < 0.01$). The increased odds were 3.7 times greater with case patients diagnosed before age 45 and 1.8 times greater with case patients diagnosed at 45 years or older. The risk was independent of gender, type of first-degree relative (father, mother, siblings, or children), site of cancer, and number of malignant lesions (single or multiple).

Fuchs et al. (3) observed prospective data from 32,085 men and 87,031 women regarding first-degree relatives with CRC. For men with a positive family history, the age-adjusted relative risk of colorectal cancer was 1.64 (95% CI, 1.04 to 2.58) and for women, 1.77 (95% CI, 1.32 to 2.37). For participants < 45 years of age who had first-degree relatives with CRC, the relative risk of CRC was 5.37 (95% CI, 1.98 to 14.6); for those 65 years of age or older, the relative risk associated with a family history approached 1.0. As in the Australian study, the risk was independent of type of affected relative (father, mother, or sibling).

The presence of a family history of a colonic adenoma may in some cases be as significant a risk factor as a positive family history of colorectal cancer. Randomly chosen participants in the National Polyp Study with newly diagnosed adenomatous polyps were interviewed for information on the history of colorectal cancer in their parents and siblings (4). The first-degree relatives of patients with adenomas had a relative risk for CRC of 1.78 (95% CI, 1.18 to 2.67). The risk of CRC was significantly higher for the siblings and parents of patients in whom adenomas were diagnosed before the age of 50 (4.08, 95% CI 1.56 to 10.68). The relative risk decreased significantly and approached 1.0 among relatives of those whose adenomas were diagnosed at 60 years or older. Based on these and other studies, routine colonoscopic screening has been recommended to first-degree relatives of patients with CRC and/or adenomatous polyps beginning at age 40 or at an age 5 to 10 years earlier than the youngest age of cancer diagnosis in the family, whichever is earlier (5–8).

There is increased evidence in the literature that suggests patients with diabetes mellitus are at increased risk for development of colon cancer. In the Nurses' Health Study (9), 118,403 female nurses have been followed through periodic health questionnaires since 1976. The relative risk of colorectal cancer was 1.43 in those with diabetes mellitus, and this risk was independent of age, body mass index, and other factors.

Ureterocolic anastomoses have been associated with an increased risk of colon cancer in the colonic region close in proximity to the insertion of the ureters (10). Regular surveillance with mucosal biopsies around the ureteric-colonic anastomoses is recommended. Pelvic irradiation has also been described as a risk factor for CRC after a 5- to 10-year latency, but it is still unclear as to whether these patients should be placed in a high-risk category in need of aggressive screening (11). Males with acromegaly also have a higher prevalence of adenomatous polyps and polyps proximal to the splenic flexure than controls (12). Such patients should thus be screened with colonoscopy rather than with flexible sigmoidoscopy.

PROTECTIVE FACTORS

In addition to the above described risk factors for colorectal cancer, some protective factors have been identified, including a diet high in fruits and vegetables (dietary fiber), a diet low in fat, regular physical activity, and hormone-replacement therapy in postmenopausal women.

DIETARY FIBER

Dietary fiber is defined as the components of edible plant tissues that are resistant to digestion by human enzymes. Dietary fiber is found in vegetables, fruits, grains, seeds, nuts, and legumes and consists of nonpolysaccharides (such as lignin) and nonstarch polysaccharides (including cellulose, pectin, and gums). There are multiple possible mechanisms by which fiber can protect against the development of colorectal cancer. Fiber increases stool bulk, thereby decreasing transit time and contact time for intraluminal carcinogens. Fiber binds with bile acids and other potential carcinogens and also lowers anaerobic fecal flora levels. Fiber also decreases fecal pH, thereby inactivating bile acids and inhibiting bacterial degradation of food constituents into potential carcinogens.

The fiber hypothesis was introduced in 1971 when Burkitt (13) recognized the relative infrequency of colon cancer in most African populations and was impressed by the high fiber and low refined carbohydrate content of the African diet and the diets found in other underdeveloped areas of the world. Since then, the majority of both observational epidemiologic and case-control studies have supported a protective effect of fiber-rich diets. It is important to note, however, that in the majority of the studies, the data do not differentiate between fiber and other nonfiber components also present in vegetables, such as vitamins and other micronutrients.

Several studies have reported a protective effect of fiber on colorectal cancer. A combined analysis of 13 case-control studies reported decreased relative risks of colorectal cancer of 0.79, 0.69, 0.63, and 0.53 for the four highest quintiles of fiber intake compared to the lowest one (14). Trock et al. (15) analyzed 37 epidemiologic studies on the relationship between colorectal cancer and fiber. Of these studies, 21 demonstrated either a strong or moderate protective effect of dietary fiber, 2 studies showed a lack of association, and the remainder were equivocal. Overall, the majority of the studies supported the protective role of dietary fiber in colorectal carcinogenesis.

The findings of cohort studies are less consistent. In the Health Professionals Follow-Up Study (16) involving >50,000 male health professionals, dietary fiber was inversely associated with risk of colorectal adenoma formation. The relative risk of colorectal cancer was reduced by 64% in men in the highest quintile of dietary fiber intake compared to those in the lowest quintile. Conversely, data from the Nurses' Health Study published in 1990 (17), covering a population of 88,751 women, failed to show any protective effect of increased dietary fiber. There was only a weak inverse association between fruit fiber consumption and colorectal cancer, but the overall trend did not attain statistical significance. When the data were reanalyzed after longer follow-up, no significant association was seen between fiber intake and the risk of colorectal adenoma or colorectal cancer in this population (18). In another large cohort study, the Iowa Women's Health Study (19), 98,030 postmenopausal women were asked to answer a self-administered questionnaire dealing with health issues and diet. This group was followed for 4 years. A weak and statistically nonsignificant inverse association was observed between dietary fiber intake and the risk of colon cancer.

In conclusion, although the majority of observational and case-control studies support the protective effect of dietary fiber on colorectal carcinogenesis, large cohort studies have failed to confirm this and suggest the protective effects may be confined to men.

DIETARY FAT AND LIFESTYLE

Other factors that have been evaluated in relation to colorectal cancer development include high dietary fat and high dietary red meat, obesity, and degree of physical activity. The highest rates of colorectal cancer are observed in Western, industrialized, and economically prosperous countries. There is a strong dose relationship between per capita fat intake (measured as total fat, total saturated fat, and cholesterol) and colorectal cancer incidence and mortality (20). In the Nurses' Health Study (17), animal fat was positively associated with the risk of colon cancer, with a relative risk of 1.89 for women in the highest as compared with the lowest quintile. There was no association for vegetable fat or for linoleic acid, the most abundant polyunsaturated fat. Processed meats and liver were also significantly associated with increased CRC risk, whereas chicken without skin and fish were associated with a decreased risk. In a case-control study of persons with colorectal adenomatous polyps, increased saturated fat, decreased fish and chicken, and increased meat-to-fish and meat-to-chicken ratios were all associated with a higher incidence of polyps among women. Increased caloric intake and increased total fat also raised the risk for recurrent polyps among women with a known history of polyps (21).

The association between physical activity, obesity, and risk for colon cancer has been extensively evaluated in both case-control and cohort studies. In the Health Professionals Follow-Up Study (22), physical activity was inversely associated with risk for colon cancer. The relative risk when comparing the highest with the lowest quintile of energy expenditure was 0.53. The analysis was adjusted for age, smoking, body mass, and intake of red meat, dietary fiber, folate, and alcohol. Body mass index (BMI) was directly associated with risk for colon cancer, independent of physical activity. The relative risk for those with waist circumference $\geqslant 43$ inches compared with those with waist circumference <35 inches was 2.56. In a study of overweight men with adenomatous polyps (23), the greatest risk of developing a high-risk adenoma was seen among those aged 50 to 68 years with the highest BMI, independent of cholesterol levels.

VITAMIN AND MINERAL INTAKE

The antioxidant micronutrients, including vitamin A, carotenoids, vitamin C, vitamin E, selenium, zinc, copper, iron, and manganese, are part of the body's natural defense against free radicals and reactive oxygen species. Although it has long been presumed that those with low levels of antioxidants are at higher risk of developing certain cancers, prospective studies have not shown a significant negative association between low levels of such micronutrients and colorectal cancer. Data from the Iowa Women's Health Study, which looked at the effect of vitamins A and C on the relative risk of developing colorectal cancer, demonstrated no protective effect. Total vitamin E intake, however, did indicate an inverse association (24). A randomized controlled trial in 864 patients testing the efficacy of β-carotene and vitamins C and E in the prevention of colorectal adenomas showed no beneficial effect at 4 years of follow-up (25). Perhaps more individuals must be studied over longer periods of time if any benefits from this type of intervention are to be detected.

Increased dietary calcium or calcium supplementation may have a protective effect in colorectal cancer. Possible mechanisms by which calcium may work include suppressing proliferation of colonic epithelium and binding to free bile acids and fatty acids, thereby reducing their carcinogenic effects. In one randomized controlled trial that included 930 subjects with a history of colorectal adenomas (26), calcium carbonate supplementation (1200 mg of elemental calcium daily) was associated with a reduction of recurrent adenomas (relative risk 0.85) seen in follow-up colonoscopy at 1 and 4 years. In a prospective study of 7472 men, the incidence of colon cancer decreased significantly with increasing intake of calcium (27). The relative risk for those with the highest calcium intake was 0.6. Other studies have not shown such protective effect, including the Health Professionals Follow-Up Study and the Nurses' Health Study (28). These findings probably reflect the difficulties of separating calcium intake from confounding factors such as caloric intake, dietary fat, and use of vitamin and mineral supplements.

Epidemiologic evidence from two prospective studies suggests that folate intake may reduce the risk of colon cancer. In the Nurses' Health Study (29), women who used multivitamins containing folic acid for 15 years or longer had a lower risk of colon cancer (relative risk of 0.25). The benefit was seen even after controlling for intake of vitamins A, C, D, and E as well as for intake of red meat, alcohol, and fiber. In the Health Professionals Follow-Up Study (30), the highest risk for colon cancer (relative risk of 3.30) was seen among those with a high alcohol, low methionine, and low folate intake.

HORMONE-REPLACEMENT THERAPY

Finally, evidence is accumulating that indicates postmenopausal hormone administration may reduce a woman's risk of colorectal cancer. In the Nurses' Health Study (31), women who reported taking hormone-replacement therapy had a relative risk of 0.65 for the development of colorectal cancer. This benefit disappeared 5 years after hormone use was discontinued. Similar findings were found in women participants in the Cancer Prevention Study II (32). More than 0.5 million women were asked to complete a questionnaire that included questions about hormone use. A negative association was observed between having ever taken estrogen and colon cancer mortality (relative risk of 0.71). The benefit was greatest in currently treated women and in those treated for more than 10 years.

ROLE OF ASPIRIN IN COLORECTAL CANCER

Several recent studies have examined whether the use of aspirin and other NSAIDs reduces the risk of developing colorectal cancer. In a prospective study of $>660{,}000$ men and women enrolled in the Cancer Prevention Study II, regular aspirin use was associated with a decreased risk of colorectal cancer (33). The relative risk among those who used aspirin 16 or more times per month for at least 1 year was 0.6 in men and 0.58 in women. These results were unchanged after adjusting for dietary fat, vegetable, fruit, and grain consumption, obesity, physical activity, and family history. In the Nurses' Health Study (34), there was a statistically significant reduction in colorectal cancer after 20 years of consistent use of aspirin. The maximal reduction in risk was observed among women who took four to six tablets per week. Different results were seen in the Physicians' Health Study (35). More than 22,000 male physicians were first randomized to receive aspirin (325 mg per day) or placebo. After 6 years, the randomization was stopped, and participants then chose by themselves to receive aspirin or placebo for the rest of the follow-up period (another 6 years). Both the randomized and observational analyses indicated no beneficial association between the use of aspirin and the incidence of colorectal cancer. It is unclear as to whether a longer period of follow-up would have led to different end results. It appears that if a beneficial effect is to be seen with aspirin, it will require prolonged and consistent use.

SCREENING FOR COLORECTAL CANCER

Virtually all colorectal cancers arise from adenomatous polyps, some of which progress from smaller to larger polyps, then to dysplasia, and finally to cancer. This progression appears to require at least 10 years to reach completion (malignancy) in most individuals (1). A major benefit of this long process is that it allows for the detection and removal of polyps before cancer develops; it also allows earlier identification of cancers, leading to removal at a lesser stage, with subsequent improvement in prognosis. But it is the former, the ability to detect and remove premalignant lesions (polyps), which truly differentiates colorectal cancer screening from the preventive strategies used for other major neoplasms. Indeed, breast examination and mammograms, pelvic examination and pap smears, and prostate examination and prostate-specific antigen (PSA) analysis are not truly preventive in that these strategies aim at detecting early cancers not premalignant lesions. Colorectal cancer screening alone stands out as a truly preventive strategy beause it aims to detect and remove lesions before the development of malignancy. Thus the overwhelming majority of all colorectal cancers could be prevented through safe, rapid, currently existing screening techniques. Unfortunately, the majority of the population are never screened, and this malignancy remains a major cause of morbidity and mortality. Even more disturbing is the realization that appropriate screening is most often never offered to patients by their health care providers.

The major colorectal cancer screening tests now available to detect polyps and early cancers are the fecal occult blood test (FOBT), sigmoidoscopy, double-contrast barium enema (DCBE), and colonoscopy.

FECAL OCCULT BLOOD TESTING

The concept of detecting cancers of the colon and rectum by testing for blood in the stool is based on the observation that neoplastic tissue, especially malignant tissue, bleeds more than normal mucosa. The amount of bleeding increases with the size of a polyp and the stage of a cancer. Testing for fecal occult blood will, therefore, lead to detection of some cancers and large polyps.

The test most widely used for detecting blood in the stool is the guaiac-based test for peroxidase activity. The positive reaction with blood results from the pseudoperoxidase activity of hemoglobin. The test is not specific for blood per se, because other substances with peroxidase activity (dietary red meat, bacteria, and hyperoxides in some fruits and vegetables) can cause false-positive reactions if they are present in the stool. The sensitivity of guaiac-based tests is increased if the test slide is rehydrated with a few drops of water before adding the hydrogen peroxide reagent. This increase in sensitivity, however, is accompanied by a reduction in specificity. Vitamin C, an antioxidant, can interfere with the reaction and cause a false-negative test. Iron supplements do not interfere with the test, but by turning the stools dark in color, iron can make the interpretation of a change in the color of the guaiac-impregnated slide difficult.

Several studies have been published which examine the benefits and limitations of FOBT screening. In a study from the University of Minnesota, 46,551 participants, aged 50 to 80 years, were randomly assigned to screening with FOBT every year, screening every 2 years, or to a control group (36). Participants were asked to submit six guaiac-impregnated paper slides with two smears from each of three consecutive stools. They were asked to avoid red meat, horseradishes (to prevent false-positive peroxidase reactions), aspirin, and vitamin C (to prevent false negative chemical reactions) for 24 h before and during the collection of the samples. Approximately 83% of the slides were rehydrated, which increased the sensitivity of the test but also the false-positive rate. Participants who tested positive underwent a diagnostic evaluation, usually with colonoscopy. A 33% decline in mortality was observed in the annually screened group and a nonsignificant 6% decline was seen in those screened every other year. Reduced mortality in the annually screened group was accompanied by improved survival in those with colorectal cancer and a shift to detection at an earlier stage of cancer. There were twice as many Dukes' stage D (metastatic) cancers in the control group as in the annually screened group, and this accounted for the improved survival in the study group. A notable feature of the Minnesota study was the effect of slide rehydration on the test results. Rehydration raised the positivity rate from 2.4 to 9.8%, increasing the number of evaluations in the study population. Rehydration increased the sensitivity of the test for colorectal cancer from 80.8 to 92.2% and decreased the specificity from 97.7 to 90.4%. The positive predictive value decreased from 5.6 to 2.2%.

Two other large, randomized, controlled trials were published that confirm that FOBT reduces colorectal cancer mortality. Both studies used nonrehydrated Hemoccult cards with biennial (every other year) screening. In the study from Denmark (37) involving 140,000 participants, aged 45 to 75 years, there was an 18% reduction in colorectal cancer mortality. In the British study (38) of a similar number of participants, mortality was decreased by 15%. Interestingly, a longer follow-up of the Minnesota study that looked at the biennial FOBT screening group showed a reduction in mortality of 21%, a remarkable increase from the original 6% reported in the 1993 article (39).

In a large controlled trial from Memorial Sloan-Kettering in New York, 21,756 patients were randomized to annual rigid sigmoidoscopy and FOBT versus annual rigid sigmoidoscopy alone (control group). Survival was significantly greater in the study group than in the control group (70% versus 48%). Colorectal cancer mortality was lower (0.36 versus 0.63) in the study group, but the trend did not achieve statistical significance. There was a statistically significant difference, however, in the distribution of Duke's staging, with a shift to earlier stage cancers in the study group (40).

In summary, FOBT reduces colorectal cancer mortality primarily by diagnosing early stage tumors. Biennial screening might be as effective as annual screening. Nonrehydrated specimens should be used. Using rehydrated cards may result in more positive tests (both true positives and false positives) and may add to the overall costs of a screening program. As a strategy, the major limitation of FOBT is its inability to detect adenomatous polyps. Thus FOBT is clearly aimed at detecting cancer after it develops but while still in an early stage. Once a positive FOBT is obtained, the patient should be promptly evaluated by colonoscopy.

SIGMOIDOSCOPY

Sigmoidoscopy as a screening modality offers important advantages over FOBT. Sigmoidoscopy allows physicians to visualize the bowel directly. If a lesion is found, it can be safely and easily biopsied. More important, sigmoidoscopy can reduce colorectal cancer mortality not only by detecting early-stage cancers but also by detecting and removing premalignant lesions (adenomatous polyps). The evidence that sigmoidoscopy reduces colorectal cancer mortality comes from a number of well-designed case-control studies. In a study from Oakland Kaiser-Permanente (41), 261 patients who died of cancer of the rectum or distal colon were matched to 868 control subjects. Data on use of screening by rigid sigmoidoscopy during the 10 years before diagnosis were analyzed for both groups. Only 8.8% of the case subjects had undergone screening by sigmoidoscopy compared to 24.2% of the controls. Screened subjects had only 30% of the risk for fatal colorectal cancer compared to unscreened subjects. Furthermore, the data suggested that screening sigmoidoscopy could reduce the risk of developing colorectal cancer for as long as 10 years. Clearly, the reduction in mortality was limited to tumors within reach of the sigmoidoscope.

In another case-control study from Wisconsin (42), the records of 66 patients who died of colorectal cancer and those of 196 controls were reviewed. Of those who died, 10% had undergone at least a single screening sigmoidoscopy over a 10-year period, as opposed to 30% of the cancer-free controls. The risk of death was reduced by

79% after a single examination. Again, the reduction in risk appeared to be limited to tumors in the rectum and distal colon (those within reach of the sigmoidoscope). In another case-control study, Muller and Sonnenberg (43) evaluated >4000 U.S. veterans dying of colorectal cancer and both living and dead controls without the disease. Sigmoidoscopy was associated with a 60% reduction in colorectal cancer mortality.

Although no large, prospective, controlled studies have been published that examine the efficacy of sigmoidoscopy as a screening method, there is strong evidence for a protective effect that results from endoscopic removal of premalignant lesions. Sigmoidoscopy does not reduce the mortality from colonic tumors above the reach of the sigmoidoscope, but sigmoidoscopy should always lead to colonoscopy if a moderate size or large adenomatous polyp is found or if any size polyp with tubulovillous or villous characteristics is identified (44). The literature is less clear in determining whether a patient who is found on sigmoidoscopy to have a small tubular adenoma should undergo colonoscopy.

Double-Contrast Barium Enema

There are no studies evaluating the effectiveness of DCBE in the prevention of colorectal cancer. The sensitivity of DCBE is 50 to 80% for polyps <1 cm, 70 to 90% for polyps >1 cm, and 55 to 85% for Dukes' stage A and B cancers (45). It is thought that DCBE might be effective in preventing colorectal cancer because it identifies lesions better than FOBT and nearly as well as colonoscopy; however, such efficacy has never been demonstrated. Because DCBE may perform less well when evaluating the more tortuous rectosigmoid area, flexible sigmoidoscopy is usually recommended to complement the radiographic evaluation. It is unclear if this combination increases the sensitivity for the detection of lesions.

COLONOSCOPY

It is quite reasonable to suspect that colonoscopy can prevent colorectal cancer deaths, because it allows for the identification and removal of premalignant lesions. There is no direct evidence, however, that colonoscopy reduces colorectal cancer mortality in people without symptoms or known polyps. Indirect evidence comes from studies that show detection and removal of polyps and detection of early cancers reduces mortality.

In a study of patients with polyps (not a screened population) in which the colon was cleared of polyps by colonoscopy, there was a large (76 to 90%) reduction in mortality compared to patients who did not have polyps removed and compared to the general population (46). Studies showing that sigmoidoscopy reduces colorectal cancer deaths in the area examined provide compelling evidence that colonoscopy, with examination of the entire colon and rectum, should also be effective (41–43).

The disadvantages of colonoscopy are its major, albeit infrequent, complications, including perforation, hemorrhage, and respiratory depression owing to oversedation. The procedure is also somewhat expensive and requires careful bowel preparation.

SUMMARY

The American Cancer Society, the National Cancer Institute, and several other advisory panels (8) recommend that screening for colorectal cancer in asymptomatic, average-risk individuals begin at age 50 and consist of annual FOBT plus flexible sigmoidoscopy every 5 years. Positive screening examinations should be promptly followed by colonoscopy or, by DCBE, preferably with flexible sigmoidoscopy as well. Most physicians prefer colonoscopic evaluation in patients with a positive screening test, because identification of a suspicious lesion on DCBE necessitates colonoscopic evaluation and possible removal.

First-degree relatives of patients who were diagnosed with an adenomatous polyp before age 60 are at increased risk for colorectal cancer; and as such, they should be offered routine colonoscopic evaluations.

Individuals with a single, elderly first-degree relative with an adenoma or colorectal cancer are not necessarily at increased risk of colorectal cancer. Such patients should undergo the same screening as average-risk individuals. However, if there are two or more affected first-degree relatives, even if elderly, or if the neoplasm has occurred in a young first-degree relative (cancer before the age of 55), routine colonoscopic examinations should be performed beginning at age 40 or 5 years earlier than the earliest cancer in the family.

REFERENCES

1. Eddy DM. Screening for colorectal cancer. Ann Intern Med 1990;113:373–384.
2. St. John JB, McDermott FT, Hopper L, et al. Cancer risk in relatives of patients with common colorectal cancer. Ann Intern Med 1993;118:785–790.
3. Fuchs CS, Giovannucci EL, Colditz GA, et al. A prospective study of family history and the risk of colorectal cancer. N Engl J Med 1994;331:1669–1674.
4. Winawer SJ, Zauber AG, Gerdes H, et al. Risk of colorectal cancer in the families of patients with adenomatous polyps. N Engl J Med 1996;334:82–87.
5. Burt RW, Bishop DT, Lynch HT, et al. Risk and surveillance of individuals with heritable factors for colorectal cancer. Bull World Health Org 1998;68:655–665.
6. Burt RW, Bishop DT, Cannon LA, et al. Dominant inheritance of adenomatous colonic polyps and colorectal cancers. N Engl J Med 1985;312:1540–1544.
7. Cannon-Albright LA, Skolnick MH, Bishop DT, et al. Common inheritance of susceptibility to colonic adenomatous polyps and associated colorectal cancers. N Engl J Med 1988;319:533–537.

8. Winawer SJ, Fletcher RH, Miller L, et al. Colorectal cancer screening: clinical guidelines and rationale. Gastroenterology 1997;112:594–642.
9. Hu FB, Manson JE, Liu S, et al. Prospective study of adult onset diabetes mellitus (type II) and risk of colorectal cancer in women. J Natl Cancer Inst 1999;91:542–457.
10. Stewart M, Macrae FA, Williams CB. Neoplasia and ureterosigmoidostomy: a colonoscopy survey. Br J Surg 1982;69:414–416.
11. Sandler RS, Sandler DP. Radiation-induced cancers of the colon and rectum: assessing the risk. Gastroenterology 1983;84:51–57.
12. Delhougne B, Deneux C, Abs R, et al. The prevalence of colonic polyps in acromegaly: a colonoscopic and pathological study in 103 patients. J Clin Endocrinol Metab 1995;80:3223–3226.
13. Burkitt DP. Epidemiology of cancer of the colon and rectum. Cancer 1971;28:3–13.
14. Howe GR, Benito E, Castelleto R, et al. Dietary intake of fiber and decreased risk of cancers of the colon and rectum: evidence from the combined analysis of 13 case-control studies. J Natl Cancer Inst 1992;84:1887–1896.
15. Trock B, Lanza E, Greenwald P. Dietary fiber, vegetables, and colon cancer: critical review and meta-analyses of the epidemiologic evidence. J Natl Cancer Inst 1990;82:650–661.
16. Giovannucci E, Stampfer MJ, Colditz G, et al. Relationship of diet to risk of colorectal cancer in men. J Natl Cancer Inst 1992;84:91–98.
17. Willett WC, Stampfer MJ, Colditz GA, et al. Relation of meat, fat, and fiber intake to the risk of colon cancer in a prospective study among women. N Engl J Med 1990;323:1664–1672.
18. Fuchs CS, Giovannucci EL, Colditz GA, et al. Dietary fiber and the risk of colorectal cancer and adenoma in women. N Engl J Med 1999;340:169–176.
19. Steinmetz KA, Kushi LH, Bostick RM, et al. Vegetables, fruit, and colon cancer in the Iowa Women's Health Study. Am J Epidemiol 1994;139:1–15.
20. Rose DP, Boyar AP, Wynder EL. International comparisons of mortality rates for cancer of the breast, ovary, prostate and colon, and per capita food consumption. Cancer 1986;58:2363–2371.
21. Neugut AI, Garbowski GC, Lee WC, et al. Dietary risk factors for the incidence and recurrence of colorectal adenomatous polyps. Ann Intern Med 1993;118:91–95.
22. Giovannucci E, Ascherio A, Rimm EB, et al. Physical activity, obesity, and

risk for colon cancer and adenoma in men. Ann Intern Med 1995;122:327–334.

23. Bayerdörffer E, Mannes GA, Ochsenkühn T, et al. Increased risk of "high risk" colorectal adenomas in overweight men. Gastroenterology 1993;104:137–144.
24. Bostick RM, Potter JD, McKenzie DR, et al. Reduced risk of colon cancer with high intake of vitamin E: the Iowa Women's Health Study. Cancer Res 1993;53:4230–4237.
25. Greenberg ER, Baron JA, Tosteson TD, et al. A clinical trial of antioxidant vitamins to prevent colorectal adenoma. N Engl J Med 1994;331:141–147.
26. Baron JA, Beach M, Mandel JS, et al. Calcium supplements for the prevention of colorectal adenomas. N Engl J Med 1999;340:101–107.
27. Stemmermann GN, Nomura A, Chyou P. The influence of dairy and nondairy calcium on subsite large bowel cancer risk. Dis Colon Rectum 1990;33:190–194.
28. Kampman E, Giovannucci E, van't Veer P, et al. Calcium, vitamin D, dairy foods, and the occurrence of colorectal adenomas among men and women in two prospective studies. Am J Epidemiol 1994;139:16–29.
29. Giovannucci E, Stampfer MJ, Colditz GA, et al. Multivitamin use, folate and colon cancer in women in the Nurses' Health Study. Ann Intern Med 1998;129:517–524.
30. Giovannucci E, Rimm EB, Ascherio A, et al. Alcohol, low-methionine-low-folate diets, and risk of colon cancer in men. J Natl Cancer Inst 1995;87:265–273.
31. Grodstein F, Martinez ME, Platz EA, et al. Postmenopausal hormone use and risk for colorectal cancer and adenoma. Ann Intern Med 1998;128:705–712.
32. Calle EE, Miracle-McMahill HL, Thun MJ, Heath CW. Estrogen replacement therapy and risk of fatal colon cancer in a prospective cohort of postmenopausal women. J Natl Cancer Inst 1995;87:517–523.
33. Thun MJ, Namboodiri MM, Heath CW. Aspirin use and reduced risk of fatal colon cancer. N Engl J Med 1991;325:1593–1596.
34. Giovannucci E, Egan KM, Hunter DJ, et al. Aspirin and the risk of colorectal cancer in women. N Engl J Med 1995;333:609–614.
35. Stürmer T, Glynn RJ, Lee IM, et al. Aspirin use and colorectal cancer: post-trial follow-up data from the Physicians' Health Study. Ann Intern Med 1998;128:713–720.
36. Mandel JS, Bond JH, Church TR, et al. Reducing mortality from colorectal

cancer by screening for fecal occult blood. N Engl J Med 1993;328:1365–1371.

37. Kronborg O, Fenger C, Olsen J, et al. Randomised study of screening for colorectal cancer with faecal-occult-blood test. Lancet 1996;348:1467–1471.

38. Hardcastle JD, Chamberlain JO, Robinson MH, et al. Randomised controlled trial of faecal-occult-blood screening for colorectal cancer. Lancet 1996;348:1472–1477.

39. Mandel JS, Church TR, Ederer F, Bond JH. Colorectal cancer mortality: effectiveness of biennial screening for fecal occult blood. J Natl Cancer Inst 1999;91:434–xxx.

40. Winawer SJ, Flehinger BJ, Schottenfeld D, Miller DG. Screening for colorectal cancer with fecal occult blood testing and sigmoidoscopy. J Natl Cancer Inst 1993;85:1311–1318.

41. Selby JV, Friedman GD, Quesenberry CP, Weiss NS. A case-control study of screening sigmoidoscopy and mortality from colorectal cancer. N Engl J Med 1992;326:653–657.

42. Newcomb PA, Norfleet RG, Storer BE, et al. Screening sigmoidoscopy and colorectal cancer mortality. J Natl Cancer Inst 1992;84:1572–1575.

43. Muller AD, Sonnenberg A. Protection by endoscopy against death from colorectal cancer. Arch Intern Med 1995;155:1741–1748.

44. Atkin WS, Morson BC, Cuzick J. Long-term risk of colorectal cancer after excision of rectosigmoid adenomas. N Engl J Med 1992;326:658–662.

45. Fork FT. Double contrast enema and colonoscopy in polyp detection. Gut 1981;22:971–977.

46. Winawer SJ, Zauber AG, Ho MN, et al. Prevention of colorectal cancer by colonoscopic polypectomy. N Engl J Med 1993;329:1977–1981.

CHAPTER 4

Hereditary Nonpolyposis Colorectal Cancer Syndromes (Lynch Syndromes)

Henry T. Lynch, M.D.,
and Jane F. Lynch, B.S.N.

HNPCC

Hereditary nonpolyposis colorectal cancer (HNPCC), also known as Lynch syndrome, is one of the most important known risk factors for the development of colorectal cancer, accounting for between 5 and 10% of the total colorectal cancer (CRC) burden. Thus in terms of actual cancer cases, HNPCC is significantly more important than familial adenomatous polyposis and the inflammatory bowel diseases combined, yet many physicians know little or nothing about the syndrome. HNPCC is an autosomal dominantly inherited cancer-prone syndrome characterized by the development of malignant neoplastic lesions in a variety of tissues, including gastrointestinal, endometrial, ovarian, and urinary. The most frequent lesion is CRC (1–3). Despite its name, HNPCC does indeed involve the

Colon and Rectal Cancer, Edited by Peter S. Edelstein, M.D.
ISBN 0-471-35145-8

development of benign adenomatous colorectal polyps (although relatively few in number compared to the polyposis syndromes), and the clinical features and pathology of the colorectal neoplastic process in HNPCC appear to follow an adenoma-to-carcinoma progression somewhat similar to that described in familial adenomatous polyposis (FAP) and sporadic cancer settings. However, several aspects of the clinical manifestations in HNPCC, as well as the molecular pathophysiologies underlying the carcinogenesis process, may be distinctive (4).

HNPCC was traditionally recognized by the familial clustering of CRC in people without obvious colonic polyposis. In 1991, the so-called Amsterdam criteria were defined by the International Collaborative Group on HNPCC to standardize inclusion criteria for multicenter studies. These criteria include all of the following: three cases of colorectal cancer verified by histology in a family, one patient being a first-degree relative of the other two; colorectal cancer in at least two generations; at least one patient was < 50 years of age at cancer diagnosis; and FAP has been excluded (5). The Amsterdam criteria were not originally designed for clinical diagnostic purposes, because they are quite restrictive and do not include extracolonic cancers. Hence, full reliance on these criteria will miss otherwise classical HNPCC families that may present with gynecologic, urologic, or other cancer types that are integral to this syndrome.

TWO LYNCH SYNDROMES

HNPCC actually represents related syndromes that are characterized by the following cardinal features: Lynch syndrome I shows an autosomal dominant inherited predilection to carcinoma of the colon, with a proximal colonic predominance (~70% proximal to the splenic flexure), an excess of synchronous and metachronous cancers (~30% frequency of metachronous cancer development within 10 years in patients who undergo limited surgical resection, such as hemicolectomy or segmental colectomy, as their initial cancer treatment), and improved survival from CRC compared to carefully stage-matched historical controls (1,6–8). Lynch syndrome II shows these identical natural history features of CRC, with the possible exception of a significantly increased risk of rectal cancer relative to Lynch syndrome I patients. In addition, the syndrome includes extracolonic cancers, foremost of which is endometrial carcinoma, followed by carcinoma of the ovary, stomach, small bowel, hepatobiliary tract, and transitional cell carcinoma of the ureter and renal pelvis (Fig. 4.1) (2), as well as sebaceous adenomas, sebaceous carcinomas, and multiple keratoacanthomas in the Muir-Torre syndrome variant (Fig. 4.2) (11,12). Carcinoma of the pancreas appears to occur in excess in selected HNPCC families. Brain tumors, particularly glioblastoma multiforme, appear in HNPCC Turcot's-like families in association with multiple colonic adenomas (13). The cutaneous signs that characterize the Muir-Torre syndrome, and the multiple colonic adenomas in the Turcot's-like variant of HNPCC, represent, so far as we know, the only premonitory signs of cancer susceptibility for HNPCC. Therefore, before recent discoveries regarding the genetic basis for HNPCC, the clinician had to make a diagnosis based exclusively on a detailed family history of the patient combined with a high index of suspicion.

In addition, in HNPCC the pathology of CRC is often distinctive, although not pathognomonic. Specifically, the CRCs in HNPCC show an excess of mucoid, signet cells, poorly differentiated medullary features, a Crohn-like reaction, and tumor-infiltrating lymphocytes (14).

SURVEILLANCE AND TREATMENT

Surveillance and management strategies for HNPCC are predicated upon its natural history. Thus the proximal predominance of CRC requires full colonoscopy so that there can be excellent visualization throughout the colon inclusive of the cecum. The excess of synchro-

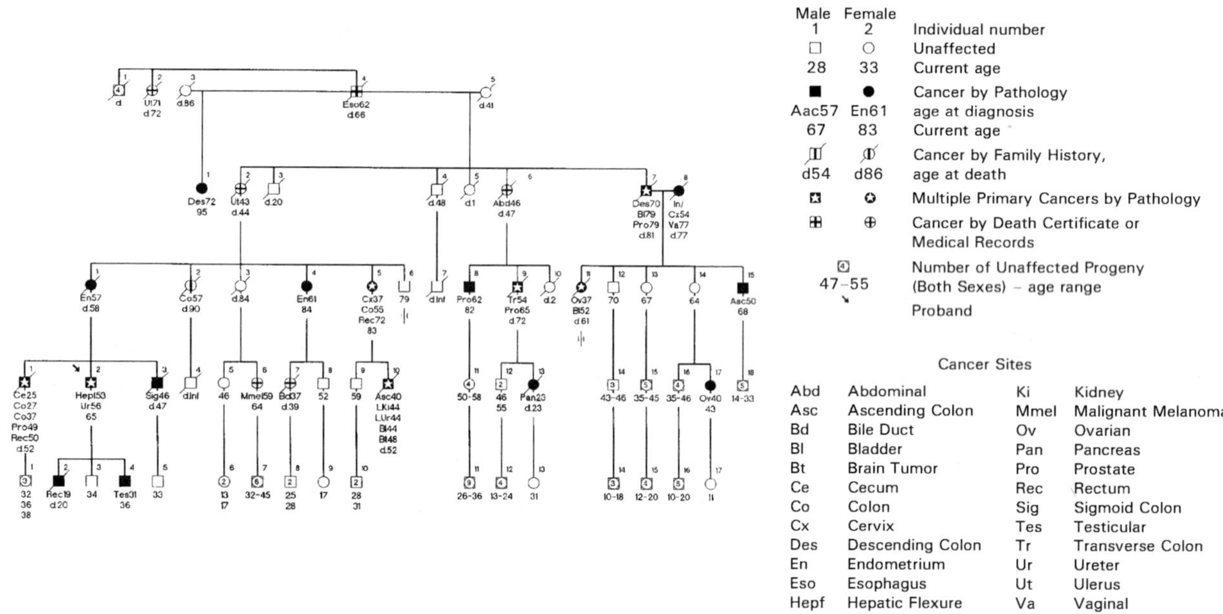

FIGURE 4.1. Pedigree of a family showing Lynch syndrome II, with diverse cancer. (Updated with permission Ref. 9.)

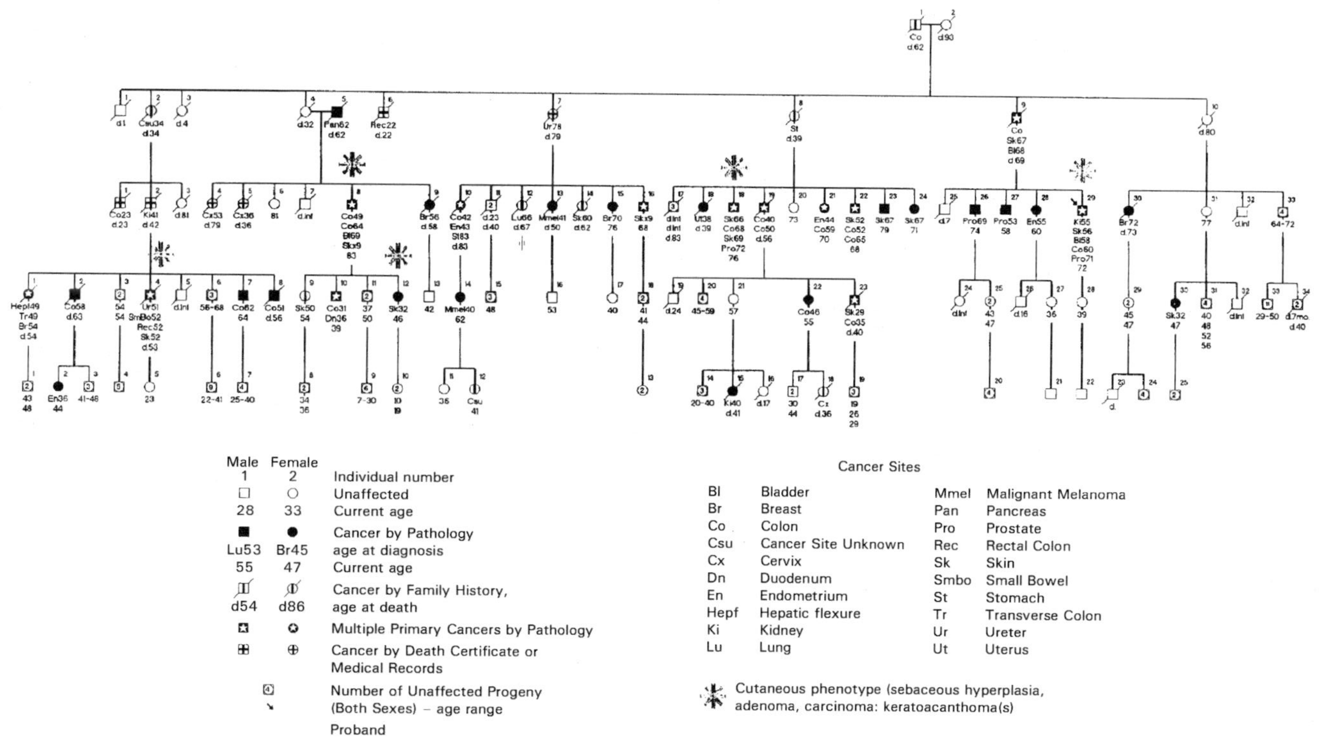

FIGURE 4.2. Pedigree of a family with a tumor spectrum consonant with Muir-Torre cutaneous phenotype in association with Lynch syndrome II variant. (Updated with permission from Ref. 10.)

nous and metachronous CRCs mandates subtotal colectomy at the time of operation for initial CRC. The scenario of a young HNPCC patient developing an incurable metachronous colon cancer only years after undergoing a limited resection for an initial colon cancer is nothing short of a preventable tragedy (metachronous cancers occur in approximately 30% of HNPCC patients within 10 years after limited initial resections). Because of the early age of onset of CRC, we initiate annual colonoscopy at age 25, and given the problem of accelerated carcinogenesis of CRC in HNPCC, we recommend that this procedure be performed annually. Because of the problem of extracolonic cancer excess in HNPCC, we recommend routine screening for endometrial carcinoma, the second most common cancer after CRC, via routine endometrial aspiration; and ovarian cancer screening is provided via regular transvaginal ultrasound evaluation. If acceptable to female patients, total abdominal hysterectomy and bilateral salpingo-oophorectomy may be recommended. Other screening recommendations may include urinalysis, urine cytology, and esophagoduodenoscopy. After subtotal colectomy, regular proctoscopy is required, because the rectum is still at risk for polyp and cancer development (approximately 12% at 12 years). For maximum compliance, it is essential that patients be well educated about the natural history of HNPCC so that they can fully appreciate the reasoning behind this intensive surveillance and management program.

HNPCC Genetics

Mismatch Repair Gene Mutations

DNA replication is a process that is frequently disrupted when base pairing is incorrect, leading to mismatched DNA sequencing. Environmental factors and errors in the enzymatic replication process itself are common causes of such DNA mismatch occurrences. Such base mispairings are normally recognized and excised and the errors corrected by a system of at least seven protein subunits. The proteins themselves are likewise encoded by genes called mismatch repair (MMR) genes. HNPCC is caused by inherited mutations in one of the Mut-related MMR genes, including *hMSH2* (15), *hMLH1* (16), *hPMS2*(17), and *hMSH6* (18), the genes encoding for the protein products that are responsible for recognizing and correcting errors that arise when DNA is replicated (4). After the inheritance of a defect in one allele of an MMR gene (a germline mutation), a somatic mutation in the remaining MMR gene allele (loss of the wild type), causes a DNA mismatch repair defect. The result is an in vivo defect that is believed to contribute to the progressive accumulation of secondary mutations throughout the genome and thereby affects crucial growth-regulatory genes that ultimately lead to cancer development. Cells in which defects at both alleles of an MMR gene have occurred may accumulate further mutations at accelerated rates, as high as a thousand times greater than that which occur in a cell with normal MMR genes. To date, more than 70 different germline mutations have been identified in MMR genes that are known to be associated with HNPCC. Detectable mutations in *hMSH2* and *hMLH1* account for roughly equal proportions of HNPCC kindreds and appear to be responsible for a majority (up to 70%) of these families (4,18). Of note, Lin et al. (19) determined that the risk of development of CRC in patients harboring *hMLH1* mutations and *hMSH2* mutations is 84 and 71%, respectively, similar to other reports suggesting an approximate 80% risk overall. Other types of mutations and/or classes of genes will likely be recognized as playing a causal role in the remaining cases of HNPCC. In addition, some of the mutation-negative families may be HNPCC phenocopies.

Once a cancer-associated germline mutation has been identified in a family, other family members are eligible for genetic counseling, DNA testing, and highly targeted surveillance and management strategies, which are in accord with the syndrome's natural history. Patients found to be mutation carriers through this process and those whose cancer status denotes that they are likely to harbor an MMR mutation are ideal candidates for chemoprevention trials.

Carcinogenesis in HNPCC

The development of colon cancer is a multistep process involving the accumulation of a succession of critical mutations. HNPCC has expanded our perception of the multistep model, and we now recognize that the specific "steps" may have a different molecular basis in different clinical settings. Carcinogenesis in HNPCC appears to involve mutations in *K-ras* and *p53* less often than in sporadic CRC. Recent findings from Losi et al. (20) are representative of this phenomenon. The authors studied 23 CRCs from HNPCC patients and compared them to 40 sporadic CRCs. They detected a *K-ras* mutation in 17% of the HNPCC cases, compared to 48% of sporadics. None of the HNPCC cases had detectable changes in both *K-ras* and *p53*, compared to 20% of sporadics.

Colonic Adenomas in HNPCC: Extraordinary Carcinogenic Potential

Although colonic adenomas are relatively sparse in HNPCC, they nevertheless harbor an exquisite proclivity to undergo carcinogenesis. This contrasts with FAP, in which there may be 1000 or more colonic adenomas, yet the CRC rates and even the average age of onset are similar to those in HNPCC. A remarkable feature of HNPCC is its extraordinarily accelerated carcinogenesis (1). This raises important implications for more frequent screening colonoscopy. Specifically, we now recommend annual colonoscopy for HNPCC germline mutation carriers.

Genetic Testing

Microsatellite Instability and HNPCC DNA regions that are composed of repeated mononucleotides and dinucleotides are known as microsatellites. Although microsatellite regions do not encode for proteins (and the true functions of which currently remain unknown), differences in length of microsatellite regions between neoplastic and normal tissue (microsatellite instability) can serve as a marker of MMR gene dysfunction and subsequent abnormal replication. Microsatellite instability (MSI) is present in as many as 86% of cancers in HNPCC patients but in only 10 to 15% of sporadic colorectal cancers (19). Aaltonen et al. (21) stress the importance of MSI as a marker for HNPCC because with the exception of the cutaneous signs in Muir-Torre syndrome, there is an absence of striking phenotypic signs of HNPCC cancer risk status, thereby forcing the diagnosis to be otherwise based solely on family history. Although the identification of a specific HNPCC germline mutation in a family merits family member testing for the identified gene defect, routine screening for germline mutations in MMR genes may be inefficient (22).

On the other hand, Aaltonen et al. noted that an initial routine search for MSI replication errors followed by direct sequencing of *hMLH1* and *hMSH2* to search for specific MMR gene defects in individuals manifesting such MSI may be an important strategy for detecting HNPCC, thereby making its diagnosis more efficient. They prospectively screened CRC specimens from 509 consecutive patients in Finland, employing microsatellite-marker analyses of tumor DNA in a search for microsatellite replication errors that are characteristic of HNPCC. Individuals identified with MSI replication errors were then screened for specific germline mutations of the MMR genes *hMSH2* and *hMLH1*. Supporting this strategy is the fact that all of the patients in the study who demonstrated MMR germline mutations had at least one of the three hallmarks of HNPCC: a family history of CRC and/or endometrial cancer, young age of cancer onset (<50 years), or multiple primary cancers. However, 3 of the 10 patients manifesting MMR germline mutations were >60 years, and 1 of the 10 lacked a family history of HNPCC cancer. Aaltonen et al. suggest that the efficiency of screening for HNPCC in patients with CRC could be improved when all young patients, those with a first-degree relative with CRC or endometrial cancer, and all patients with multiple primary cancers, particularly where the pattern includes CRC and endometrial cancer, are analyzed for MSI. Their findings disclosed that

> 8 percent, 16 percent, and 3 percent of the 509 patients would have fallen into these respective categories, but because of overlap among the groups, only 24 percent would have been analyzed for replication errors. Among these patients, there would have been 20 with replication errors (4 percent of patients), and mutation analysis would have led to the identification of the same 10 patients who were identified with the other approach

Thus Aaltonen et al. suggest that with patients with CRC whose family histories or clinical profiles suggest HNPCC should be tested for MSI and individuals whose tumors have MSI replication errors should be referred for specific MMR genetic testing, placing microsatellite-marker analysis at a different point in the testing algorithm and narrowing its role.

Lynch and Smyrk (23), commenting on the Aaltonen et al. paper, suggest that the low yield of routine MSI testing (only 10 to 15% of CRCs have MSI replication errors and only 10% of those are the result of HNPCC) indicates that this approach is not justifiable in clinical practice. However, it may be important to know the microsatellite status in individuals with CRC for reasons not connected directly to HNPCC in that it appears that many CRC patients demonstrating MSI replication errors, even those without HNPCC, have a better prognosis, and their response to chemotherapeutic agents may also differ (24). Furthermore, Lynch and Smyrk also believe that once suspicion of HNPCC has been raised on the basis of family history or other clinical pathologic clues, the absence of microsatellite instability should not be used as an exclusionary criterion for further specific genetic testing, with emphasis placed more strongly on the family history, which is one of the most important messages gleaned from the Aaltonen et al. report.

MICROSATELLITE INSTABILITY AND SPORADIC CRC It must be appreciated that 10 to 15% of putative sporadic CRCs (non-HNPCC patients) demonstrate MSI replication errors (25). This subset of sporadic CRCs with MSI is of interest in that, as in the case of HNPCC, these cancers often develop at an earlier age, have a predilection for the right colon, frequently display certain similar pathologic features (an excess of mucinous histology and signet cells, poor differentiation), and appear to have a better prognosis than sporadic CRCs lacking such microsatellite features (7). Interestingly, tumors from young sporadic CRC patients are more likely to demonstrate MSI than those of older patients. Liu et al. (26) found MSI in 18 of 31 (58%) CRCs from patients <35 years old, compared to 12% of patients >35 years. Breivik et al. (27) argue that the association between younger age and MSI is also linked to gender, and that young males in particular are likely to harbor MSI-high tumors.

TESTING FOR GERMLINE MUTATIONS OF MMR GENES Given the low prevalence of HNPCC, it is not feasible to test all CRC patients for mutations in MMR genes. One might instead test only individuals whose clinical presentation raises the possibility of HNPCC or those with a suspicious family history. As an example of the first approach, Beck et al. (28) looked for germline mutations in "adenoma-formers," patients with multiple or early-onset adenomas. The rationale for testing this population was the authors' suspicion that HNPCC patients may develop adenomas earlier and more often than the general population. This belief was supported by a St. Mark's Hospital study showing a greater frequency of multiple adenomas in HNPCC than in the general population (29), and by the work of Jass and Stewart (30) who found significantly more adenomas in HNPCC patients <50 years of age than in age-matched autopsy controls. Beck et al. studied 25 patients who formed adenomas at a young age or had multiple adenomas. The patients were 19 to 78 years old (mean age of 51) and had from 1 to greater than 100 adenomas (mean of 15). A germline mutation in an MMR gene was identified in only 1 patient, suggesting that MMR genetic testing based solely on early or multiple colonic adenoma formation is not an effective HNPCC screening approach.

Tomlinson et al. (31) likewise used young age as a trigger for gene testing, but in this case studying 50 patients under the age of 45 years who had developed CRC but were without a family history of CRC or any other HNPCC-related cancer. Germline changes in *hMSH2* or *hMLH1* (the two MMR genes most commonly mutated in HNPCC) were discovered in only 3 patients (6%). These variants were believed to represent new or low penetrant mutations, or perhaps genetic polymorphisms. Thus as was the case with early or multiple adenoma formation, specific MMR genetic screening based solely on early age at diagnosis of CRC was not efficient.

FAMILY HISTORY AS A BASIS FOR DNA TESTING Whether a suspicious family history alone is adequate to support specific MMR genetic analysis has also been addressed. Wijnen et al. (32) studied families with familial clustering of CRC, but not fulfilling Amsterdam criteria. They found mutations of *hMSH2* or *hMLH1* in only 8% of these families and concluded that the Amsterdam criteria have practical value in selecting those families most likely to reward gene testing. Indeed DNA testing has been performed based on family history using either the Amsterdam criteria or a less strict clinical definition of HNPCC. Weber et al. (33) studied 32 families from the eastern United States with a strong family history of CRC (31 met Amsterdam criteria). The authors found germline mutations of *hMSH2* in 3 families and of *hMLH1* in 2 more, for a total yield of 16%. Viel et al. (34) analyzed DNA from 17 Italian HNPCC families who met Amsterdam criteria, finding *hMSH2* mutations in 2 of the families and *hMLH1* mutations in 5, for a total yield of 41%. Wijnen found germline MMR mutations in 49% of Amsterdam criteria families, and Heinimann et al. (35) found such mutations in 64% of Swiss families meeting Amsterdam criteria. Thus basing genetic analysis solely on the overstrict Amsterdam criteria (which exclude families with extracolonic malignancies, more likely to have *hMSH2* mutations) also appears inadequate, probably missing a significant number of families that truly suffer from HNPCC and deserve MMR gene testing.

Still other investigators have reported different experiences. Beck et al. (36) studied 10 families with clustering of CRC or endometrial cancer in successive generations. Germline mutations of MMR genes were discovered in 6 (60%) of these families (3 with *hMLH1* and 3 with *hMSH2*). Similarly, Wang et al. (37) investigated 9 incomplete HNPCC families (defined by the authors as meeting two of the three Amsterdam criteria) and found mutations of *hMLH1* in 3 and an *hMSH2* mutation in another, giving a yield of 44%.

Genuardi et al. (38) investigated a series of 32 Italian putative HNPCC individuals who were selected on the basis of family history of CRC and/or extracolonic tumors, early onset of CRC, and presence of multiple primary cancers in the same individual. *hMLH1* and *hMSH2* mutation analysis disclosed truncating mutations in 4 cases (12.5%), 3 of which involved *hMSH2* and one *hMLH1*. The authors also noted 2 missense *hMLH1* variants of uncertain significance. Of interest was the fact that all pathogenetic mutations identified were associated with early age at onset (<40 years) as well as proximal CRC involvement. The authors' contention was supported in that

> constitutional MMR mutations can also occur in individuals without the classical HNPCC pattern. Moreover, evaluation of the clinical parameters associated with MMR mutations indicates that early onset combined with CRC location in the proximal colon can be definitively considered suggestive of

MMR-related hereditary CRC and should be included among the guidelines for referring patients for genetic testing.

In conclusion, we believe that family history remains the principal basis for identifying families that may benefit from gene testing. Such history should include age at diagnosis and the location of tumors within the colon. Furthermore, genetic testing should not be limited only to families meeting Amsterdam criteria. Endometrial carcinoma and other extracolonic malignancies that are integral to HNPCC (small bowel, stomach, ovary, renal pelvis, and ureter) should be taken into consideration when deciding whether a family should be tested.

Correlations Between Genotype And Phenotype

It appears that there is justification at the molecular level for the long-standing observation that HNPCC can be divided into Lynch syndrome I (colon cancer only) and Lynch syndrome II (colonic and extracolonic cancers). It may be that the basis for this separation resides in the specific MMR gene affected (*hMLH1* versus *hMSH2* versus others). However, it appears more likely that phenotypic differences are actually more directly influenced by the specific type of mutation occurring in the MMR gene rather than solely on the specific gene affected.

Vasen et al. (39) studied cancer risk in 124 individuals known to carry a germline *hMLH1* mutation and 86 patients with known mutations of *hMSH2*. The lifetime risk of CRC was 80% in both groups. However, Lin et al. (19) described a significant difference in the lifetime risk of extracolonic tumors, with a 48% risk of such malignancies in patients with *hMSH2* mutations compared to 11% in those harboring *hMLH1* mutations. Vasen et al. found that both groups had a greatly increased risk for small bowel carcinoma (relative risk of 100). Endometrial carcinoma appeared to be more common in people with *hMSH2* mutations (61% versus 42%), although the difference was not statistically significant. Increased risk for cancer of the renal pelvis, ureter, stomach, and ovary was seen only in carriers of *hMSH2* mutations.

It is likely that the specific nature of the MMR gene mutation contributes more to the resultant phenotype than does the specific gene affected. Jäger et al. (40) described an *hMLH1* intron 14 splice donor mutation in 5 Danish HNPCC families. This mutation resulted in a "silenced" allele, i.e., no abnormal protein was generated. Families with this mutation had a natural history similar to 16 other HNPCC families with respect to CRC, but only two extracolonic cancers were seen (one endometrial, one ampulla of Vater) compared to 44 in the other families. The extracolonic:colorectal cancer ratio was approximately 1 : 11 in families with the intron 14 splice donor site mutation compared to 1 : 2 in the other families. The authors argue that the silenced allele results in less severe disease (fewer extracolonic lesions) owing to the absence of a dominant negative effect.

Beck et al. (36) observed that cancer families not meeting the Amsterdam criteria who have germline MMR mutations often have missense mutations. They speculate that missense mutations result in less severe disease or lower penetrance (thus not meeting the stricter clinical criteria) owing to less pronounced structural changes of the encoded protein.

These observations signify the importance of cataloging the specific gene mutations found in HNPCC families and then critically comparing mutations to phenotypic expression. A major effort in this regard was performed by Peltomäki et al. (41) who provided phenotypic details of 126 HNPCC mutations: 75 involved *hMLH1*, 48 involved *hMSH2*, 1 affected *hPMS1*, and 2 affected *hPMS2*. Most *hMSH2* mutations in the database were frameshift (60%) or nonsense (23%), and most *hMLH1* mutations were frameshift (40%) or missense (31%) alterations. The authors argue that such databases are crucial to deciphering the connection between genotype and phenotype. Further, they point out that kindreds sharing the same mutation but living in different circumstances will provide an opportunity to assess the contribution of environmental factors to colorectal carcinogenesis.

hMSH6: A Newly Recognized Mismatch Repair Gene Involved in HNPCC

Miyaki et al. (18) studied five Japanese HNPCC families in whom germline mutations of *hMSH2* and *hMLH1* were not found. They discovered a germline mutation of *hMSH6* in one family, and found such mutations in family members with colonic, endometrial, ovarian, and pancreatic cancers. Interestingly, this family did not meet Amsterdam criteria, showing instead a predominance of endometrial and ovarian carcinomas.

Transforming Growth Factor β2 Receptor Gene

The unifying theme of the mutations that contribute to carcinogenesis in HNPCC (and in sporadic CRC with defective MMR) seems to be that they involve genes with microsatellites. Because the human genome includes >100,000 microsatellites, there are a large number of potential targets for mutation. The best-studied of these is the transforming growth factor β2 receptor (TGF-β2R) gene. It appears that mutation of this receptor allows escape from inhibitory controls by interfering with binding between TGF-β and the receptor. Mutations of TGF-β2R are more common in HNPCC than in sporadic CRC. Two studies provided supportive evidence. Akiyama et al. (42) studied 14 adenomas and 13 CRCs from 10 HNPCC patients. Mutational alterations in the poly A repeat (microsatellite region) of the TGF-β2R gene were seen in 57% of the adenomas and 85% of the carcinomas. Similarly, Tannergard et al. (43) found mutated

TGF-β2R in 28 of 42 (67%) CRCs from HNPCC patients, compared to 10% in sporadic CRC. It is important to realize that 10 to 15% of sporadic CRCs show microsatellite instability, and thus it would also be likely for some of them to show the TGF-β2R mutation.

INFLAMMATORY BOWEL DISEASE AND HNPCC

Pokorny et al. (44) studied DNA in 126 unrelated individuals, of whom 45 had Crohn disease, 36 manifested ulcerative colitis, and 45 control subjects did not have intestinal disease. The authors identified a novel genetic and clinical association between *hMLH1* and inflammatory bowel disease (IBD). Specifically, they identified two genetic markers within and one near the DNA MMR gene and found two categories of haplotypes associated with the family history of Crohn disease and ulcerative colitis. Pokorny et al. indicated that there was a "significant association of *hMLH1* exon 15/D3S1611 haplotype with colonic Crohn's disease, as opposed to ulcerative colitis, which may prove to be useful in distinguishing ulcerative colitis from Crohn's disease of the colon." This knowledge may, therefore, be useful for identifying individuals at high risk of developing IBD.

Commenting on this work, Sandborn (45) notes that genetic instability at microsatellite sequences of DNA in patients with ulcerative colitis and CRC, similar to those found with HNPCC, had been previously reported. The study by Pokorny et al. raises the question of whether family members of HNPCC kindreds are at risk for IBD.

A study of phenotypic aspects of a family with HNPCC reported an excess of macrophages and crypt atrophy in the colonic mucosa in 50% of patients enrolled in an endoscopic surveillance program (46). Subsequently, a member of this family, considered not at risk for HNPCC by genetic analysis, developed ulcerative colitis. Caruso et al. (47) speculate that the earlier findings of an excess of macrophages and crypt atrophy in the colonic mucosa of patients in an HNPCC family may represent a subclinical phenotype of IBD. These observations are intriguing and merit intensive research directed toward molecular genetic studies on families with IBD.

Immunology, Tumor-Infiltrating Lymphocytes, and CRC

The implications of the presence of lymphocytes infiltrating colorectal malignancies on pathologic examination are undergoing extensive study. For example, Ropponen et al. (48) evaluated clinical follow-up data on 276 CRC patients from Finland between 1976 and 1986 for a mean of 14 years. Clinical findings were correlated with tumor-infiltrating lymphocytes (TILs) and with histologic and quantitative factors, including nuclear parameters and volume-corrected mitotic index. Of interest was the fact that

> in univariate survival analysis, TNM classification, Dukes' stage, histological grade, and TILs were significant predictors of survival. TNM classification, Dukes' stage, and TILs also predicted recurrence-free survival. In multivariate analysis, TILs were an independent prognostic factor of survival in all cases, as well as in patients with T1-4N0-3M0 and T1-4N1-3M1. TILs also independently predicted recurrence-free survival.

It was concluded that TILs harbor important prognostic information in CRC, and TIL analysis may prove useful in the evaluation of patients under consideration for adjuvant therapy. There are preliminary data showing a statistically significant excess of TILs in CRC specimens from HNPCC. Furthermore, and highly pertinent to Lynch syndrome, cancers with DNA microsatellite instability showed a high frequency of lymphocyte infiltration, and the prognosis of patients with MSI was better (49,50).

In an attempt to examine immunologic factors in CRC in general, Barth et al. (51) examined TIL, expression of interleukin 2 (IL-2), IL-4, tumor necrosis factor α (TNF-α), interferon γ (IFN-γ), granulocyte-macrophage colony-stimulating factor (GM-CSF), IL-10, and TGF-β as well as tumor cell expression of IL-10 and TGF-β in situ in 49 primary CRCs and in 20 metastases using immunochemistry. Lymphocytes were found to infiltrate primary colon carcinomas more frequently than metastases. Furthermore, the percentage of colon cancers expressing each of the different cytokines by > 20% of TILs was variable. Interestingly, expression of TNF-α by even a small proportion ($\geq$3%) of the TILs in a colon carcinoma specimen was associated with better overall survival ($P = .01$) compared to patients with little or no TIL TNF-α expression (5-year survival 82% vs. 47%). Although IL-10 was expressed by colon carcinoma cells and TILs, it is likely that IL-10 played an important immunosuppressant role. Noteworthy is the finding that TNF-α and IL-4 are more commonly expressed by colon carcinoma TILs and are both associated with improved survival. It was concluded that differences exist between the human microenvironment of primary tumors and cancer metastases.

GENDER DIFFERENCES AND TUMOR RATIOS

It is important to note that gender differences in the expression of tumor ratios may exist. Dunlop et al. (52) identified 67 HNPCC gene carriers whose risk to age 70 for all cancers was 91% for males and 69% for females. Of clinical importance was the finding that the risk of developing CRC was significantly greater for males than for females (74% vs. 30%; $P = .006$). The risk of uterine cancer was 42%, greater than the risk of CRC in females (53). Lin et al. (19) similarly determined that extracolonic neoplasms developed in 69% of females harboring *hMSH2* mutations but in only 34% of males with *hMSH2* genetic alterations. This significant difference was offered as an explanation for the finding of significantly greater risk of CRC development in *hMSH2* males (96%) than females (39%). These findings emphasize the importance of broadening cancer surveillance to include the extraintestinal organ systems at risk, with special attention focused on the uterus.

ANTICIPATION

Voskuil et al. (54) studied the phenomenon of anticipation in determining whether successive generations of HNPCC families had earlier onset of disease. They found that

> at young ages, HNPCC family members experience an up-to-150 times higher risk for colorectal cancer than the general population. This risk difference declines from age 60 onwards. The earlier age of onset in successive HNPCC generations does not appear to be a biological feature of HNPCC, but reflects a secular time trend in cancer occurrence in these families, similar to that in the general population.

Tsai et al. (55) found no evidence for the effect of parental gender on the age of diagnosis in offspring of either gender in HNPCC. They did not find a secular trend toward younger-onset CRC. They concluded that there was no evidence for genetic anticipation or genomic imprinting of age of diagnosis among their sample of HNPCC families.

COST-EFFECTIVENESS OF SCREENING

Vasen et al. (56) developed a model for estimating the potential effects in terms of life expectancy and health care costs of surveillance for carriers of an HNPCC-mutated MMR gene. Colonoscopy was performed every 2 to 3 years; these patients were compared to a group who did not receive CRC surveillance. Estimates were then determined for a lifetime risk of developing CRC in concert with the stage distribution of the cancer among symptomatic individuals derived from the Dutch HNPCC Registry. Results indicated that gene carriers under surveillance had an increase in life expectancy of 7 years and that the cost of surveillance was less than the cost of no surveillance. These investigators concluded that CRC surveillance of HNPCC gene carriers was effective, and they recommended that governmental agencies and health insurance organizations support such surveillance.

Genetic Counseling in HNPCC

The Creighton Cancer Genetic Research Team provided DNA testing and genetic counseling to 199 bloodline relatives in five *hMLH1* and two *hMSH2* families (57,58). The patients' stated major reason for coming forward for genetic counseling and DNA testing was to be able to inform their children and other loved ones of their gene mutation status. A statistically significant finding was that patients overestimated their risk for inheriting the HNPCC mutations. There was also a high rate of interest in prophylactic colectomy as well as prophylactic total abdominal hysterectomy and bilateral salpingo-oophorectomy among women with one of the germline mutations for HNPCC. Many of the family members were very concerned about insurance discrimination, and a number declined DNA testing for fear that their results would ultimately fall into the hands of their third-party insurance carriers and subject them to discrimination. The overwhelming majority of patients who were tested and came for disclosure of their DNA results requested that this information not be sent to their family physicians, fearing that it might find its way into their medical records and, should they apply for insurance in the future, could then become known to a particular company.

SUMMARY

HNPCC is one of the most common known risk factors for the development of colorectal cancer and extraintestinal malignancies, yet many health care providers know little or nothing about the Lynch syndromes. Initially, a high index of suspicion on the part of the physician evaluating a young patient with gastrointestinal symptoms, particularly in the setting of a family history significant for colorectal and/or extraintestinal malignancies, may allow for the diagnosis of cancer when it would not otherwise be entertained at such an age. Not only does the early diagnosis of colorectal cancer improve the patient's outcome, but the further determination of whether or not the patient does indeed have HNPCC is vital not only for that specific individual but also for his or her entire kindred. The discovery of MMR germline mutations in HNPCC (and in other hereditary disorders involving cancer and/or noncancer health problems) is very recent; thus much is still to be learned about translating this information into the clinical practice setting. Because current genetic testing does not detect every specific inherited mutation in many HNPCC patients, clinical suspicion should still lead to aggressive cancer surveillance in the index patient and his or her relatives. However, for many, genetic analysis following appropriate counseling will allow for rapid identification of mutations and testing of relatives.

Treatment for HNPCC patients diagnosed with colon cancer should not be limited to partial resections, because of the high incidence of synchronous and metachronous lesions; a subtotal colectomy should be the patient's initial surgical treatment. Follow-up surveillance of the remaining colon and rectum and screening for the other common extraintestinal HNPCC malignancies should be aggressively implemented. The extent of surgery indicated for HNPCC patients diagnosed with rectal cancer is currently debatable, because the risk of developing metachronous cancers in the remaining large intestine after proctectomy is unknown.

Patient education via a knowledgeable physician and genetic counselor is of significant benefit in patient care and surveillance. We believe that knowledge about HNPCC, including its molecular genetic diagnosis, implications for genetic counseling, patient and family surveillance, and management opportunities, is still emerging. Greater physician education is needed regarding all facets of hereditary cancer, including a basic understanding of DNA testing and genetic counseling.

REFERENCES

1. Lynch HT, Smyrk T, Lynch J. An update of HNPCC (Lynch syndrome). Cancer Genet Cytogenet 1997;93:84–99.
2. Watson P, Lynch HT. Extracolonic cancer in hereditary nonpolyposis colorectal cancer. Cancer 1993;71:677–685.
3. Marra G, Boland CR. Hereditary nonpolyposis colorectal cancer: the syndrome, the genes, and historical perspectives. J Natl Cancer Inst 1995;87:1114–1125.
4. Kinzler KW, Vogelstein B. Lessons from hereditary colon cancer. Cell 1996;87:159–170.
5. Vasen HFA, Mecklin J-P, Khan PM, Lynch HT. The International Collaborative Group on Hereditary Nonpolyposis Colorectal Cancer (ICG-HNPCC). Dis Colon Rectum 1991;34:424–425.
6. Lynch HT, Smyrk T. Hereditary nonpolyposis colorectal cancer (Lynch syndrome): an updated review. Cancer 1996;78:1149–1167.
7. Watson P, Lin K, Rodriguez-Bigas MA, et al. Colorectal carcinoma survival among hereditary nonpolyposis colorectal cancer family members. Cancer 1998;83:259–266.
8. Albano WA, Recabaren JA, Lynch HT, et al. Natural history of hereditary cancer of the breast and colon. Cancer. 1982;50:360–363.
9. Lynch et al. Dis Colon Rectum 1991;34:891–895.
10. Lynch et al. Br J Dermatol 1985;113:295–301.
11. Lynch HT, Lynch PM, Pester JA, Fusaro RM. Sebaceous neoplasia and visceral cancer (Torre's syndrome) and its relationship to the cancer family syndrome. In: Lynch HT, Fusaro RM, eds. Cancer-associated genodermatoses. New York: Van Nostrand Reinhold, 1982:366–393.

12. Lynch HT, Fusaro RM. Muir-Torre syndrome: heterogeneity, natural history, diagnosis, and management. Probl General Surg 1993;10:1–14.

13. Hamilton SR, Liu B, Parsons RE, et al. The molecular basis of Turcot's syndrome. N Engl J Med 1995;332:839–847.

14. Jass JR, Cottier DS, Jeevaratnam P. Pathology of hereditary nonpolyposis colorectal cancer with clinical and molecular genetic correlations. In: Baba S, ed. New strategies for treatment of hereditary colorectal cancer. Tokyo: Churchill Livingstone, 1996:29–39.

15. Fishel R, Lescoe MK, Rao MRS, et al. The human mutator gene homolog *MSH2* and its association with hereditary nonpolyposis colon cancer. Cell 1993;75:1027–1038.

16. Bronner CE, Baker SM, Morrison PT, et al. Mutation in the DNA mismatch repair gene homologue *hMLH1* is associated with hereditary nonpolyposis colon cancer. Nature 1994;368:258–261.

17. Nicolaides NC, Papadopoulos N, Liu B, et al. Mutations of two PMS homologues in hereditary nonpolyposis colon cancer. Nature 1994;371:75–80.

18. Miyaki M, Konishi M, Tanaka K, et al. Germline mutation of *MSH6* as the cause of hereditary nonpolyposis colorectal cancer. Nat Genet 1997;17:271–272.

19. Lin KM, Shashidharan M, Thorson AG, et al. Cumulative incidence of colorectal and extracolonic cancers in *MLH1* and *MSH2* mutation carriers of hereditary nonpolyposis colorectal cancer. J Gastrointest Surg 1998;2:67–71.

20. Losi L, Ponz de Leon M, Jiricny J, et al. *K-ras* and *p53* mutations in hereditary non-polyposis colorectal cancers. Int J Cancer (Pred Oncol) 1997;74:94–96.

21. Aaltonen LA, Salovaara R, Kristo P, et al. Incidence of hereditary nonpolyposis colorectal cancer and the feasibility of molecular screening for the disease. N Engl J Med 1998;338:1481–1487.

22. Brassett C, Joyce JA, Froggatt NJ, et al. Microsatellite instability in early onset and familial colorectal cancer. J Med Genet 1996;33:981–985.

23. Lynch HT, Smyrk TC. Identifying hereditary nonpolyposis colorectal cancer. N Engl J Med 1998;338:1537–1538.

24. Fink D, Nebel S, Norris PS, et al. The effect of different chemotherapeutic agents on the enrichment of DNA mismatch repair-deficient tumour cells. Br J Cancer 1998;77:703–708.

25. Lothe RA, Peltomaki P, Meling GI, et al. Genomic instability in colorectal

cancer: relationship to clinicopathological variables and family history. Cancer Res 1993;53:5849–5852.

26. Liu B, Farrington SM, Petersen GM, et al. Genetic instability occurs in the majority of young patients with colorectal cancer. Nature Med 1995;1:348–352.
27. Breivik J, Lothe RA, Meling GI, et al. Different genetic pathways to proximal and distal colorectal cancer influenced by sex-related factors. Int J Cancer (Pred Oncol) 1997;74:664–669.
28. Beck NE, Tomlinson IP, Homfray TF, et al. Frequency of germline hereditary non-polyposis colorectal cancer gene mutations in patients with multiple or early onset colorectal adenomas. Gut 1997;41:235–238.
29. Hodgson SV, Harocopos C, Gaglia P. Screening results in a family cancer clinic: five years experience. Anticancer Res 1993;13:2581–2586.
30. Jass JR, Stewart SM. Evolution of hereditary non-polyposis colorectal cancer. Gut 1992;33:783–786.
31. Tomlinson IPM, Beck NE, Homfray T, et al. Germline HNPCC gene variants have little influence on the risk for sporadic colorectal cancer. J Med Genet 1997;34:39–42.
32. Wijnen J, Khan PM, Vasen H, et al. Hereditary nonpolyposis colorectal cancer families not complying with the Amsterdam criteria show extremely low frequency of mismatch-repair-gene mutations. Am J Hum Genet 1997;61:329–335.
33. Weber TK, Conlon W, Petrelli NJ, et al. Genomic DNA-based *hMSH2* and *hMLH1* mutation screening in 32 Eastern United States hereditary nonpolyposis colorectal cancer pedigrees. Cancer Res 1997;57:3798–3803.
34. Viel A, Genuardi M, Capozzi E, et al. Characterization of *MSH2* and *MLH1* mutations in Italian families with hereditary nonpolyposis colorectal cancer. Genes Chromosomes Cancer 1997;18:8–18.
35. Heinimann K, Müller H, Weber W, Scott RJ. Disease expression in Swiss hereditary non-polyposis colorectal cancer (HNPCC) kindreds. Int J Cancer (Pred Oncol) 1997;74:281–285.
36. Beck NE, Tomlinson IPM, Homfray T, et al. Genetic testing is important in families with a history suggestive of hereditary non-polyposis colorectal cancer even if the Amsterdam criteria are not fulfilled. Br J Surg 1997;84:233–237.
37. Wang Q, Desseigne F, Lasset C, et al. Germline *hMSH2* and *hMLH1* gene mutations in incomplete HNPCC families. Int J Cancer 1997;73:831–836.
38. Genuardi M, Anti M, Capozzi E, et al. *MLH1* and *MSH2* constitutional mutations in colorectal cancer families not meeting the standard criteria

for hereditary nonpolyposis colorectal cancer. Int J Cancer 1998;75:835–839.

39. Vasen HFA, Wijnen JT, Menko FH, et al. Cancer risk in families with hereditary nonpolyposis colorectal cancer diagnosed by mutation analysis. Gastroenterology 1996;110:1020–1027.
40. Jäger AC, Bisgaard ML, Myrhoj T, et al. Reduced frequency of extracolonic cancers in hereditary nonpolyposis colorectal cancer families with monoallelic *hMLH1* expression. Am J Hum Genet 1997;61:129–138.
41. Peltomäki P, Vasen HFA, International Collaborative Group on Hereditary Nonpolyposis Colorectal Cancer. Mutations predisposing to hereditary nonpolyposis colorectal cancer: database and results of a collaborative study. Gastroenterology 1997;113:1146–1158.
42. Akiyama Y, Iwanaga R, Saitoh K, et al. Transforming growth factor *β* type II receptor gene mutations in adenomas from hereditary nonpolyposis colorectal cancer. Gastroenterology 1997;112:33–39.
43. Tannergard P, Liu T, Weger A, et al. Tumorigenesis in colorectal tumors from patients with hereditary non-polyposis colorectal cancer. Hum Genet 1997;101:51–55.
44. Pokorny RM, Hofmeister A, Galandiuk S, et al. Crohn's disease and ulcerative colitis are associated with the DNA repair gene *MLH1*. Ann Surg 1998;225:718–725.
45. Sandborn WJ. Inflammatory bowel disease and hereditary nonpolyposis colorectal cancer: is there a genetic link? Gastroenterology 1998;114:608–609.
46. Cristofaro G, Lynch HT, Caruso ML, et al. New phenotypic aspects in a family with Lynch syndrome II. Cancer 1987;60:51–58.
47. Caruso ML, Cristofaro G, Lynch HT. HNPCC-Lynch syndrome and idiopathic inflammatory bowel disease. A hypothesis on sharing of genes. Anticancer Res 1997;17:2647–2650.
48. Ropponen KM, Eskelinen MJ, Lipponen PK, et al. Prognostic value of tumour-infiltrating lymphocytes (TILs) in colorectal cancer. J Pathol 1997;182:318–324.
49. Kim H, Jen J, Vogelstein B, Hamilton SR. Clinical and pathological characteristics of sporadic colorectal carcinomas with DNA replication errors in microsatellite sequences. Am J Path 1994;145:148–156.
50. Jass JR, Cottier DS, Jeevaratnam P, et al. Diagnostic use of microsatellite instability in hereditary non-polyposis colorectal cancer. Lancet 1995;346:1200–1201.
51. Barth RJ Jr, Camp BJ, Martuscello TA, et al. The cytokine microenviron-

ment of human colon carcinoma: lymphocyte expression of tumor necrosis factor-alpha and interleukin-4 predicts improved survival. Cancer 1996;78:1168–1178.

52. Dunlop MG, Farrington SM, Carothers AD, et al. Cancer risk associated with germline DNA mismatch repair gene mutations. Hum Mol Genet 1997;6:105–110.

53. Lynch HT, Cavalieri RJ, Lynch JF, Casey MJ. Gynecologic cancer clues to Lynch syndrome II diagnosis: a family report. Gynecol Oncol 1992;44:198–203.

54. Voskuil DW, Vasen HFA, Kampman E, et al. Colorectal cancer risk in HNPCC families: development during lifetime and in successive generations. Int J Cancer 1997;72:205–209.

55. Tsai Y-Y, Petersen GM, Booker SV, et al. Evidence against genetic anticipation in familial colorectal cancer. Genet Epidemiol 1997;14:435–446.

56. Vasen HFA, van Ballegooijen M, Buskens E, et al. A cost-effectiveness analysis of colorectal screening of hereditary nonpolyposis colorectal carcinoma gene carriers. Cancer 1998;82:1632–1637.

57. Lynch HT, Watson P, Shaw TG, et al. Clinical impact of molecular genetic diagnosis, genetic counseling and management of hereditary cancer: Part I. Cancer family studies. Cancer, in press.

58. Lynch HT, Watson P, Shaw TG, et al. Clinical impact of molecular genetic diagnosis, genetic counseling and management of hereditary cancer: Part II. HNPCC as a model. Cancer, in press.

CHAPTER

5

FAMILIAL ADENOMATOUS POLYPOSIS

CLIFFORD KO, M.D.,
AND PATRICIA L. ROBERTS, M.D.

Familial adenomatous polyposis (FAP) is an inherited autosomal dominant disease characterized by the presence of at least 100 adenomatous polyps in the colon and rectum. In mild or "attenuated" FAP and in young children, <100 polyps may be found. In such circumstances, the presence of multiple adenomas and a positive family history are sufficient to make the diagnosis of FAP. Although case reports in the eighteenth and nineteenth centuries described patients with multiple colorectal polyps, Cripps (1) is credited with first reporting the polyposis condition. In 1890, Handford (2) subsequently described how these disseminated adenomatous polyps would eventually progress to malignancy. In regard to terminology, FAP with or without extracolonic manifestations is now considered the proper term to use when describing this disease and should replace older terms, including Gardner syndrome, Turcot syndrome, familial polyposis coli, and familial multiple polyposis.

Colon and Rectal Cancer, Edited by Peter S. Edelstein, M.D.
ISBN 0-471-35145-8

The incidence of FAP is 1 in 7,000 to 1 in 16,000, and the prevalence is 1 in 25,000 (3). Colorectal cancers in patients with FAP account for approximately 1% of all newly diagnosed colorectal cancers. Because of the autosomal dominant inheritance, offspring of patients with FAP have a 50% chance of inheriting the genetic defect. As such, appropriate patient surveillance, in part through the assistance of polyposis registries, is essential. Approximately 20% of patients with FAP have no family history and presumably are patients with spontaneous genetic mutations (4).

The significant feature of FAP is that at least one of the adenomatous polyps will progress to invasive carcinoma if left untreated. The natural history of this disease is well documented with the data from the Polyposis Registry of St. Mark's Hospital in London. Bussey (5) described the natural course for the average untreated patient with FAP. Adenomas generally appear in patients by the age of 25 years and symptoms by age 33 years. The mean age at detection of adenomas is 36 years. In untreated patients, a diagnosis of invasive cancer is made at a mean of 39 years, and death from carcinoma occurs by age 42 years (5).

Because FAP will eventually progress to invasive cancer in all patients, the optimal therapy for patients with FAP is prophylactic colectomy after the diagnosis has been confirmed and ideally before an invasive cancer has developed.

Clinical Manifestations, Screening, and Surveillance

On presentation, patients may or may not have symptoms. Ideally, with the help of polyposis registries, patients and their family members are made aware of their disease (or predilection for FAP) and thus undergo appropriate screening. "Informed" family members are the patients who usually do not have symptoms on presentation. Of more importance, they are seen before the development of invasive cancer. Screening with flexible sigmoidoscopy is usually initiated between the ages of 10 and 16 years (6). No consensus exists on the exact age to begin screening.

Patients who are inadequately screened are the ones who generally have symptoms on presentation. Bleeding is most common (80%), followed by diarrhea (70%). Other more ominous presenting complaints include weight loss, anemia, and intestinal obstruction, implying the presence of malignancy (7). Of patients who have symptoms on presentation, 27 to 66% already have a cancer in the colon or rectum or both (8, 9).

Screening for FAP is performed by flexible sigmoidoscopy. By definition, the polyps in FAP are almost always within reach of the flexible sigmoidoscope, and therefore, the sensitivity is high. Moreover, biopsy specimens may be obtained with this technique, which provides histologic proof of adenomatous polypoid disease. When adenomas are seen on sigmoidoscopy, colonoscopy establishes the severity of the disease and helps plan prophylactic surgery (10). When adenomas are found, surgery is usually carried out when the patient reaches the beginning of the third decade.

During screening and when treating patients with FAP, it is important to recognize the variability of the size and location of the polyps. Depending on innumerable factors, the polyps in FAP can vary in size from barely visible 1- to 2-mm mucosal lesions to lesions of 1 cm or larger (Fig. 1). With regard to location, the left colon tends to have a higher density of polyps than the right colon (5), and the risk of carcinoma developing is highest in the rectum and the sigmoid colon. Although it had been assumed that the rectum was often involved with polyps, it is not unusual to find that the rectum is relatively or even totally spared (11). This fact has significant implications when planning which surgical resection to perform.

In addition to the colorectal manifestations of FAP, this entity can also present with one of its many associated extracolonic manifestations, including desmoid tumors, gastric or duodenal polyps, osteomas, epidermoid cysts, and others (discussed later).

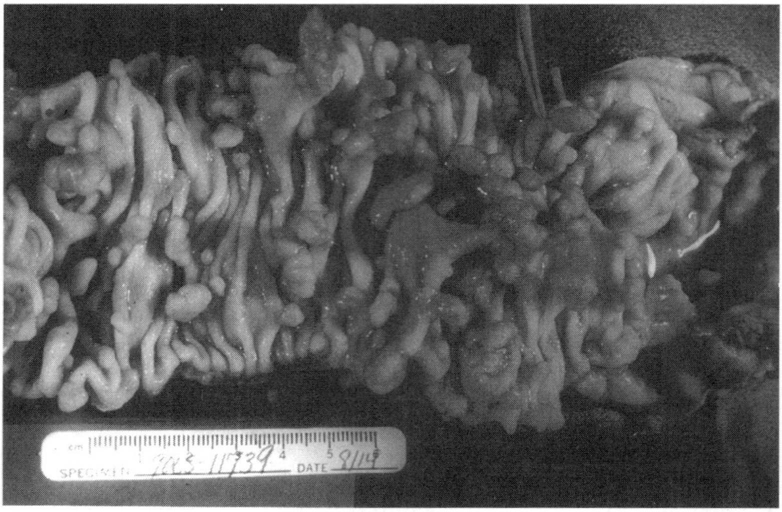

FIGURE 5.1. Colectomy specimen showing multiple polyps in a patient with FAP.

SURGICAL OPTIONS

Although the surgical options for patients with FAP include total abdominal colectomy with ileorectal anastomosis, total proctocolectomy with permanent ileostomy or continent ileostomy (Kock pouch), and total proctocolectomy with ileal pouch–anal anastomosis, the ileorectal anastomosis and ileal pouch–anal anastomosis are the two most commonly performed procedures for FAP. Factors, including the number of rectal polyps, the presence of cancer, sphincter function, the presence of extracolonic disease, and the willingness of the patient to comply with a follow-up program, influence the selection of the most appropriate surgical procedure for a given patient. The goal of surgery is to attempt to stop the progression of colorectal adenoma to cancer.

TOTAL ABDOMINAL COLECTOMY WITH ILEORECTAL ANASTOMOSIS

Total abdominal colectomy with ileorectal anastomosis is usually reserved for patients with a relatively small number of rectal polyps.

Although the operation removes the diseased colon, the rectum is left in place, and patients are at risk for the development of rectal cancer. Patients who elect to undergo ileorectal anastomosis should be compliant and committed to follow-up visits at 6- to 12-month intervals for sigmoidoscopic surveillance. Ileorectal anastomosis avoids the need for pelvic dissection, with the resultant risk of sexual or urinary dysfunction and for a stoma. These points, along with the fact that the procedure generally is associated with a good functional result, make this surgical approach an attractive option for young, asymptomatic patients.

The risk of rectal cancer in patients who have undergone an ileorectal anastomosis increases with age and is not eradicated by compliance with a surveillance program or by the use of sulindac to suppress adenoma growth. Before the age of 50 years, the risk of development of rectal cancer is approximately 8%, and this rate rises to 30% at age 60 years (12). Although rectal cancer ultimately occurs in 30% of patients, only approximately 25% of those patients who develop a malignancy die of the rectal cancer (13). The most common causes of death in patients with FAP who have undergone ileorectal anastomosis are periampullary cancers and desmoid tumors.

Some surgeons have recommended operation based on factors relating to the severity of polyposis and have considered total abdominal colectomy and ileorectal anastomosis a reasonable option when the number of rectal polyps is few, in patients who are compliant with surveillance, when overall disease is mild (<1000 polyps), when incurable colon cancer is present, and in patients who are asymptomatic (10).

ILEAL POUCH–ANAL ANASTOMOSIS

The ileal pouch–anal anastomosis (IPAA) has become an increasingly popular surgical option for patients with both ulcerative colitis and FAP. Some centers recommend IPAA for all patients with FAP to avoid the risk of rectal cancer after ileorectal anastomosis.

The procedure is usually performed in two stages, with an initial colectomy and rectal resection, the creation of an ileal pouch with an anastomosis to the anus, and with the creation of a loop ileostomy. In selected patients, the operation may be performed in one stage with omission of the loop ileostomy. A great deal of controversy surrounds the best way to anastomose the ileal pouch to the anus. To remove the most rectal mucosa, a mucosectomy and hand-sewn anastomosis to the anus are necessary; however, this procedure may be associated with high leakage rates (fecal incontinence), particularly at night. In addition, recent data suggest that compared with stapled anastomoses, hand-sewn anastomoses may be associated with a higher pelvic sepsis rate (14). Alternatively, a stapled anastomosis with preservation of the anal transitional zone may leave small quantities of viable rectal mucosa intact and at risk for the development of adenomatous and malignant transformation.

Patients who undergo an ileoanal pouch procedure have a higher risk for the development of complications than patients who undergo an ileorectal anastomosis. These include the risk of severe functional pouch failure requiring the re-establishment a permanent ileostomy, the risk of moderate functional pouch failure (greater than five or six bowel movements a day), the risk of minor degrees of incontinence to stool, and the small risk of sexual or urinary dysfunction common to all procedures involving rectal resection. Neoplastic polyps may also develop within the ileoanal pouch; for this reason, lifelong surveillance should be considered (15).

Reasonable indications for IPAA in patients with FAP include a large number of rectal polyps, large-size rectal polyps, severe dysplasia of the rectum, severe overall disease (>1000 polyps), symptomatic disease, and curable cancers of the colon or rectum (10).

Proctocolectomy with Permanent Ileostomy

Proctocolectomy and ileostomy remove the diseased colon and rectum and thus entirely eliminate the risk of colorectal cancer. The operation is carried out with minimal complications; however, there is a small but not insignificant risk of sexual and urinary dysfunction in men, and patients are left with a permanent stoma. Young patients, particularly those who have a diagnosis of familial adenomatous polyposis but are still asymptomatic, are often reluctant to accept the potential physical and psychosocial problems associated with a permanent ileostomy.

The procedure is indicated in patients who have already had a failed IPAA or in patients who have FAP on presentation and a low rectal cancer in whom adequate distal tumor clearance precludes construction of an ileoanal pouch.

Continent Ileostomy (Kock Pouch)

The Kock pouch involves the creation of an ileal pouch with an internal one-way valve constructed from the terminal ileum itself and with an ileostomy situated flush with the abdominal wall skin. With a well-constructed Kock pouch (once enlarged), the patient does not have to wear an appliance, and the stoma, being situated low on the abdominal wall, is less noticeable. The continent pouch is intubated and evacuated by the patient at regular intervals using a specialized catheter. This surgical procedure is considerably more complex than proctocolectomy and Brooke ileostomy and is associated with a high complication rate, particularly related to dysfunction ("slipping") of the nipple valve. Significant complications related to the nipple valve may occur and require revision and even pouch excision in up to 20% of patients. Pouchitis, similar to that associated with the ileoanal pouch procedure, may also occur, although it is much more common in patients undergoing resection for ulcerative colitis than for familial adenomatous polyposis. It is usually successfully treated with a short course of antibiotics.

The Kock pouch is probably best suited for patients who have undergone proctocolectomy and standard Brooke ileostomy and later wish to have a continent stoma or for patients in whom an ileal pouch–anal anastomosis cannot technically be performed owing to patient body habitus or a short mesentery.

Medical Management

For patients who have undergone total abdominal colectomy and ileorectal anastomosis, the use of a specific NSAID, sulindac, has been demonstrated to decrease the number of polyps within the rectal remnant. Sulindac, at a dose of 150 mg, is administered twice daily. The effect of sulindac is dose related and unfortunately is neither complete nor long lasting. Furthermore, a decrease in polyp counts does not absolutely eliminate the risk for the development of cancer, and at least three cases of rectal cancer have been reported in patients who were taking sulindac. Hence, the use of sulindac may lull the patient and the clinician into falsely believing that colorectal cancer will not develop in patients who are taking the drug. Although use of sulindac for duodenal adenomas and desmoid tumors has also been described, the effect is not nearly as well established as in the colorectal polyps.

Other agents have been used to decrease rectal polyps, including antioxidant vitamins and calcium. Orally administered calcium has been shown to reduce epithelial cell turnover in patients with FAP; however, no effect on the number or size of rectal polyps has been demonstrated (16).

Familial Adenomatous Polyposis Registry

The inherited colorectal cancer registry is a database that maintains records of patients and their families with inherited colorectal cancers. The purpose of having such a registry is threefold: to provide better patient care, to provide and further patient and physician education, and to facilitate research (10). For the patient with FAP, a significant amount of care needs to be coordinated, including screening, surveillance, and treatment for colorectal polyps as well as for extracolonic manifestations of the disease. Because so many aspects of this disease are often confusing or unknown to the patient, having the registry is an important resource to assist patients with their own care. The effect of the FAP registry was best explained by Spigelman and Thomson (9) who reported that 66% of unmonitored FAP patients have an invasive cancer on presentation but that the percentage plummets to only 5% when FAP patients are routinely monitored.

The second role for the registry is to provide and further education for the patient, patient's family, and the physician. Registry personnel are a consistent and knowledgeable source of information on polyposis. Interacting and learning from the registry staff may take a variety of forms, including personal communications, public lectures, brochures, and newsletters (10). Because this disease is inherited by 50% of offspring, the entire family should become educated about FAP and the implications of the disease. The registry personnel are an optimal source of such education.

As for health care providers, there have been important, recent advances in the understanding of colorectal cancer genetics and its relationship to clinical care. Education for health care providers is thus essential in regard to the most recent clinical recommendations and protocols for counseling, screening, surveillance, and treatments. Although we agree that disseminating accurate information to patients with FAP and their families is crucial, apparently it does not always achieve its desired goals. In one study of the clinical utility of commercial genetic testing and the physician or genetic counselor who requested it, Giardiello et al. (17) found that although 83% of patients had a valid indication to undergo the test, counseling before and after testing was inadequate in 80% of patients. Many of the ordering physicians or genetic counselors did not themselves understand the limitations of the test, and consequently, almost one third of the patients would have received incorrect interpretations of their results. These findings are of concern, especially for patients with a false-negative result (which occurs in approximately 20% of cases). Giardiello et al. recommended that the health care provider ordering the tests first be appropriately prepared to offer adequate and correct information concerning the tests. Personnel at the polyposis registry are an excellent educational resource for health care providers.

The polyposis registry is a powerful contributor to research in many of the numerous areas of FAP investigation, including basic science, clinical series, epidemiology, and outcome studies. In the 1990s, such research furthered our understanding of colon and rectal cancer at the genetic and molecular levels both for FAP as well as for sporadic colorectal tumors (discussed later).

PREDICTIVE GENETIC TESTING

Important recent developments in the diagnosis of FAP include the use of predictive genetic testing (18). The appropriate application of the adenomatous polyposis coli (APC) genetic test can confirm the diagnosis of FAP, justify heightened surveillance, and assist with treatment and family planning (17). Because of the complexity of the various techniques for genetic analysis, detecting germline mutations is not a simple matter. Although numerous methods are available for detecting genetic mutation, the major technique presently used for detecting the APC mutation is the in vitro synthesized-protein assay (19).

The in vitro synthesized-protein assay (also known as the protein-truncation assay) was introduced commercially in 1994 and can identify an APC gene mutation in affected members in approximately 80% of families with FAP. When the mutation within a family is already known, direct gene testing can detect the mutation with virtually 100% accuracy. The protein-truncation assay takes advantage of the fact that nearly all APC mutations result in a shorter protein product. The assay technique involves in vitro synthesis of the APC protein using the RNA code from the patient's cells. Electrophoresis of the protein product will then demonstrate a truncated protein product in the presence of the APC mutation. Subsequently, in the samples that demonstrate an alteration, the specific area of the genetic mutation can be identified and directly sequenced using radiolabeling or automated fluorescent dye sequencing. The advantage of the in vitro synthesized-protein assay is that it is rapid and sensitive. The test requires only a single sample of blood, and the results are available within 2 weeks. At present, this method is the standard test for FAP predictive genetic testing.

How much should a health care provider rely on the results of a single test? Some experts in the field will perform two genetic tests, 2 to 3 years apart (6). If the results of the tests are negative, screening still needs to be performed but at less frequent intervals. On the other hand, if both genetic tests are positive and the gene locus is confirmed, the diagnosis can be accepted 100% of the time. A positive result does not reduce the need for screening endoscopy because the phenotype (i.e., the development of the polyps) must still be identified.

Similar to the problems associated with genetic testing in other diseases, numerous financial and ethical implications are inherent in FAP genetic testing. Two issues not yet resolved are whether the test will be reimbursed by third-party payers and whether obtaining insurance coverage will be affected by a positive result confirming a genotypic mutation.

THE GENETICS OF FAP

The study of FAP has greatly contributed to the understanding of colorectal cancer genetics. Most of this understanding has occurred in the past decade. Historically, adenomatous polyposis was first observed in the eighteenth century. Its inherited nature was recognized by 1900. However, it was not until the mid-1980s that the understanding of the molecular pathogenesis began. Herrera et al. (20) demonstrated a deletion in the long arm (q) of chromosome 5. This report led other researchers (21,22) to identify genetic sequence markers that were linked to FAP on chromosome 5q21. In 1991, the APC gene was identified, sequenced, and proved to cause FAP (23, 24).

The APC gene is long and consists of 15 exons, or coding sequences, which encode a protein of 2844 amino acids. The 15th exon is the largest, having a substantially longer genetic code than the other 14 exons combined. Generally, a tendency exists for the severity of FAP to be greater with mutations in the higher numbered exons. Most of the 200 different APC mutations that have been associated with FAP are found in exon 15 (25).

The genetic defect in FAP occurs in the APC gene whose transcribed protein normally functions as a gatekeeper within the colorectal epithelium. In general, gatekeeper genes are responsible for maintaining a constant cell number by maintaining a balance between cell replication and cell death (apoptosis). When a gatekeeper gene is mutated, this defect leads to a permanent imbalance favoring cell division over cell death. This scenario seems to occur with mutations of the APC gene. When an APC mutation is present, a consequential imbalance favoring cell division over cell death occurs. This alteration is believed to play a role in neoplastic initiation.

At the molecular and protein level, the APC gene functions by encoding a protein located on the basolateral membrane of colorectal epithelial cells. Expression of this protein is increased as the mucosal cell migrates up the colonic crypt (26,27). Although the primary sequence of the APC gene has not yet offered much insight into its characteristics and function, identification of various proteins that interact with the APC protein has provided some important clues. The most telling insights into APC function come from studies of the interaction between the APC protein and β-catenin (28–30). β-

Catenin, a protein that has multiple functions, including cell-to-cell adhesion, nuclear transport, and cell signaling, is presumably an essential protein for transcriptional activity during cellular division. Under normal circumstances, when the APC gene is not mutated (the genetic wild type), the APC protein interacts with β-catenin, leading to inhibition of transcription and thus inhibiting cellular division. Subsequently, this inhibition is thought to lead to cellular apoptosis (31). On the other hand, when the APC gene is mutated, the translated mutated APC protein does not adequately bind with β-catenin. This inadequate binding permits the β-catenin protein to function continuously, thereby resulting in constitutive transcription for that cell. This mechanism is thought to be crucial in early epithelial transformation of the cell, i.e., in cancer initiation (29).

For an invasive cancer to develop, there are two phases: cancer initiation and cancer progression. Although the APC mutation initiates the neoplastic process, other mutations are still required to continue the progression. It is not clear how many more mutations are required for a colorectal tumor to become an invasive malignancy, but the number of additional mutations likely ranges from 6 to 12. Such mutations include *K-ras, DCC,* and *p53*. If these other mutations occur before the development of the APC gene mutation, the neoplastic process will not be initiated efficiently. It is not the accumulation of genetic mutations but rather the order of mutation accrual that determines the propensity for neoplasia. Moreover, only a distinct subset of genetic mutations, those that can affect cell growth, can actually result in the development of cancer (32). The APC mutation appears to be the predominant genetic alteration in the initiation of colorectal cancer development.

Extracolonic Manifestations

In addition to the colorectal polyps found in patients with FAP, numerous extracolonic manifestations have been recognized. A partial list is provided in Table 5.1. At the genetic level, the role the APC mutation plays in the development of extracolonic manifestation remains unknown. At the clinical level, however, the effects of extracolonic manifestations in patients with FAP are significant with respect to both morbidity and mortality. In fact, in most recent series death from desmoid tumors and from duodenal cancers is more frequent than from carcinomas of the colon and rectum (33).

DUODENAL POLYPS

The presence of duodenal polyps has been reported to occur in as many as 90% of patients with FAP, usually in the periampullary region. Whether bile contributes to the development of polyps remains unproved. Polyps in the duodenum tend to be white and sessile and are often small. The risk of subsequent duodenal cancer in patients with FAP is much greater than in the normal population. The lifetime incidence of duodenal cancer in the normal population ranges from 0.01 to 0.04%, whereas in patients with FAP, the incidence of duodenal cancer is as high as 12% (34,35).

TABLE 5.1. EXTRACOLONIC MANIFESTATIONS OF FAP[a]

Benign	Malignant
Adrenal adenoma	Adrenal carcinoma
Cholangioadenoma	Cholangiocarcinoma
Thyroid adenoma	Thyroid carcinoma
Osteoma	Osteogenic sarcoma
Duodenal adenoma	Duodenal carcinoma
Small bowel adenoma	Small bowel carcinoma
Hepatic adenoma	Hepatoblastoma
Pancreatic adenoma	Pancreatic carcinoma
Epidermoid cysts	Medulloblastoma
Congenital hypertrophy of retinal pigmented epithelium	Glioblastoma
Desmoid	

[a]Reprinted with permission from Ref. 10.

Similar to polyps in the colon and rectum, symptoms do not present until late in their progression, and thus many duodenal tumors are advanced at the time of initial diagnosis. These complaints include unexplained abdominal pain, weight loss, jaundice, anemia, melena, and vomiting. Diagnosis is made with a combination of endoscopic ultrasonography (EUS), CT, and endoscopic retrograde cholangiopancreatography (ERCP) with biopsy. No single test is perfect. Kalantzis et al. (36) reported the sensitivity of EUS to be as high as 92% in the diagnosis of benign tumors of the upper GI tract, but tissue sampling is not possible. Ryan et al. (37) found that management of duodenal villous tumors may be difficult even if biopsy techniques are available. This difficulty is mainly the result of the false-negative biopsy rate, which can be as high as 56%. The technical aspects of managing duodenal polyps can also be challenging. Endoscopic snare removal is often difficult because of the sessile nature of the lesions. If the polyps are near the ampulla of Vater, electrocoagulation can result in ampullary scarring or stricturing or both. Nevertheless, for early stage duodenal adenomatous polyps, endoscopic removal is routinely attempted. Surgical management is generally determined by polyp size, type, and location and by whether the polyp demonstrates villous changes, severe dysplasia, rapid growth, or induration upon endoscopic probing (38). Surgical options include wide local excision with or without reconstructive sphincteroplasty or pancreatoduodenectomy (Whipple procedure). Local polyp excision can be performed with low morbidity, but this approach has been associated with a high recurrence rate (39) and a significant potential for complications (40). However, pancreatoduodenectomy should be considered only when there is evidence of invasive carcinoma of the duodenum (6).

There is no definitive medical treatment for duodenal polyps. In some studies, sulindac has been demonstrated to reduce the mucosal proliferation in FAP-associated polyps. Although the use of sulindac has received increasing attention for duodenal polyps, its efficacy is still debated (12,41,42). Trying to prevent the onset of duodenal cancer in a patient with FAP cannot be achieved solely by medical means such as sulindac. At the present time, primary management of patients with duodenal polyps should be endoscopic or surgical removal.

The prevalence and mortality rates associated with duodenal polyps and cancers, respectively, are significant. A retrospective survey of 10 polyposis registries revealed a 30% incidence of duodenal carcinomas in 1225 patients with FAP (35). The St. Mark's Hospital Registry reported on its series of FAP patients who had undergone colectomy and ileorectal anastomosis. The number of deaths from duodenal carcinoma was more than twice that from cancer within the retained rectal stump (43). Likewise, Arvanitis et al. (44) reported that the major causes of death in patients with FAP after (procto)colectomy were desmoid tumor (31%), duodenal carcinoma (22%), and rectal carcinoma (8%).

The exact screening and surveillance protocols for gastroduodenal polyps are debated. Marcello et al. (45) recommended that when results of the initial screening are negative, surveillance upper endoscopy should be performed every 2 to 3 years unless upper gastrointestinal tract symptoms develop. When the duration of known polyposis disease reaches 15 to 20 years or the patient reaches age 50, yearly upper endoscopic examinations are warranted because of the higher likelihood of malignant transformation. Physicians at St. Mark's Hospital begin endoscopic screening of patients at age 25 years. The subsequent surveillance intervals range from 6 months to 5 years, depending on the degree of polyposis (46). The severity of duodenal polyposis can be scored objectively using the staging system developed by Spigelman et al. (38), which relies on clinical and histologic assessment of the duodenal lesions.

GASTRIC POLYPS

Gastric lesions associated with FAP are generally benign. FAP-associated gastric tumors include fundal gland polyposis, hyperplastic polyps, adenomas, and rarely, invasive adenocarcinoma. The prevalence reported in the literature ranges from 30 to 100%; the most common lesion is hyperplastic polyps in the fundus (45,47). Seow-Choen et al. (42) found that sulindac reduces mucosal cell proliferation in the gastric epithelium more effectively than in the duodenum. By default, screening of the stomach is performed on the same schedule as of the duodenum.

DESMOID TUMORS

Desmoid tumors originate from fibroaponeurotic tissue. They are classically benign because they have no metastatic potential. Their presence, however, can be disabling and even lethal owing to their focally invasive and frequently aggressive growth (48). Desmoid tumors occur in 10 to 14% of patients with FAP; 50% are found within the mesentery, 34% within the abdominal wall, and 14% in other anatomic locations (49). In patients with polyposis, 80% of desmoid tumors occur postoperatively. The most common desmoid symptom in FAP patients is a painful abdominal mass, which occurs in approximately 50% of patients. Symptoms are generally secondary to obstruction (bowel or ureteral), direct pressure from the tumor, or bleeding into the tumor (50). Methods of diagnosis include CT and MRI. The latter is able to provide equal or better definition of the soft tissues while sparing the patient the radiation effects associated with CT. Desmoid tumors may also be asymptomatic and found incidentally at the time of unrelated surgery.

If the tumor is superficial, small, or contained within the abdominal wall, complete surgical excision offers the best chance for cure. For tumors that have infiltrated the mesentery, complete excision is rarely possible. Unfortunatly, mesenteric desmoid tumors are rarely small enough or sufficiently well localized to permit complete resection without compromise of a significant amount of bowel (Fig. 5.2). Recurrence has been noted in as many as 65 to 80% of patients (50). Predictors of local failure include young age

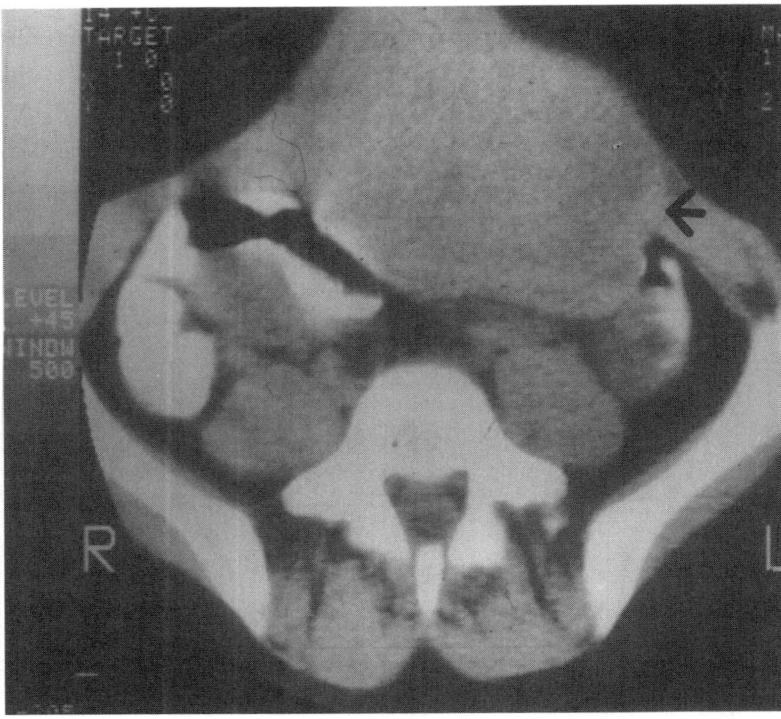

FIGURE 5.2. Massive mesenteric desmoid tumor (*arrow*) in a patient with FAP who had previously undergone total abdominal colectomy and ileorectal anastomosis.

(between 1 and 30 years), presentation with recurrent disease, partial or limited tumor margin excision, positive margin of resection, and failure to administer radiation therapy for obvious residual disease (51).

In many patients, the mesenteric desmoid tumors will remain the same size or will have both periods of growth and periods of remission. Approximately 10% will grow rapidly and approximately 7% will resolve (10). Pharmacologic therapy with sulindac with or without the use of tamoxifen has been attempted for unresectable mesenteric desmoid tumors. Sulindac may retard the growth or cause regression of such tumors. For lesions that continue to grow despite the use of sulindac and/or tamoxifen, further chemotherapy may be used. An antisarcoma regimen of doxorubicin and dacarbazine may be effective. Moslein and Dozois (52) reported successful tissue responses in nine patients who were given the antisarcoma chemotherapy regimen of doxorubicin and dacarbazine. A complete response was demonstrated in four patients and a partial response in five patients.

The presence of a mesenteric desmoid tumor may limit surgical options (53), as in the case of patients who have undergone total abdominal colectomy and ileorectal anastomosis and are contemplating conversion to an ileoanal pouch. A mesenteric desmoid tumor may make such an ileoanal pouch operation technically impossible because a sufficient length of mesentery may not be achievable to allow the pouch to reach the anus.

EPIDERMOID CYSTS

Epidermoid cysts usually occur on the back. Patients with FAP develop such cysts all over their bodies, including the face, scalp, and arms. Cysts reportedly occur in approximately 50% of patients with FAP (54). In the general population, epidermoid cysts are rarely present in children. These cysts have, however, been reported to occur before the development of colorectal polyps in young patients with FAP. Leppard and Bussey (54) recommended that any child with an epidermoid cyst should undergo yearly sigmoidoscopy from age 14 years and until at least the age of 30 years to adequately rule out FAP.

OSTEOMAS

Osteomas are benign lesions found most commonly in the facial bones, usually the mandible. Symptoms are routinely secondary to local growth of the tumor. As with any of the other extracolonic FAP manifestations, osteomas may be identified before development of colorectal polyps in patients with FAP (3). Although some physicians have routinely ordered screening Panorex dental films on FAP patients, this practice is not currently recommended.

EYE LESIONS

The most common eye lesion associated with FAP is congenital hypertrophy of the retinal pigmented epithelium (CHRPE). On ophthalmic examination, the appearance of CHRPE is described as a round or oval pigmented retinal lesion with a surrounding pale halo (Fig. 5.3). The incidence of CHRPE in patients with FAP ranges from 50 to 79% compared to 5 with 7% in the general population (3,

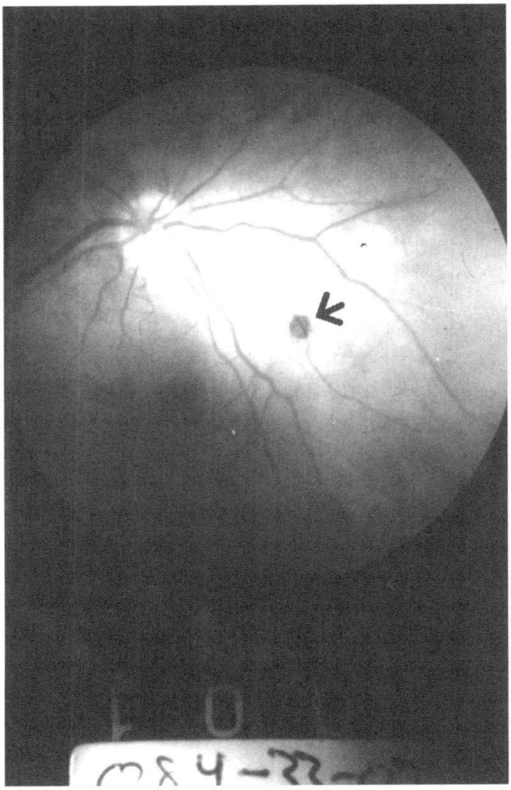

FIGURE 5.3. Congenital hypertrophy of the retinal pigmented epithelium (*arrow*).

55). The sensitivity of CHRPE for FAP is 79%, with a specificity of 95% (3). CHRPE can be present before colorectal polyps develop.

Brain Neoplasm

Tumors of neuroepithelial origin can be seen in association with familial polyposis. Turcot syndrome is the familiar eponym given to this association. Turcot et al. (56) initially described two siblings with polyposis and cerebral tumors (glioblastoma and medullary medulloblastoma, respectively). One interesting aspect concerning the polyposis in patients with cerebral tumors is that the mode of inheritance and the genetic makeup of the disease may be different from those in the more common FAP patient (57). Some authors believe the disease's inheritance in patients in whom brain neoplasms develop is recessive in nature, and often generations will be skipped. Moreover, genetic testing in these patients has demonstrated no involvement of the APC gene. The phenotypic expression is also different. There are generally a fewer number (20 to 100) of adenomatous colorectal polyps, the polyps tend to be larger in size (> 3 cm), and colon cancer may develop earlier (second or third decade) (58). If a patient with polyposis fits this phenotypic pattern, diagnostic studies should be entertained to evaluate that patient for the presence of a brain tumor. Clearly, the overwhelming majority of patients with FAP do not require such routine diagnostic studies.

References

1. Cripps W. Two cases of disseminated polyps of the rectum. Trans Pathol Soc Lond 1882;33:165–166.
2. Handford H. Disseminated polyps of the large intestine becoming malignant. Trans Pathol Soc Lond 1890;41:133–135.
3. Campbell WJ, Spence RA, Parks TG. Familial adenomatous polyposis. Br J Surg 1994;81:1722–1733.
4. Rustin RB, Jagelman DG, McGannon E, et al. Spontaneous mutation in familial adenomatous polyposis. Dis Colon Rectum 1990;33:52–55.

5. Bussey HJ (1975). Familial polyposis coli. Family studies, histopathology, differential diagnosis, and results of treatment. Baltimore: Johns Hopkins University Press, 1975.
6. Fazio VW, Church J, Cohen Z, Hawley P. Symposium: familial polyposis. Contemp Surg 1995;47:46–58.
7. Corman ML. Colon and rectal surgery. Philadelphia: Lippincott, 1998.
8. Jang YS, Steinhagen RM, Heimann TM. Colorectal cancer in familial adenomatous polyposis. Dis Colon Rectum 1997;40:312–316.
9. Spigelman A, Thomson JP. Introduction, history and registry. In Phillips RK, Spigelman A, Thomson JP, eds. Familial adenomatous polyposis and other polyposis syndromes. London: Arnold, 1994;9–14.
10. Church JM, Williams BR, Casey G. Moleclular genetics and colorectal neoplasia: a primer for the clinician. New York: Igaku-Shoin, 1996.
11. Dick JA, Owen WJ, McColl I. Rectal sparing in familial polyposis coli. Br J Surg 1984;71:664.
12. Nugent KP, Farmer KC, Spigelman AD, et al. Randomized controlled trial of the effect of sulindac on duodenal and rectal polyposis and cell proliferation in patients with familial adenomatous polyposis. Br J Surg 1993;80:1618–1619.
13. Nugent KP, Phillips RK. Rectal cancer risk in older patients with familial adenomatous polyposis and an ileorectal anastomosis: a cause for concern. Br J Surg 1992;79:1204–1206.
14. Ziv Y, Fazio VW, Church JM, et al. Stapled ileal pouch anal anastomoses are safer than handsewn anastomoses in patients with ulcerative colitis. Am J Surg 1996;171:320–323.
15. Church JM, Oakley JR, Wu JS. Pouch polyposis after ileal pouch-anal anastomosis for familial adenomatous polyposis. Report of a case. Dis Colon Rectum 1996;39:584–586.
16. Thomas MG, Thomson JP, Williamson RC. Oral calcium inhibits rectal epithelial proliferation in familial adenomatous polyposis. Br J Surg 1993;80:499–501.
17. Giardiello FM, Brensinger JD, Petersen GM, et al. The use and interpretation of commercial APC gene testing for familial adenomatous polyposis. N Engl J Med 1997;336: 823–827.
18. Petersen GM. Genetic counseling and predictive genetic testing in familial adenomatous polyposis. Semin Colon Rectal Surg 1995;6:55–60.
19. Powell SM, Petersen GM, Krush AJ, et al. Molecular diagnosis of familial adenomatous polyposis. N Engl J Med 1993;329:1982–1987.

20. Herrera L, Kakati S, Gibas L, et al. Gardner syndrome in a man with an interstitial deletion of 5q. Am J Med Genet 1986;25:473–476.

21. Bodmer WF, Bailey CJ, Bodmer J, et al. Localization of the gene for familial adenomatous polyposis on chromosome 5. Nature 1987;328:614–616.

22. Leppert M, Dobbs M, Scambler P, et al. The gene for familial polyposis coli maps to the long arm of chromosome 5. Science 1987;238:1411–1413.

23. Groden J, Thliveris A, Samowitz W, et al. Identification and characterization of the familial adenomatous polyposis coli gene. Cell 1991;66:589–600.

24. Nishisho I, Nakamura Y, Miyoshi Y, et al. Mutations of chromosome 5q21 genes in FAP and colorectal cancer patients. Science 1991;253:665–669.

25. Bonneton C, Larue L, Thiery JP. The APC gene product and colorectal carcinogenesis. C R Acad Sci [III] 1996;319:861–869.

26. Smith KJ, Johnson KA, Bryan TM, et al. The APC gene product in normal and tumor cells. Proc Natl Acad Sci U S A 1993;90: 2846–2850.

27. Miyashiro I, Senda T, Matsumine A, et al. Subcellular localization of the APC protein, immunoelectron microscopic study of the association of the APC protein with catenin. Oncogene 1995;11:89–96.

28. Rubinfeld B, Souza B, Albert I, et al. Association of the APC gene product with beta-catenin. Science 1993;262: 1731–1734.

29. Korinek V, Barker N, Morin PJ, et al. Constitutive transcriptional activation by a beta-catenin-Tcf complex in APC-/- colon carcinoma. Science 1997;275:1784–1787.

30. Sparks AB, Morin PJ, Vogelstein B, Kinzler KW. Mutational analysis of the APC/beta-catenin/Tcf pathway in colorectal cancer. Cancer Res 1998;58:1130–1134.

31. Morin PJ, Vogelstein B, Kinzler KW. Apoptosis and APC in colorectal tumorigenesis. Proc Natl Acad Sci U S A 1996;93:7950–7954.

32. Kinzler KW, Vogelstein B. Lessons from hereditary colorectal cancer. Cell 1996;87:159–170.

33. Belchetz LA, Berk T, Bapat BV, et al. Changing causes of mortality in patients with familial adenomatous polyposis. Dis Colon Rectum 1996;39:384–387.

34. Jones TR, Nance FC. Periampullary malignancy in Gardner's syndrome. Ann Surg 1977;185:565–573.

35. Jagelman DG, DeCosse JJ, Bussey HJ. Upper gastrointestinal cancer in familial adenomatous polyposis. Lancet 1997;1:1149–1151.

36. Kalantzis N, Laoudi F, Kallimanis G, et al. The role of endoscopic ultrasonography in diagnosis of benign lesions of the upper GI tract. Eur J Surg Oncol 1993;19:449–454.

37. Ryan DP, Schapiro RH, Warshaw AL. Villous tumors of the duodenum. Ann Surg 1986;203:301–306.

38. Spigelman AD, Williams CB, Talbot IC, et al. Upper gastrointestinal cancer in patients with familial adenomatous polyposis. Lancet 1989;2:783–785.

39. Penna C, Phillips RK, Tiret E, Spigelman AD. Surgical polypectomy of duodenal adenomas in familial adenomatous polyposis:Experience of two European centres. Br J Surg 1993;80:1027–1029.

40. Soravia CB, Haber G, Cohen Z, Gallinger S. Management of advanced duodenal polyposis in familial adenomatous polyposis. J Gastrointest Surg 1997;1:474–478.

41. Richard CS, Berk T, Bapat BV, et al. Sulindac for periampullary polyps in FAP patients. Int J Colorectal Dis 1997;12:14–18.

42. Seow-Choen F, Vijayan V, Keng V. Prospective randomized study of sulindac versus calcium and calciferol for upper gastrointestinal polyps in familial adenomatous polyposis. Br J Surg 1996;83:1763–1766.

43. Kashiwagi H, Spigelman AD, Debinski HS, et al. Surveillance of ampullary adenomas in familial adenomatous polyposis [Letter]. Lancet 1994; 344:1582.

44. Arvanitis ML, Jagelman DG, Fazio VW, et al. Mortality in patients with familial adenomatous polyposis. Dis Colon Rectum. 1990;33:639–642.

45. Marcello PW, Asbun HJ, Veidenheimer MC, et al. Gastroduodenal polyps in familial adenomatous polyposis. Surg Endosc 1996;10:418–421.

46. Wallace MH, Phillips RK. Upper gastrointestinal disease in patients with familial adenomatous polyposis. Br J Surg 1990;85:742–750.

47. Utsunomiya J, Maki T, Iwama T, et al. Gastric lesions of familial polyposis coli. Cancer 1974;34:745–754.

48. Clark SK, Phillips RK. Desmoids in familial adenomatous polyposis. Br J Surg 1996;83:1494–1504.

49. Heiskanen I, Jarvinen HJ. Occurrence of desmoid tumours in familial adenomatous polyposis and results of treatment. Int J Colorectal Dis 1996;11:157–162.

50. Church JM. Desmoid tumors in patients with familial adenomatous polyposis. Semin Colon Rectal Surg 1995;6:29–32.

51. Posner MC, Shiu MH, Newsome JL, et al. The desmoid tumor. Not a benign disease. Arch Surg 1989;124:191–196.

52. Moslein G, Dozois RR. Desmoid tumors associated with familial adenomatous polyposis. Perspect Colon Rectal Surg 1998;10:109–126.

53. Penna C, Tiret E, Parc R, et al. Operation and abdominal desmoid tumors in familial adenomatous polyposis. Surg Gynecol Obstet 1993;177:263–268.

54. Leppard B, Bussey HJ. Epidermoid cysts, polyposis coli and Gardner's syndrome. Br J Surg 1975;62:387–393.

55. Talbot IC. Pathology. In: Phillips RK, Spigelman AD, Thomson JP, eds. Familial adenomatous polyposis and other polyposis syndromes. London: Arnold, 1994;15–25.

56. Turcot J, Despres JP, St Pierre F. Malignant tumors of the central nervous system associated with familial polyposis of the colon. Report of two cases. Dis Colon Rectum 1959;2:465–468.

57. Bret MC, Hershman MJ, Glazer G. Other manifestations of familial adenomatous polyposis. In: Phillips RK, Spigelman AD, Thomson JPS, eds. Familial adenomatous polyposis and other polyposis syndromes. London: Arnold, 1994;143–158.

58. Itoh H, Ohsato K. Turcot syndrome and its characteristic colonic manifestations. Dis Colon Rectum 1985;28:399–402.

CHAPTER

6

Cancer in Inflammatory Bowel Disease

Nasser Al-Sanea, M.D.
and Andrew A. Shelton, M.D.

Cancer Risk and Risk Factors

There is no controversy concerning the association between ulcerative colitis and the development of colorectal cancer. Crohn and Rosenberg (1) first reported on this relationship in 1925. However, the magnitude of that increase in risk is controversial. It appears that early estimates of the long-term cancer risk in ulcerative colitis patients were overstated (up to 60% at 30 years). These erroneous estimates were the result of a number of biases. Before the advent of colonoscopy, prophylactic colectomy was often advocated after 10 years of known disease to protect against the development of colorectal cancer (2,3). Colectomy was thus performed on a significant number of patients with chronic ulcerative colitis well before 30 years of disease, and therefore, the risk of cancer was based on extrapolation of survival curves (4,5). Additional confounding factors included generalization of data from referral center populations, inclusion of patients with cancer at the time of referral,

Colon and Rectal Cancer, Edited by Peter S. Edelstein, M.D.
ISBN 0-471-35145-8

inability to identify a true denominator of patients at risk for malignancy, and limited numbers of patients followed long term.

Not all patients suffering from ulcerative colitis are at equal risk for the development of colorectal cancer. Well-accepted risk factors include duration of disease greater than 8 to 10 years and colitis extending proximal to the splenic flexure (6–9). Patients with pancolitis have a relative risk of colorectal cancer estimated to be 4.3 to 29 times that of the general population compared to the 1.5 to 3.0 times risk of patients with only left-sided colitis (10). Patients with isolated proctitis are at no additional risk for the development of cancer. Other factors that have been positively correlated with the risk of colorectal cancer are the presence of sclerosing cholangitis and a family history of colorectal cancer (11,12). Interestingly, severity of disease has not been found to be associated with an increased risk. This is important, because risk continues even in those with only minimally active disease. A reasonable estimate of the incidence of cancer development in patients with ulcerative colitis is 0.5 to 1.0% per year after 8 to 10 years of disease (13,14).

SURVEILLANCE STRATEGIES

The increased risk of cancer in ulcerative colitis has led to the development of surveillance strategies designed to identify patients at particularly increased risk. To date, these programs have focused on dysplasia as a premalignant marker.

DYSPLASIA

Warren and Sommers (15) first proposed epithelial dysplasia as a precursor to carcinoma in ulcerative colitis in 1949. In 1967, Morson and Pang (16) first suggested that the presence of dysplasia in a rectal mucosal biopsy could be used as a marker for carcinoma elsewhere in the colon. Dysplasia is defined as an unequivocal neoplastic transformation of the epithelium. It is based on the recognition of characteristic microscopic features in routine histologic sections. Interpretation of such images is a subjective exercise for the pathologist and has historically been plagued by significant interobserver and intraobserver variability. However, the development of standardized diagnostic criteria by the Inflammatory Bowel Disease-Dysplasia Morphology Study Group in 1983 provided a common ground among pathologists. Three basic diagnostic categories were put forth: negative for dysplasia, indefinite for dysplasia, and positive for dysplasia. Biopsies reported as positive for dysplasia are further subdivided into low-grade dysplasia and high-grade dysplasia. Low-grade dysplasia is characterized by nuclear enlargement, crowding, and mild stratification that is generally limited to the basal half of the epithelial cells. High-grade dysplasia usually displays a greater degree of nuclear pleomorphism, marked nuclear stratification with nuclei extending to the luminal aspect of the epithelial cells, and budding of crypts. When a spectrum of dysplastic change is observed, a biopsy is usually graded according to the most severe area. Dysplasia is clearly a precursor to malignancy. Low-grade dysplasia is accompanied by carcinoma elsewhere in the colon in 15 to 20% of cases. High-grade dysplasia is associated with a 40 to 45% incidence of synchronous cancer. Patients with dysplasia associated with abnormal appearing raised mucosa, or dysplasia-associated lesion or mass (DALM), have an approximately 50% incidence of synchronous cancer. Progression to high-grade dysplasia can be expected in 29 to 54% of patients with low-grade dysplasia (17–19).

COLONOSCOPIC SURVEILLANCE

The finding of mucosal dysplasia in the setting of ulcerative colitis is clearly associated with an increased risk of synchronous or future colorectal cancer. These findings have led most authorities today to recommend that patients who have had colitis extending proximal to the splenic flexure for more than 8 to 10 years undergo surveillance colonoscopy on an annual or biannual basis. Random mucosal biopsies are taken at 10-cm intervals. Biopsies of any suspicious areas or lesions are also taken. Proctocolectomy is indicated if dysplasia of any degree is identified.

Although such routine colonoscopic surveillance is currently standard practice, the limitations of such an approach must be clearly understood by both the physician and the ulcerative colitis patient. These limitations include interobserver variability, sampling error, poor negative predictive value, and failure to prevent colon cancer.

Although there are objective descriptors for the distinction between high- and low-grade dysplasia, there is a subjective component that can depend on the interest and experience of the examining pathologist. Agreement for the diagnosis of high-grade dysplasia is generally good. There is, however, significant interobserver variablility even among experienced pathologists concerning the diagnosis of low-grade dysplasia, concensus on the diagnosis can be as low as 40 to 60% (20). In addition, reactive atypia can be difficult to differentiate from dysplasia. Inflammation and epithelial regeneration are associated with varying degrees of nuclear enlargement, hyperchromasia, increased mitotic activity, reduced cytoplasmic maturation, and mucin depletion. Thus dysplasia in the setting of active inflammation can be a difficult diagnosis and must always be viewed with caution.

Dysplastic epithelium most commonly occurs in areas of normal-appearing mucosa, and therefore, colonoscopic surveillance relies on obtaining random biopsies at defined intervals. It has been estimated that two random biopsies taken every 10-cm actually samples only 0.2% of the surface area of the colon. It has further been estimated that 320 randomly spaced biopsies taken at 10-cm intervals would be necessary to reasonably guarantee that a patch of dysplasia 2-cm in diameter (3.14-cm^2) would be sampled (21). Thus a major problem with this surveillance strategy is based on the tremendously limited sampling performed.

The negative predictive value of dysplasia is low. Between 20 and 25% of cancers occur in the absence of detectable dysplasia. Taylor et al. (22) took random biopsies (32 biopsies) at eight anatomically defined sites in 50 colectomy specimens containing cancer. Dysplasia was absent in 26%. Possible explanations for the lack of dysplasia to still be associated with malignancy include sampling error, destruction of the dysplastic epithelium by tumor, or a possible nondysplastic alternate pathway for the development of cancer.

An unfortunate but critically important fact is that the detection of dysplasia does not reliably identify patients before they develop invasive cancer. If low-grade dysplasia is present, cancer may be expected to be found in up to 20% of colectomy specimens. If high-grade dysplasia or DALM is the indication for colectomy, the risk of synchronous malignancy rises to 40 to 45%. Of these cancers, 50% will have lymph node or distant metastases at the time of diagnosis.

Finally, there have been no prospective, randomized trials demonstrating a significant benefit of routine colonoscopic surveillance in reducing deaths from colorectal cancer in patients with long-standing ulcerative colitis. It has been estimated that 4700 patients would need to be followed for 20 years to demonstrate a 50% reduction in mortality from colorectal cancer (23). Colonoscopy has a very high cost-to-effectiveness ratio. In a review of 11 studies, 3807 colonoscopies were done to detect only eight cancers; 476 colonoscopies were performed for each cancer detected (24).

Despite all these limitations to dysplasia-based colonoscopic surveillance, and although a prospective randomized trial of surveillance colonoscopy will likely never be done, retrospective studies comparing patients undergoing regular surveillance to those not followed endoscopically have suggested a benefit to regular colonoscopic examinations with biopsies. A retrospective study by Choi et al. (25) of 41 patients with ulcerative colitis and colorectal cancer demonstrated a 77% five-year survival in patients undergoing regular colonoscopic evaluation compared to 36% for those not examined regularly. The investigators noted that the cancers tended to be diagnosed at an earlier stage in the regularly scoped patients. Although the study is plagued by all of the drawbacks inherent to retrospective studies, other authors have demonstrated similar results (26,27)

FUTURE PROSPECTS

A number of other premalignant markers have been proposed as alternatives to the use of dysplasia in the surveillance of patients with long-standing pancolitis. These include aneuploidy, abnormal mucin production, and the presence of tumor-suppressor gene mutations.

ANEUPLOIDY

Aneuploidy is defined as abnormal cell DNA content and is easily determined after biopsy by the readily available technique of flow cytometry. Clonal expansion of aneuploid cell lines is found in 50 to 70% of sporadic colorectal cancers and in a high percentage of cancers occurring in the setting of chronic ulcerative colitis (28–30). The frequency of aneuploidy also increases with increasing grades of dysplasia. Aneuploidy by itself does not represent a specific genetic event essential for the development of cancer, but rather represents genetic instability that characterizes "premalignant mucosa."

ABNORMAL MUCIN PRODUCTION

Mucins are large molecular-weight glycoproteins that are secreted by colonic goblet cells. Abnormal mucins are seen in colons harboring either inflammation or neoplasia. There are increased amounts of one subtype of mucins, sialomucins, in the colonic mucosa of patients with ulcerative colitis and an even greater increase in the presence of dysplasia. These mucin changes are present even before to the development of dysplasia or cancer. However, because a predominance of sialomucins is also seen with active inflammation, mucin analysis is not sufficiently specific to allow for use as a surveillance tool. The use of monoclonal antibody or immunohistochemical staining for sialosyl-Tn (STn) antigen—produced within the colonic mucosa of sporadic colorectal cancers and adenomatous, but not hyperplastic, polyps—holds some promise as a surveillance tool. Up to 85% of cells with high-grade dysplasia will stain positive for STn, and it may, therefore, be a useful premalignant marker for ulcerative colitis patients at greater risk for malignant transformation (31,32).

P53

The tumor-suppressor gene *p53* may also be useful for surveillance in ulcerative colitis patients. *p53* mutation is a relatively late event in the adenoma to carcinoma sequence of sporadic colorectal cancer (33). Studies have shown, however, that *p53* mutations occur relatively early in the sequence of carcinogenic events leading to cancer development in the setting of ulcerative colitis. Archival biopsies of 35 patients with ulcerative colitis and cancer demonstrated *p53* mutations in 27 patients. Intervals between *p53* mutation and the development of low-grade dysplasia, high-grade dysplasia, and cancer were 8, 26, and 38 months, respectively (30,34).

TREATMENT

Proctocolectomy is indicated when biopsies reveal cancer or dysplasia of any degree. Treatment of cancer arising in the setting of ulcerative colitis involves adherence to standard oncologic principles, including complete excision of the primary tumor and high ligation of the involved mesenteric vessels with wide mesenteric clearance. Total mesorectal excision should be performed if a rectal cancer is known or suspected. Rectal cancer is not a contraindication to a continence-preserving procedure, provided that a standard rectal cancer resection can be performed without injuring the anal sphincter mechanism. Thus only in the case of a very distal rectal cancer, for which abdominoperineal resection would be performed in a patient without ulcerative colitis, is proctocolectomy with permanent ileostomy required. In the presence of rectal cancer, consideration should be given to possible neoadjuvant therapy based on endorectal ultrasound and CT scan staging. Endorectal ultrasonography may, however, be difficult in the setting of active proctitis, risking overstaging of the primary lesion. For the colon in the setting of ulcerative colitis, some favor a staged procedure with delayed creation of an ileoanal pouch after initial total abdominal colectomy plus appropriate adjuvant therapy, followed by a period of observation. Most patients, however, can undergo restorative proctocolectomy as the initial operation for both the ulcerative colitis and the associated malignancy (35–38). An exception is the patient with unresectable distant metastases who requires only palliative resection.

There is some controversy about whether the double-stapled technique is adequate when performing a restorative proctocolectomy for dysplasia or cancer. When using the double-stapled technique, a very short cuff of at-risk mucosa is left behind in the patient, between the pouch proximally and the anal canal distally. Studies have found dysplasia in the mucosal cuff in up to 25% of patients operated on for cancer and up to 10% of patients operated on for dysplasia (39–42). Because of this, complete mucosectomy with a hand-sewn anastomosis is often recommended when the indication for proctocolectomy and ileal pouch formation is either cancer or dysplasia. However, after complete mucosectomy, minute residual islands of viable rectal mucosa have been identified between the rectal muscular cuff and the ileal pouch serosa or at the anastomotic line in up to 20% of patients after mucosectomy (43). When behind the pouch, these diseased rectal mucosal islands are completely hidden from endoscopic view. Of note, only four cases of colorectal cancer after proctocolectomy and ileal pouch anal anastomosis have been reported, all of which occurred after complete rectal mucosectomy and hand-sewn anastomosis (44–47).

CROHN DISEASE

The risk for cancer in inflammatory bowel disease is not limited to patients with chronic ulcerative colitis but is also seen in those with Crohn disease. In contrast to ulcerative colitis, however, a majority of patients with Crohn disease will undergo surgery either for complications or for medical intractability some time during the course of the disease. Therefore, the study and understanding of the long-term cancer risk in Crohn disease patients undergoing chronic medical treatment has been quite limited.

Adenocarcinomas are seen both in small bowel Crohns disease and in Crohn colitis. An increased incidence of small bowel cancer was reported in bypassed intestinal segments in 1975 (48). This practice is now to be condemned given the alternatives of resection or strictureplasty. Small intestinal cancers often appear radiographically as smooth strictures (49). Thus without the addition of histologic evaluation, such lesions can be difficult if not impossible to differentiate from the benign, fibrotic, inflammatory strictures seen commonly on imaging studies of Crohn patients. For this reason, biopsy of a stricture is recommended at time of surgical strictureplasty.

Patients with long-standing, extensive Crohn colitis are clearly at increased risk for the development of colorectal cancer. This risk is estimated to be 8% after 20 years of disease (50). However, patients with Crohn colitis are likely to undergo surgical resection for the treatment of either complications or disease intractability, so the actual number of patients with colorectal cancer complicating the colitis is fewer than is seen with ulcerative colitis (51). It is thought that cancer in Crohn disease follows the same dysplasia-cancer sequence that occurs in ulcerative colitis. Regular surveillance colonoscopy and multiple biopsies for dysplasia, such as is performed for ulcerative colitis patients, is thus warranted in patients with long-standing, extensive Crohn colitis.

Conclusion

Early detection of colorectal cancer in patients with ulcerative colitis is often difficult. Diagnosis of frank carcinoma may be delayed because symptoms such as altered bowel habits, rectal bleeding, abdominal pain, and weight loss are attributed to the colitis rather than to a superimposed carcinoma. Furthermore, patients with quiescent disease may not seek follow-up, yet their risk of cancer development continues unabated. Surveillance colonoscopy is not invariably reliable for detection of dysplasia, and colonic tumors arising in ulcerative colitis can be difficult to detect during colonoscopy because of active inflammation, friability, bleeding, and pseudopolyp formation. An additional problematic factor is that cancers developing amid ulcerative colitis are often flat, infiltrating, scirrhous lesions that are not obvious to the endoscopist's eye. The use of genetic markers holds some promise for identifying patients at higher risk for malignant transformation, but for now these tests are probably subject to the same sampling problems as dysplasia analysis. The good results of restorative proctocolectomy give both the patient with long-standing pancolitis and the physician an acceptable alternative to the surveillance strategy with its associated limitations and imperfections. Although there are only limited data concerning the true malignant potential of Crohn disease, the evidence seemingly supports a surveillance strategy for selected Crohn colitis patients that mimics the approach used for ulcerative colitis patients, although surgical options for treatment of dysplasia or cancer in the Crohn patient are more limited.

REFERENCES

1. Crohn BB, Rosenberg H. The sigmoidosccpic picture of chronic ulcerative colitis (non-specific). Am J Med Sci. 1925;170:220–227.
2. Devroede GJ, Taylor WF, Sauer WG, et al. Cancer risk and life expectancy of children with ulcerative colitis. N Engl J Med 1971;285:17–21.
3. Hultén L, Kewenter J, Åhrén C. Precancer and carcinoma in chronic ulcerative colitis: a histopathologic and clinical investigation . Scand J Gastroenterol 1972;7:663–669.
4. Ransoff DF. Colon cancer in ulcerative colitis. Gastroenterology 1988;94:1089–1091.
5. Lashner BA. Colorectal cancer in ulcerative colitis patients: survival curves and surveillance. Cleve Clin J Med 1994;61:272–275.
6. Willenbucher R. Inflammatory bowel disease. Semin Gastrointest Dis, 1996;7:1–13.
7. Greenstein A, Sachar DB, Pucillo A, et al. Cancer in universal and left sided ulcerative colitis: clinical and pathological features. Mt Sinai Med J 1979;46:25–32.
8. Gyde SN, Prior P, Allan RN, et al. Colorectal cancer in ulcerative colitis: a cohort study of primary referrals from three centers. Gut 1988;29:206–217.
9. Sugita, Sachar DB, Bodian C, et al. Colorectal cancer in ulcerative colitis. Influence of anatomical extent and age at onset on colitis-cancer interval. Gut 1991;32:167–169.
10. Choi PM, Kim WH. Colon cancer surveillance. Gastroenterol Clin North Am 1995;24:671–687.
11. Ekbom A, Helmick C, Zack M, Adami HO Ulcerative colitis and colorectal cancer. A population-based study. N Engl J Med 1990;323:1228–1233.
12. Broome U, Lindberg G, Lofberg R. Primary sclerosing cholangitis in ulcerative colitis: a risk factor for the development of dysplasia in DNA aneuploidy. Gastroenterology 1992;102:1877–1880.
13. Ransohoff D, Riddell R, Levin B. Ulcerative colitis and colonic cancer: problems in assessing the diagnostic usefulness of mucosal dysplasia. Dis Colon Rectum 1985;28:383–388.
14. Sachar DB, Greenstein AJ. Cancer in ulcerative colitis: good news and bad news. Ann Intern Med 1981;95:642–644.
15. Warren S, Sommers S. Pathogenesis of ulcerative colitis. Am J Pathol, 1949;25:637–645.

16. Morson BC, Pang LS. Rectal biopsy as an aid to cancer control in ulcerative colitis. Gut 1967;8:423–434.

17. Nixon JB, Burdick JS, Mirza AH. Premalignant changes in ulcerative colitis. Semin Surg Oncol, 1995;11:386–1193.

18. Bernstein CN, Shanahan F, Weisteine WM. Are we telling patients the truth about surveillance colonoscopy and ulcerative colitis? Lancet 1994;343:71–74.

19. Connell WR, Talbot IC, Harpaz N, et al. Clinicopathological characteristics of colorectal carcinoma complicating ulcerative colitis. Gut 1994;35:1419–1423.

20. Dundas SAC, Kay R, Beck S, et al. Can histopathologists reliably assess dysplasia in chronic inflammatory bowel disease? J Clin Pathol 1987;40:1282–1286.

21. Riddell RH. Grading dysplasia. Eur J Cancer 1995;31A:1169–1170.

22. Taylor BA, Pemberton JH, Carpenter HA, et al. Dysplasia in chronic ulcerative colitis: implications for colonoscopic surveillance. Dis Colon Rectum 1992;35:950–956.

23. Provenzale D, Kowdley KV, Arora S, Wong JB. Prophylactic colectomy or surveillance for chronic ulcerative colitis? A decision analysis. Gastroenterology 1995;109:1188–1196.

24. Axon AT. Colonic surveillance in ulcerative colitis is not essential for every patient. Eur J Cancer 1995:31A:1183–1186.

25. Choi PM, Nugent FW, Shoetz DJ, et al. Colonoscopic surveillance reduces mortality from colorectal cancer in ulcerative colitis. Gastroenterology 1993:105:418–424.

26. Rozen P, Baratz M, Fefer F, Gilat T. Low incidence of significant dysplasia in a successful endoscopic surveillance program of patients with ulcerative colitis. Gastroenterology 1995;108:1361–1370.

27. Giardiello F, Gurbuz A, Bayless T, et al. Colorectal cancer in ulcerative colitis: survival in patients with and without colorectal cancer symptoms. Inflammatory Bowel Disease 1996;2:6–10.

28. Befrits R, Hammarberg C, Rubio C, et al. DNA aneuploidy and histologic dysplasia in long-standing ulcerative colitis: a ten-year follow-up study. Dis Colon Rectum 1994:37:313–320.

29. Lofberg R, Brostrom O, Karlen P, et al. DNA aneuploidy in ulcerative colitis: reproducibility, topographic distribution, and relationship to dysplasia. Gastroenterology 1992;102:1149–1152.

30. Rubin CE, Haggitt RC, Burmer GC, et al. DNA aneuploidy in colonic biopsies predicts future development of dysplasia in ulcerative colitis. Gastroenterology 1992;103:1611–1620.

31. Izkowitz SH, Marshall A, Kornbluth A, et al. Sialosyl-Tn antigen: initial report of a new marker of malignant progression in long-standing ulcerative colitis. Gastroenterology 1995;109:490–497.

32. Izkowitz SH, Young E, Dubois D, et al. Sialosyl-Tn antigen is prevalent and precedes dysplasia in ulcerative colitis: a retrospective case-control study. Gastroenterology 1996;110:694–704.

33. Brentnall TA, Crispin DA, Rabinovitch PS, et al. Mutations in the *p53* gene: an early marker for neoplastic progression in ulcerative colitis. Gastroenterology 1994;107:369–378.

34. Lashner BA, Shapiro BD, Goldblum JR. Evaluation of the usefulness of testing for *p53* mutations in colorectal cancer surveillance for ulcerative colitis. Am J Gastroenterol 1999;94:456–462.

35. Ziv Y, Fazio VW, Strong SA, et al. Ulcerative colitis and coexisting colorectal cancer: recurrence rate after restorative proctocolectomy. Ann Surg Oncol 1994;1:512–515.

36. Wiltz O, Hashmi HF, Schoetz DJ Jr, et al. Carcinoma and the ileal pouch-anal anastomosis. Dis Colon Rectum 1991;34:805–809.

37. Stelzner M, Fonkalsrud EW. The endorectal ileal pullthrough procedure in patients with ulcerative colitis and familial polyposis with carcinoma. Surg Gynecol Obstet 1989;169:187–194.

38. Shelton AA, Lehman RE, Schrock TR, Welton ML. Retrospective review of colorectal cancer in ulcerative colitis at a tertiary center. Arch Surg, 1996;131:806–810.

39. Tsunoda A, Talbot IC, Nichols RJ. Incidence of dysplasia in the anorectal mucosa in patients having restorative proctocolectomy. Brit J Surg, 1990;77:506–508.

40. King DW, Lubowski DZ, Cook TA. Anal canal mucosa in restorative proctocolectomy for ucletative colitis. Br J Surg 1989;76:970–972.

41. Thompson-Fawcett MW, Mortensen NJ. Anal canal transition zone and columnar cuff in restorative proctocolectomy. Br J Surg 1996;83:1047–1055.

42. Ziv Y, Fazio VW, Sirimarco MT, et al. Incidence, risk factors, and treatment of dysplasia in the anal transition zone after ileal pouch anal anastomosis. Dis Colon Rectum 1994;37:1281–1285.

43. O'Connell PR, Pemberton JH, Weiland LH, et al. Does rectal mucosa regenerate after ileoanal anastomosis? Dis Colon Rectum 1987;30:1–5.

44. Rodriguez-Sanjuan JC, Polavieja MG, Naranjo A, Castillo J. Adenocarcinoma in an ileal pouch for ulcerative colitis [Letter]. Dis Colon Rectum 1995;38:779–80.

45. Puthu D, Rajan N, Rao R, et al. Carcinoma of the rectal pouch following restorative proctocolectomy. Report of a case. Dis Colon Rectum 1992;35:257–260.

46. Stern H, Walfisch S, Mullen B, et al. Cancer in an ileoanal reservoir: a new late complication? Gut 1990;10:1161.

47. Ravitch MM. The reception of new operations. Ann Surg, 1984;200:231–246.

48. Greenstein AJ, Janowits HD. Cancer in Crohn's disease: the danger of the bypassed loop. Am J Gastroenterol, 1975;64:122–124.

49. Wide JM, Loughran CF, Shocker BS. Crohn's disease, calculi, and cancer: a report of two cases. Clin Radiol, 1996;51:651–653.

50. Gillen CD, Walmsely RS, Prior P, et al. Ulcerative colitis and Crohn's disease: a comparison of the colorectal cancer risk in extensive colitis. Gut 1994;35:1507–1508.

51. Choi PM, Zelig MP. Similarity of cancer in Crohn's disease and ulcerative colitis: implications for carcinogenesis and prevention. Gut 1995;36:153–154

PART

II

ADENOCARCINOMA OF THE COLON

CHAPTER

7

PRESENTATION AND PRETREATMENT EVALUATION OF PATIENTS WITH ADENOCARCINOMA OF THE COLON

RAYMOND M. SHAHEEN, M.D., AND PETER S. EDELSTEIN, M.D.

In many ways, the signs and symptoms of colon cancer and rectal cancer overlap and mimic one another, and often the initial evaluation process leading to the diagnosis of cancer is the same regardless of the location of the tumor within the large bowel. Similarly, the preoperative evaluation of patients, during which an individual's fitness to undergo surgery is assessed, is virtually identical whether the patient harbors a colonic or a rectal lesion. Despite all of these similarities, it is crucial to recognize that adenocarcinoma of the colon and adenocarcinoma of the rectum have distinct and unique features in terms of their natural history, specifically in terms of local recurrence risk. Thus radiation, an adjuvant treatment rarely used for colon cancers, is a mainstay in the treatment for a majority of rectal cancer patients. Furthermore, operative intervention for rectal cancer carries greater risks and has a significantly greater effect on

Colon and Rectal Cancer, Edited by Peter S. Edelstein, M.D.
ISBN 0-471-35145-8

the patient's postoperative quality of life than does surgery for colon cancer, especially in cases in which a permanent stoma is required. Finally, local tumor excision and endocavitary irradiation are important techniques used to cure some rectal tumors, but these approaches play no role in the treatment of colonic lesions.

Thus given the significant differences in the natural history, treatment options, and effect on quality of life between patients with colon cancers and those with rectal cancers, the pretreatment evaluation of patients with tumors in these two locations actually does vary in several important ways. First, the initial treatment for patients suffering from cancer of the colon involves surgical resection in virtually all cases, the exception being the extremely rare situation in which, at initial diagnosis, a colon cancer patient has overwhelming metastatic disease or is deemed as an unacceptably high risk for any operative intervention and when, in addition, the primary colonic lesion does not require surgical palliation. The vast majority of colon cancer patients, however, do not have stage IV (metastatic) disease and, whether symptomatic or not, do require initial operative resection in an attempt to cure them and/or prevent the development of significant complications (such as obstruction). Determination for use of adjuvant chemotherapy and (much less frequently) adjuvant radiation therapy is based on findings both at surgery and at pathologic examination of the operative specimen. Even for patients who do initially present with metastatic disease, whose primary tumors have usually reached a size at which they are symptomatic, colonic resection almost always offers the best chance at palliation.

The same arguments do not hold true for rectal cancers. As is discussed in other chapters, pretreatment staging for patients diagnosed with rectal cancer serves several purposes. Staging identifies patients who may be cured through less-invasive, safer approaches, such as endocavitary irradiation and transanal excision. Furthermore, staging identifies patients who will benefit from neoadjuvant therapy before surgical intervention, whether to increase the chance of resectability, to spare the anal sphincter and avoid a colostomy, or to improve postoperative function of the neorectum (among other reasons). Thus when performed before instituting treatment, staging of rectal cancers, unlike staging of colon cancers, dramatically affects the types and ordering of treatment modalities used and the patient's functional outcome. Fortunately, endorectal ultrasonography has dramatically improved our ability to accurately stage rectal cancers before treatment.

Therefore, for adenocarcinoma of the colon only limited cancer staging is necessary (or even possible) before operation. In fact, the use of preoperative CT scan staging to identify the minority of patients with metastatic disease, is, we believe, greatly overused in patients with no clinical or laboratory signs to suggest liver involvement, especially (as is discussed) given the significantly better results obtained with intraoperative ultrasound of the liver. Thus much of the focus of the pretreatment evaluation for patients with colon cancer revolves around identifying the general colonic location of the lesion, excluding any synchronous neoplasms of the large bowel (adenomatous or malignant), and evaluating the patient's extraintestinal systems (cardiac, pulmonary, renal, hepatic) in terms of surgical risk.

This chapter focuses only on patients suffering from adenocarcinoma of the colon. Patient presentation and pretreatment evaluation are addressed. Similar issues for patients harboring rectal adenocarcinomas are discussed in chapter 11.

Patient Presentation

Patients with adenocarcinoma of the colon may present in a variety of ways. Although they may demonstrate signs and symptoms referable to their tumors (Table 7.1), many patients are completely asymptomatic. Most colon cancer patients will present in a nonurgent manner, but some present urgently or emergently. Possessing

TABLE 7.1. PRESENTING SIGNS AND SYMPTOMS OF COLON CANCER[a]

Signs	Symptoms
Positive fecal occult blood test stools	Blood per rectum (hematochezia or melena)
Palpable abdominal mass	Change in bowel habits (diarrhea and/or constipation)
Abdominal distension	Narrowing of stool caliber or size
Unintentional objective weight loss	Abdominal pain and/or obstructions symptoms
Microcytic anemia	Decrease or loss of appetite
Elevation of carcinoembryonic antigen	Fatigue, weakness, malaise
Overt cachexia	

[a] Adapted with permission from Ref. 1.

a clear understanding of these variable presentations is crucial to patient management, because the clinical situation at initial presentation greatly affects the time deemed available for a thorough preoperative assessment of medical comorbidities. Therefore, relative to patients with nonurgent presentations, individuals presenting urgently or emergently may not undergo as complete a preoperative evaluation, increasing the potential for minor and major perioperative complications.

Asymptomatic patients who are diagnosed with colon cancer may be generally categorized into three groups. The first includes patients with a normal risk for development of colorectal cancer and who are diagnosed as a result of routine screening measures recommended for the general population, such as fecal occult blood testing or flexible sigmoidoscopy. The second group includes patients with an increased risk for the development of colorectal cancer based on factors such as a personal history of adenomatous polyps or a strong family history of colorectal malignancy. Generally, these patients are diagnosed as a result of routine surveillance such as colonoscopy. The third group includes patients who are incidentally diagnosed during evaluations for other medical conditions, such as those who are incidentally found to be anemic (and subsequently diagnosed with colon cancer) while being evaluated for an unrelated medical condition or complaint. Although these three groups may be distinct in how their asymptomatic colon cancers were initially diagnosed, their tumors share a similar natural history owing to diagnosis at an earlier disease stage than is usually seen in patients with symptomatic cancers. And associated with this earlier diagnosis, there is a trend toward improved prognosis in patients who are asymptomatic at the time of diagnosis of their colon cancer.

Along with several classic signs, symptomatic patients may present with either systemic or localizing complaints, as illustrated in Table 7.1. In regard to obstructive symptoms, patients may experience abdominal bloating, cramping pain, nausea, vomiting, constipation and/or diarrhea, and decreased caliber (even "pencil thin") stools. Furthermore, in obstructed patients, there is a relationship between the colonic location and the morphology and size of the tumor. For a number of reasons, tumors of the right colon tend to reach a greater size before causing obstructive symptoms than those of the left colon. One factor is colonic luminal size, which is significantly greater in the cecum and ascending colon than in the left colon. Furthermore, stool within the right colon is liquid, whereas more distally it is much more solid and, therefore, more easily obstructed. Finally, the morphologic features of colon cancer vary, depending on location. Cecal and ascending colon lesions are usually exophytic masses that fungate into the large, liquid-filled lumen and, as such, must achieve a significant size to produce obstructive symptoms. Left colonic cancers frequently grow in an annular, napkin-ring pattern, producing circumferential obstruction of the narrower, solid stool-filled left colon even when small. Thus in terms of one major set of symptoms, obstructive symptoms (including constipation and diarrhea), left-sided lesions tend to present at an earlier stage than those in the right colon.

As history has revealed, the clinical signs and symptoms of adenocarcinoma of the colon may be easily overlooked or misinterpreted by both patient and physician because of their commonality and their lack of specificity. For example, blood in the stool is frequently attributed to hemorrhoids, and patients may insist that their weight loss is intentional, caused by dieting. However, the results of a significant delay in the diagnosis of colon cancer can be disastrous. Thus even such seemingly benign patient complaints must trigger a compulsive but sensible workup, including a detailed personal and family history and a thorough physical examination (including digital rectal examination with fecal occult blood testing). All "normal risk" patients age 50 and older should have annual occult blood testing, flexible sigmoidoscopy every 5 years, and endoscopic evaluation at an earlier point if warranted based on new signs or symptoms.

PRETREATMENT EVALUATION AFTER DIAGNOSIS

Two important goals of pretreatment evaluation after the initial diagnosis of colon cancer is made are to identify the location of the primary lesion and to rule out synchronous colonic adenomas or cancers. However, as noted earlier, there is currently no role for neoadjuvant therapy before surgical resection in patients with colon cancer, and for the majority of patients (as will be discussed), preoperative CT scanning for staging is both unnecessary and inferior to intraoperative liver ultrasonography. Thus the need for preoperative disease staging is quite limited. The third major pretreatment goal is to optimize patient care by identifying risk factors for perioperative complications and to then take the appropriate steps to reduce those risks.

EVALUATION OF THE COLON AND RECTUM

The incidence of synchronous colorectal cancers (two large intestinal adenocarcinomas existing at the same time) is 2 to 3% in patients suffering from the sporadic form of the disease (it is considerably greater in those at increased risk, such as in patients with hereditary nonpolyposis colorectal cancer). A colon cancer patient's risk of harboring a synchronous adenomatous polyp, however, is significantly greater, possibly even as high as 50%. Thus it is crucial that, before surgery, patients diagnosed with colon cancer have their entire colon and rectum evaluated to identify synchronous lesions that require attention either before or at the time of definitive resection. Although the entire colon and rectum is usually evaluated at the same time that the cancer is initially diagnosed (usually by colonoscopy), some distal cancers are diagnosed on sigmoidoscopy, and the proximal colon is never visualized. In such cases, either a barium enema or a complete colonoscopy should be performed before resection. A more difficult situation occurs when a tumor obstructs the colonic lumen, preventing the passage of the colonoscope more proximally. In such cases, choosing between the few options must be based on an evaluation of the individual patient and the tumor. If the obstruction is indeed high grade, proximal evaluation with a barium enema is probably not worth the risks of converting the situation into a complete obstruction with barium impacted proximal to the lesion. If, however, the obstruction is not high grade but only tight enough to prevent passage of the colonoscope, consideration should be given to repeat endoscopy with a pediatric colonoscope or to radiographic enema with either barium or a water-soluble contrast material (which may miss smaller proximal mucosal lesions but at least should not miss larger masses). If proximal colonic evaluation is not feasible, the patient may need to first undergo colonic resection (with intraoperative palpation of the proximal colon) and then undergo endoscopic evaluation of the unexamined proximal bowel after recovery from surgery. In the vast majority of such cases, synchronous cancers will not be missed on intraoperative palpation, and proximal adenomas will likely be amenable to postoperative colonoscopic excision.

Given the infrequency of isolated pulmonary colon cancer metastases at initial presentation (< 1%) and given the need for at least palliative surgery in the vast majority of stage IV colon cancer patients, ordering a chest radiograph simply as part of preoperative disease staging is probably not warranted. However, a simple chest x-ray is virtually always a part of the preoperative cardiopulmonary evaluation (as discussed later), and this plain x-ray is adequate to exclude pulmonary metastases as well.

A significantly more controversial issue concerns the need for evaluation of the liver before embarking on colonic resection in patients with no clinical or laboratory abnormalities that suggest hepatic metastases. Once again, the vast majority of stage IV colon cancer patients have significant symptoms referable to their primary tumor, such as bleeding, obstruction, and pain. And again, in almost all patients, despite the secondary malignant involvement of the liver, death from liver disease is not imminent, and there is a strong desire on the part of both the patient and the doctor to palliate the colonic symptoms. Far and away the most effective means of palliation is surgical resection, and unlike stage IV patients suffering from rectal cancer, colonic resection is a relatively rapid and safe process. Thus the determination of liver metastases will not likely deter either the patient or the surgeon from proceeding with bowel resection, it will only change the nature of the procedure from one with curative to one with palliative intent. Thus, because it is significantly superior to preoperative abdominal CT scanning for the evaluation of liver metastases, intraoperative ultrasonography (IOUS) of the liver is the evaluatory staging procedure of choice.

Yet proponents of preoperative CT scanning of colon cancer patients argue that knowledge of liver metastases allows for the preoperative planning of liver resection at the time of colon resection. However, the criteria allowing for liver resection at the time of primary colon resection are very stringent (e.g., a total resection volume no greater than that of the left lateral segment, rapid colon resection with minimal blood loss), and most surgeons will readily admit that combined curative colon and liver resections are few and very far between. Our own recent retrospective review of 88 colon cancer patients who underwent routine preoperative CT scanning for staging (when liver metastases were not suspected based on clinical or laboratory abnormalities) revealed the following: 0 cases for which the preoperative CT scan directly altered the operative procedure performed, 11% false-positive CT scan results, and 6% false-negative CT scan results. The false-negative results are of concern because this imaging technique missed metastatic lesions identified at surgery by either palpation or IOUS of the liver. The false positives are problematic because they tend to require the addition of IOUS when palpation fails to identify the suspicious CT lesion. Of greater concern was 1 case in which a patient was told to forego colon resection because of liver metastases identified on CT imaging. He sought a second opinion, and at the time of colon resection, no liver metastases were found on palpation or on IOUS, the suspicious CT lesion in fact turning out to be a benign hemangioma. Perhaps most impressive is that in no cases did preoperative liver findings on CT scanning in any way alter the surgical procedure performed. The overwhelming majority of patients had no evidence of liver metastases. In all cases, of those who did have radiographic findings suspicious for tumor spread, the metastases were clearly identifiable by intraoperative palpation or by IOUS. Even in this subset with stage IV disease, few patients met the criteria to undergo anything greater than a biopsy at the time of their colon resection (owing to overwhelming hepatic involvement). And in the few patients who actually had potentially curable liver disease and also met the criteria for synchronous resection, preoperative knowledge was unnecessary, because the limited resection was identified by IOUS and simply carried out after completion of the colon resection.

Thus for patients who are diagnosed with colon cancer and have no findings on physical examination or on blood liver function testing to suggest metastatic spread to the liver, preoperative CT scan imaging to evaluate the liver for metastatic disease is not indicated. Instead, at the time of colon resection, IOUS of the liver should be obtained. This study is (at least in our institution) less costly than CT imaging, requires < 10 min to perform adequately, and carries no significant risk to the patient. If a suspicious lesion is identified on IOUS, a core-needle or wedge biopsy can be performed under ultrasound guidance at the time of operation.

For patients who do have findings suspicious for metastatic involvement of the liver (e.g., hepatomegaly, jaundice, elevated alkaline phosphatase), it seems more reasonable to perform a preoperative CT scan. In a few of these cases, CT will demonstrate such overwhelming malignant hepatic replacement that colon resection may not be the most appropriate form of palliation. Other nonemergent situations in which early CT scan imaging has a role in treatment planning include colon cancer patients suspected of having complications of the tumors, such as contained perforations or abdominal wall invasion, and those suspected of having large, bulky sigmoid or rectosigmoid lesions that may be impinging on or obstructing the left ureter (in which case ureteral stent placement before resection may be beneficial).

CARCINOEMBRYONIC ANTIGEN

Since the 1960s, carcinoembryonic antigen (CEA) has been evaluated as a putative tumor marker. Although elevated CEA serum levels may be seen in patients with several different tumor types and even in patients with some benign conditions, the highest concentrations are found in patients with colon and rectal carcinoma. Unfortunately, only 6 to 12% of patients with localized colon cancer have elevated serum levels, and thus CEA evaluations are not useful for screening normal patient populations. For patients with colon cancer, however, preoperative CEA levels have clinical use for predicting prognosis, establishing a point of reference for postoperative evaluations (usually the level falls precipitously after successful surgical resection), and following patients after primary resection. Elevated CEA levels after primary resection occur in 70 to 80% of patients with recurrences and can be used to detect these recurrences up to 6 months before they become clinically evident. Radiologic studies, such as CT, MR, and PET scan imaging may be obtained to determine the extent and location of recurrent disease based on recurrent postoperative CEA elevation, and even second-look laparoscopy or laparotomy can be performed if such radiographic studies fail to identify recurrent disease. Other adjuncts to localizing subclinical recurrences include CEA-directed monoclonal antibodies; however, their role in clinical practice remains to be defined.

OTHER BLOOD TESTS

Preoperative evaluation of the patient's hematocrit or hemoglobin should be obtained, because many patients present with microcytic anemia, which has perioperative morbidity implications. Baseline BUN and creatinine may also be of benefit, particularly in patients suspected of having mild to moderate renal insufficiency, by making the surgeon and anesthesiologist aware of the problem so they can prevent further renal insult during the perioperative period. Likewise, basic liver function analysis is indicated in patients whose history or examination suggests hepatic insufficiency, such as previous hepatitis or alcoholism. In such cases, a preoperative evaluation of prothrombin time (PT) may also be invaluable in identifying a coagulopathy resulting from hepatic insufficiency.

Other routine preoperative laboratory evaluations besides CEA, such as liver and biliary function tests (aspartate aminotransferase, alanine aminotransferase, alkaline phosphatase, and bilirubin), are of less clear benefit in patients with no clinical findings that suggest hepatic metastases. It is highly unlikely that malignant metastatic spread to the liver significant enough to produce elevations of hepatic enzymes or bilirubin will be resectable for cure. As argued earlier concerning preoperative CT imaging, surgery with IOUS and curative or palliative colon resection is an appropriate initial approach to colon cancer patients who are not suspected of harboring liver metastases. Some physicians believe that alkaline phosphatase (ALP) is significantly more sensitive and is, therefore, a reasonable preoperative test. If the level is elevated, abdominal CT imaging is performed. Indeed, although CEA levels have replaced ALP measurements as a method of postoperative surveillance for hepatic metastases, in the preoperative setting ALP levels appear to more specifically indicate liver involvement. Interestingly, patients found preoperatively to have elevated serum ALP levels but who at surgery do not actually have demonstrable liver metastases are at no greater risk of later developing liver metastases than patients with normal preoperative levels. In patients who do have symptoms or physical findings suspicious of liver metastases, performing liver function analysis is appropriate, because those with abnormalities may well harbor such extensive malignant hepatic replacement that nonoperative palliative treatment may be warranted.

Cardiovascular Assessment

Many patients with colon cancer are at an increased risk of having concomitant cardiovascular disease given the entities' shared association with advanced patient age. Therefore, some form of preoperative cardiovascular evaluation is indicated in the majority of colon cancer patients. At its least, this assessment should include a detailed cardiovascular history and physical examination, with attention to well-established risk factors. With the exception of young, asymptomatic patients with normal histories and physical examinations, an ECG should be performed (Table 7.2). Extreme importance should also be given to the commonly associated signs and symptoms of cardiovascular disease, such as marginal exercise

TABLE 7.2. RISK FACTORS FOR PERIOPERATIVE CARDIAC COMPLICATIONS[a,b]

History
Age > 70 years
Myocardial infarction within previous 6 months*
General metabolic status
Abnormal arterial or venous blood gas analysis
Potassium and/or HCO_3^- abnormalities
Abnormal hepatic or renal function
Bedridden
Cardiovascular examination
S_3 gallop*
Moderate to severe aortic valvular stenosis
Jugular venous distention
Electrocardiogram
Presence of PACs
> 5 PVCs/min
Rhythm other than sinus (with or without PACs or PVCs)
Emergent performance of operation

[a] Adapted with permission from Ref. 1.
[b] *, most significant risk factors.
PACS, premature atrial contractions; *PVCs*, premature ventricular contractions.

tolerance, decompensated congestive heart failure, pulmonary rales, angina, persistent systemic hypertension, symptoms of transient ischemic attacks or cerebrovascular accidents, and carotid bruits and cardiac arrhythmias on auscultation.

For the minority of patients presenting emergently (such as with a malignant complete large bowel obstruction or colonic perforation), a thorough evaluation may not be attainable before surgery. But for those patients whose cancers do not require urgent or emergent operation, identification of significant clinical risk factors for perioperative cardiovascular complications can be invaluable in determining which patients are most likely to benefit from more in-depth assessment and treatment before embarking on surgical resection of the cancer.

A systemic approach to cardiovascular evaluation should include several aspects. For patients who have undergone coronary revascularization procedures within the previous 5 years and have remained free of cardiovascular symptoms, no evaluation other than a history, physical examination, and ECG is indicated. For patients who have developed recurrent symptoms after revascularization and for symptomatic patients who have not undergone revascularization, the cardiac evaluation should proceed, usually in the form of an exercise treadmill test (ETT), a dobutamine echocardiogram, or a coronary angiogram (in the case of previously revascularized, symptomatic patients). Subsequent medical or interventional management should be based on the results of these studies and is best guided with the assistance of a cardiologist. Given the absolute need for surgical resection to avert colonic obstruction or perforation (an urgent case), however, a timely balance between risk factor modification or intervention and expedient colon resection must be achieved.

For patients demonstrating uncontrolled systemic hypertension, nonurgent and nonemergent surgery should be postponed to allow for medical treatment of blood pressure persistently elevated above 195 mm Hg systolic or 110 mm Hg diastolic. Failing to correct such hypertension may increase the risk of perioperative myocardial infarction, cerebrovascular accident, or hypertensive crisis. Preoperative antihypertensives should be continued throughout the perioperative period. This is especially important for α_2 (such as clonidine) and β_1 blockade agents to avoid severe postoperative rebound hypertension.

For patients with historical or clinical evidence of transient ischemic attacks (TIAs), as evidenced by amaurosis fugax (transient monocular or partial blindness) or other temporary focal neurologic abnormalities, nonemergent surgical cancer resection should be postponed to allow for proper neurovascular evaluation. In most institutions, a carotid artery duplex imaging study is the initial assessment procedure of choice (in some centers, the experience with MR angiography is extensive and has supplanted carotid duplex imaging as the initial evaluatory study). If duplex study results are indeterminate, either a four-vessel carotid artery angiogram (which carries minimal but not insignificant risks) or an MR angiogram can be performed. Serious consideration of carotid endarterectomy should be given to patients who show symptoms from their carotid disease and who have identifiable, correctable vessel stenosis. However, the role of carotid endarterectomy for asymptomatic artery stenosis is controversial, given that such lesions rarely contribute to cerebrovascular events during uncomplicated abdominal surgery. If the need for carotid endarterectomy in an asymptomatic patient is unclear or if the patient has a symptomatic stenosis, consultation with an experienced vascular surgeon is indicated. In most cases, the patient can undergo a successful carotid surgery and can then safely proceed with resection of the colon cancer after a delay of only 2 weeks.

PULMONARY ASSESSMENT

The goals of pulmonary assessment in patients who are preparing to undergo abdominal surgery are to prepare and educate each patient regarding what measures need to be taken postoperatively to promote optimal pulmonary function (such as incentive spirometry, pulmonary toilet, early postural changes, and ambulation), to identify risk factors for perioperative complications, and to intervene perioperatively so that these risks are reduced or minimized.

From a pulmonary view, patients may be separated into two major groups in terms of the risk of postoperative complications. The first group includes patients with no clinically obvious preoperative pulmonary dysfunction based on history and physical examination. Although these patients generally do not require any further workup other than a chest radiograph (which may itself be unnecessary in younger patients), a patient with a history of gastroesophageal reflux disease (GERD) is usually assessed by an anesthesiologist as at greater risk for perioperative aspiration. Thus patients with known GERD or symptoms suspicious for GERD (such as heartburn) may undergo induction with anesthetic agents and techniques (such as rapid-sequence induction) that differ from those used for non-GERD patients. To facilitate optimal postoperative pulmonary recovery, these patients should all be instructed in pulmonary toilet (coughing, deep breathing) and incentive spirometry and should be encouraged to change position and ambulate as soon as safely possible. The need for adequate patient analgesia to promote improved pulmonary function after abdominal surgery cannot be overemphasized. In many centers, epidural analgesia and patient-controlled analgesia (PCA) has virtually replaced the use of nurse-dependent PRN narcotic administration.

The second group of patients includes those in whom obvious chronic pulmonary dysfunction exists or in whom significant risk factors are present. This group is made up of individuals with chronic obstructive pulmonary diseases (COPD), such as emphysema, chronic bronchitis or asthma, restrictive lung disease secondary to significant obesity or severe pectus excavatum, and long-term smokers. These patients are all less able to tolerate the inherent decreased functional residual capacity (FRC) associated with anesthesia, mechanical ventilation, and postoperative abdominal pain secondary to the development of atelectasis. Several measures can be taken preoperatively to optimize the perioperative management of such patients and consequently to reduce their risks for the development of atelectasis, aspiration, bronchopneumonia, and acute respiratory distress syndrome (ARDS). Such preoperative tactics include aggressive teaching of pulmonary toilet and incentive spirometry, ceasing (or at worst significantly reducing) smoking, performing spirometry and pulmonary function tests (PFTs), obtaining a baseline arterial blood gas analysis (often extremely useful in assisting in postoperative extubation decisions but also often not drawn preoperatively), maintaining bronchodilator therapy, and considering a short course of oral antibiotics for several days preoperatively if tenacious or purulent sputum is associated with chronic bronchitis. Mucolytics and expectorants are of no value preoperatively and can actually paradoxically induce bronchospasm. In these higher-risk patients, the counsel of a pulmonologist (especially when using PFTs) is often of considerable benefit. Most commonly, PFTs are performed to measure static lung volumes, flow rates, compliance, and resistance. Forced expiratory volume in 1 sec (FEV_1) and the forced vital capacity (FVC; the volume expired from maximal inspiration to maximal expiration) are the two most routinely used values and are commonly represented as a ratio (FEV_1/FVC).

Postoperative measures include many of the same therapies, such as pulmonary toilet, incentive spirometry, continuation of bronchodilator therapy, and avoidance of mucolytics. In addition, early extubation, early postural changes and ambulation, excellent pain management, nasogastric tube decompression and/or H_2-blockade to decrease the risk and severity of early aspiration (sucralfate is preferred in many centers as prophylaxis against stress gastritis without changing gastric luminal pH and subsequently promoting bacterial overgrowth), and the careful use of fluids and blood product transfusion (which increase the risk of ARDS) are extremely important.

NUTRITIONAL ASSESSMENT

Significant protein and caloric malnutrition is a common risk factor for the development of postoperative complications in patients who undergo surgical resection of their colon cancer. Such nutrition-related complications include delayed wound healing, wound infection, sepsis, prolonged ileus, and even death owing to severe preoperative depletion of both skeletal muscle mass and visceral protein. It is, therefore, essential that all nonemergent patients diagnosed with colon cancer routinely undergo some form of nutritional assessment before embarking on surgical resection.

Of course, much of nutritional assessment can be completed through patient inspection, routine physical examination, and a few appropriate questions concerning weight changes, appetite, and diet. But for cancer patients whose examination or history clearly demonstrates or even suggests possible malnutrition, more objective anthropomorphic measurements can be obtained, such as patient height and body weight (even obese patients can be malnourished), arm muscle circumference, and triceps skinfold thickness (TST). These tests are readily available, are easily obtained, and can be compared to well-published age-matched normal values. Other parameters should be considered as well, many of which are rapidly and easily obtained: serum levels for albumin, transferrin, and prealbumin and patient response to delayed hypersensitivity reactions (DHR) skin testing to *Candida albicans* or mumps.

No single parameter is sufficiently specific or sensitive enough to reliably predict which colon cancer patients are at significant risk for malnutrition-associated postoperative complications. The prognostic nutrition index (PNI), was developed as an approach for incorporating several of these factors into a prognostic aid. The equation for calculating an individual patient's PNI is:

$$\begin{aligned}158\% &- (16 \times \text{albumin in mg/dL}) - (0.78 \times \text{TST in mm}) \\ &- (0.2 \times \text{transferrin in mg/dL}) \\ &- (5.8 \times 1 \text{ for anergy to DHR or } \times 2 \text{ for normal reaction to DHR})\end{aligned}$$

Some prospective trials have demonstrated that the preoperative PNI can stratify patients into those at low (PNI$<$ 40%), intermediate (PNI$=$ 40 to 50%), and high (PNI$>$ 50%) risk for the development of postoperative complications after gastrointestinal surgery.

These objective criteria can be used to form a plan for preoperative nutritional repletion therapy in patients with colon cancer deemed at high risk for postoperative complications based on their suboptimal nutritional status. The majority of high-risk malnourished patients can safely have their colon cancer resection delayed by 1 to 2 weeks while they receive nutritional therapy (preferably enterally, but in rare cases parenterally). Although cumulative evidence suggests that a 7- to 10-day repletion period significantly diminishes the risk of postoperative complications in high-risk patients, the evidence for nutritional repletion therapy in moderate and low-risk patients remains controversial.

Conclusions

Two aspects of the preoperative evaluation of patients diagnosed with adenocarcinoma of the colon must be addressed. The more clear-cut issue, assessing and diminishing the risks of surgery and anesthesia, may involve minor or extensive evaluations of cardiac, vascular, pulmonary, hepatic, renal, and nutritional status through a variety of techniques. Some results (e.g., severe carotid or coronary artery disease) may require therapeutic intervention before surgical resection of the colon cancer. Others (e.g., mild renal insufficiency) may simply require awareness on the part of the surgeon and the anesthesiologist to prevent further injury during the perioperative period.

The second aspect of preoperative evaluation, the staging of the malignant disease, is more controversial. In patients whose symptoms or physical examination suggests metastatic disease (almost always hepatic), further analysis is indicated in the form of blood tests and/or radiographic imaging. The rationale for this approach is that there are relatively rare patients whose metastatic disease is so advanced at presentation and whose symptoms owing to the primary colonic tumor are so mild that nonoperative palliative treatment (usually chemotherapy), or no specific treatment, is truly in the patient's best interest given their extremely limited life expectancy. However, in the overwhelming majority of colon cancer patients, there is no clinical evidence (and even no laboratory evidence) to suggest stage IV disease even when hepatic metastases are present. Furthermore, preoperative knowledge of hepatic lesions suspicious for metastases on CT scan imaging in no way obviates the need for palliative colonic resection, given that most of the primary lesions are or will become symptomatic long before the patient succumbs to malignant hepatic failure. This approach is further supported by our experience that preoperative CT suspicion of hepatic metastases in no way altered the surgery performed in any of our analyzed patients.

Thus in colon cancer patients who have no clinical suspicion of metastatic disease, we recommend complete colonoscopy and CEA analysis before surgical exploration, along with cardiovascular, pulmonary, renal, hepatic, and nutritional tests for evaluation of perioperative risk as based on each individual patient's clinical status. During surgery, every patient should undergo IOUS of the liver. Any suspicious hepatic lesions should be biopsied. In the extremely rare case in which the acceptable very limited hepatic resection can be performed for cure (as identified by ultrasound), such a resection should proceed only after a rapid, uncomplicated resection of the colon primary. CT imaging of the liver should be reserved for patients in whom there is clinical suspicion of hepatic involvement and in centers in which IOUS is unavailable.

REFERENCES

1. Goldman L, Caldera DL, Nussbaum SR, et al. Multifactorial index of cardiac risk in noncardiac surgical procedures. N Engl J Med 1977;297:845–850.

CHAPTER

8

TREATMENT OF COLON CANCER

HANNAH-NGOC HA AND BARD C. COSMAN

Colon cancer affects approximately 100,000 patients per year in the United States, and an estimated 50,000 die of the disease (1), making it the number two cancer killer overall. If diagnosed early, colon cancer is curable by operation. Although 70% of patients who present with colon cancer may have a curative resection, only 50% of these will actually be cured by surgery (2), and the rest eventually die of the disease. This underscores the fact that the best "cure" for all colon and rectal cancer is through prevention via endoscopic surveillance and polypectomy. As is the case for cervical neoplasia, each colorectal adenocarcinoma must be viewed as a screening failure, and each case should stimulate us to redouble our efforts to provide adequate endoscopic screening programs in our own institutions.

Although adenocarcinoma of the colon is similar in terms of cause and histopathology to that of the rectum, which occurs approximately half as frequently, the behavior and treatment of the two malignancies are distinct, and this chapter's focus is limited to colon, not rectal, cancer. Rectal cancer behaves differently in

Colon and Rectal Cancer, Edited by Peter S. Edelstein, M.D.
ISBN 0-471-35145-8

regard to local spread, recurrence and pattern of metastasis and thus is treated in a different fashion, and both radiation and local treatment options are commonly exercised. Given the low morbidity of performing major colon resections, local treatment of colon tumors alone is not performed for colon cancer, and radiation is almost never employed because of the infrequency of local recurrence following surgical resection. Thus adenocarcinoma of the colon is a unique, and in many ways simpler, cancer to treat from the viewpoint of the physician.

This chapter's discussion of colon cancer treatment mimics the organization in approaching a typical case of the disease, in which a patient with recently diagnosed colon cancer presents to the surgeon for curative or palliative resection. First we discuss preoperative evaluation, then preparation for surgery, followed by the operation itself (both therapeutic and diagnostic aspects), postoperative care, possible adjuvant treatment, and finally postoperative patient follow-up. Special considerations in each of these areas will be discussed.

PREOPERATIVE EVALUATION

Patients with colon cancer require preoperative cancer staging as well as evaluation of comorbid conditions and nutritional status. Comorbidity and nutritional status are assessed by history and physical examination, supplemented by routine, risk-reducing tests such as ECG for older patients. Hemoglobin or hematocrit is useful to determine the degree of anemia and provide a baseline for operative consideration of transfusion. Although pathologic staging remains the most important determinant of prognosis (3), control of postoperative morbidity is also decisive of outcome. Elderly patients (usually defined as > 70) should have the same options as younger patients. A more extensive preoperative evaluation of cardiac, pulmonary, and renal function may be considered, because some preoperative intervention for reduction of operative risk may be warranted in up to 60% of older patients (4). We use age as a surrogate marker for comorbidity, a common and useful, if not entirely justifiable, practice. Although treating the elderly may incur higher costs or charges, their 3-year survival is equal to that of younger patients (5).

Available preoperative staging tests include abdominal CT scan, liver ultrasound, chest radiography, liver function tests, blood carcinoembryonic antigen (CEA) level, and colonoscopy. One should keep in mind, however, that the upcoming operation is the ultimate staging procedure for the abdomen, and available preoperative tests should be compared not only to one other but, more important, to the operation, viewing the latter as a diagnostic and a therapeutic maneuver. Thus abdominal CT should not be obtained unless the patient is a very poor operative candidate, because liver metastases are best diagnosed at the time of operation using intraoperative liver ultrasonography.

It is important to remember that complete tumor staging is best accomplished during surgery; and staging can wait until the time of the operation given that the primary colon cancer will likely produce obstruction or hemorrhage and, therefore, requires resection even in the patient harboring unresectable metastatic liver disease. Thus, because the primary lesion should be removed for cure or palliation in virtually every case, the liver (and the rest of the peritoneal cavity) is best evaluated intraoperatively. The same reasoning applies to transcutaneous hepatic ultrasound, which adds nothing to preoperative staging unless the patient is not a candidate for laparotomy, in which case transcutaneous ultrasound is still inferior to CT scanning. Liver function tests are also unnecessary, both because the liver will be evaluated at the time of operation and also given that liver function tests may be normal in the presence of extensive liver metastases. A preoperative chest x-ray to evaluate the heart and lung fields may be reasonable, but it is unnecessary when ordered primarily to search for isolated pulmonary metastases, which are extremely rare in colon cancer. CEA should be measured because if elevated preoperatively, it may serve as a marker of recurrence postoperatively. CEA levels may correlate with tumor stage as well as prognosis, but again there is no substitute for the pathologic staging one obtains during surgery (6,7).

A complete colonoscopy is the one essential in the preoperative evaluation for colon cancer. It is useful for localizing the tumor, obtaining tissue for diagnosis (although every suspicious lesion should be removed regardless of biopsy result), and most important, for finding synchronous cancers and polyps. Synchronous colon cancer is found in 3 to 9% of patients, and the location of the lesions dictates the operative resection required (8,9). The entire colon must be examined and cleared of polyps, because the incidence of synchronous adenomatous polyps in patients with colon cancer is approximately 30% (8,10).

Neoadjuvant Therapy

There is no role for neoadjuvant therapy before the typical colon resection for cancer (11). However, in the rare case in which preoperative physical examination suggests a large fixed lesion (the vast majority of colon cancers are nonpalpable in the awake patient), it is reasonable to perform an abdominal CT scan to identify any tumor involvement of the abdominal wall and/or contiguous essential organs. If such locally aggressive behavior is detected, then direct surgical attack might result in incomplete resection, and it is prudent to reduce the tumor bulk with radiation, with or without concomitant 5-fluorouracil as a radiosensitizer. Radiation has been safely administered to large fixed lesions, and concerns about small bowel radiation damage are balanced by the overwhelming consideration of local unresectability. These cases are rare, and there are no large studies proving that neoadjuvant tumor downsizing is advantageous; however, complete resections of previously unresectable lesions have been reported, and this approach seems clinically sound.

SURGICAL PREPARATION

There have been many studies of mechanical and antibiotic bowel preparation for elective colonic surgery (12–15). The role of mechanical bowel preparation alone to reduce perioperative infection remains unclear, but a standard of care has evolved to include either low-volume cathartics (such as Fleet's Phospho-Soda) or rapid lavage with a large volume (usually 4 L) of polyethylene glycol (GoLYTELY, Colyte). This mechanical flushing is usually accompanied by a clear liquid diet during the day before the operation. There is clear evidence favoring prophylactic intravenous antibiotic administration within 1 hr before surgical incision: In one study, the rate of septic complications in patients receiving no prophylactic antibiotic for colonic operations was 30%, and the rate with an antibiotic was 12% (16). The antibiotic should cover at least skin gram-positive bacteria, but most recommendations include coverage for gram-negative coliforms and anaerobes as well, such as a second-generation cephalosporin (cefoxitin or cefotetan) or the combination of a first-generation drug (cefazolin) and metronidazole. Preoperative oral antibiotics decrease the incidence of wound infection but only in the absence of intravenous antibiotics (17). However, combinations of oral and intravenous antibiotics are commonly used: A survey of 350 colon and rectal surgeons found that all used mechanical bowel preparation, and 88% used both oral and intravenous antibiotics (18).

Positioning the patient in the modified Lloyd-Davies position (low lithotomy) allows access to the anus for intraoperative proctoscopy or colonoscopy and for testing of the integrity of a low anastomosis, an unproven but probably valuable maneuver. We use this position routinely for all colon operations except right hemicolectomy, for which the supine position is adequate. Sequential compression devices should be placed on the legs before induction of anesthesia for prevention of deep venous thrombosis (DVT). Various standard and low molecular weight heparin regimens may be equivalent or better for preventing DVT in these patients whose risk factors include malignancy, abdominal and pelvic surgery, and lithotomy position; however, this rapidly changing area is beyond the scope of this chapter.

SURGICAL DIAGNOSTIC MANEUVERS

The operation includes the most valuable staging procedures, namely, removal of the tumor and nodal basin for pathologic examination and examination of the liver and peritoneal cavity for evidence of metastatic disease. Again, the superiority of operative staging in patients who virtually all require colonic resection regardless of tumor stage is the basis of the argument favoring an extremely limited preoperative evaluation (typically colonoscopy, CEA, chest x-ray, hemoglobin, and ECG). The current practice of radical excision is unlikely to be improved on as a staging procedure for tumor and lymph nodes, and the only remaining improvement is in the area of metastasis detection.

Intraoperative identification of metastases in the abdomen is useful prognostically and in the selection of patients for adjuvant therapy: As many as 20% of patients having planned curative resection are found to be incurable at surgery (19). The majority of incurable cases are the result of multiple liver metastases (60%), and the remainder are based on intraperitoneal spread and extensive lymph node metastases. Although intraoperative palpation of the liver can detect even tiny surface lesions, it is poor for detecting small intrahepatic metastases.

Intraoperative ultrasonography (IOUS) is more accurate for detecting liver metastases than preoperative CT scanning, preoperative ultrasound, or intraoperative bimanual palpation. Occult hepatic metastases were detected by only IOUS in 5 to 10% of all patients undergoing colon cancer resection (20), and the operative plan was changed based on IOUS findings in 42% of patients (21). In patients with T1 or T2 lesions, IOUS may be less useful than in patients with T3 or T4 lesions, because occult hepatic metastases are rare in less advanced tumors. However, one does not determine the degree of invasion intraoperatively, so it is sensible to have a blanket policy of performing IOUS (if available) at the time of colon resection. Like all metastasis-detection techniques, IOUS has a significant false-negative rate of 5 to 21%. We believe that, despite its flaws, surgeon-performed IOUS is currently clearly the best method for evaluating the liver and thus should become a standard part of initial curative surgery to resect colon cancer. Surgeon-performed IOUS should be no more controversial than intraoperative endoscopy, an accepted part of operations in the gastrointestinal tract, and it no more threatens the radiologists' turf than intraoperative endoscopy threatens the gastroenterologists'. Cost-conscious administrators in capitated systems should be willing to pay for the single extra transducer and formal specific training for the surgeon, because surgeon-performed IOUS pays for itself in short order by obviating preoperative CT scanning (which, when positive, often leads to further evaluation by IOUS anyway) and the attendant specialist consultation.

Another tool for assessing the extent of colorectal cancer is radioimmuno-guided surgery (RIGS): Radiolabeled monoclonal antibodies recognize tumor antigens, and a probe detects the radioactivity intraoperatively. RIGS can certainly detect occult tumor deposits missed by CT scanning and intraoperative palpation (19,22–25) and has been reported to alter operative treatment in 25% of patients (26,27). This seems excessive given that curative and palliative resections for colon cancer are virtually identical both in technique and in complication rates. Like IOUS, RIGS is potentially most useful for detecting metastases, not for therapeutic excision but for postoperative adjuvant therapy. In one study, RIGS upstaged 26% of patients from stage I to II (no adjuvant treatment) to stage III to IV (postoperative chemotherapy) (27). Plagued by unacceptable false-positive rates and a lack of clear clinical utility, RIGS has been the "technique of the future" since 1984, and it currently has no clear role in clinical surgery.

THERAPEUTIC PRINCIPLES OF SURGERY

The primary goal of radical resection is, of course, total cure; but surgery also aims to decrease local recurrence and prolong disease-free and overall survival in those who are not cured. Therapeutic principles include en-bloc resection of the tumor with adequate margins, resection of draining lymph nodes for staging, and intraoperative assessment of the liver and peritoneal cavity for staging.

The skin incision may be vertical midline or transverse. Like the performance of an anastomosis (discussed below), the type of incision to use has been extensively debated, and it appears to best be left to the choice of the operating surgeon. Vertical midline incisions allow for a more rapid entrance into the abdominal cavity and subsequent closure but are more prone to herniation and tend to end at a level superior to that of the equivalent transverse incision, thus predisposing the patient to greater pain and pulmonary complications associated with upper abdominal incisions. Transverse incisions require more time for peritoneal access and final closure, make intraoperative liver ultrasound more technically challenging to perform, and are more frequently associated with rectus muscle hematomas (a rare surgical complication that can be fairly morbid); but they lead to fewer incisional hernias. We favor transverse incisions, except when the endoscopist's localization of the tumor is in question, as is almost always the case in transverse colon lesions. For such cases, and when takedown of both flexures may be required, we use a midline approach, the "incision of indecision."

A 5-cm margin of resection of unstretched, uninvolved colon has often been recommended because local extension is usually circumferential, and submucosal spread rarely exceeds 4 cm (28). However, what appears to be 5 cm in vivo may reduce to only 2 cm after resection (29), and it will shrink even further after immersion in formalin. In locally advanced cancers that are adherent to other organs (most commonly the small bowel and sigmoid colon), en-bloc resection is advantageous. Separation of adherent tumor from adjacent organs results in a high local recurrence rate. En-bloc resection of locally adherent T4N0 and T4N1 colon cancers carries the same 5-year survival as that of stage-matched, nonadherent tumors (30).

Lymph node involvement and the number of involved nodes are the strongest predictors of prognosis and frequently dictate adjuvant treatment of colon cancer. A standard lymph node dissection involves resection of the lymphatic channels that follow the named artery of the section of colon in which the tumor arises (ileocolic, right colic, middle colic, left colic, inferior mesenteric, or sigmoidal). The anatomic resection depends on the location of the tumor and the pattern of lymphatic drainage and vascular supply of that segment. More extensive lymphatic resection is unnecessary. However, limited resections that do not include these N3 level lymph nodes are inadequate.

For creation of the anastomosis after resection, in most cases the crux of the operation, there is long-standing debate between advocates of stapling and manual suturing. A recent meta-analysis of randomized, controlled trials addressed mortality, technical problems, leak rate, wound infection, stricture, and cancer recurrence and found that both types of anastomosis were nearly identical across the board, except that stapling yielded slightly higher rates of stricture and technical problems (31). The cost difference depends on the value of operating room time, a notoriously slippery factor: Stapled anastomoses are probably more rapid in most hands, saving operative time, whereas hand-sewn anastomoses use much less expensive materials. Thus the surgeon can still justify making whichever type of anastomosis he or she is comfortable with. More important is to use segments of proximal and distal bowel that still possess adequate vascular supplies after the cancer resection.

SURGICAL PROCEDURES

CANCER OF THE RIGHT COLON

Tumors arising from the cecum and ascending colon are resected by a right hemicolectomy. The ileocolic, right colic, and the right branch of the middle colic vessels are divided. Some authors recommend removing the last 10 cm of the terminal ileum, which does not seem necessary oncologically (the principle is to remove the cancer with adequate margins of the organ in which it arises, namely the colon) and involves the loss of a very valuable absorptive segment of small bowel. We recommend taking as little of the small bowel as possible. An ileum–proximal transverse colon anastomosis is created. Tumors arising from the hepatic flexure are resected by an extended right hemicolectomy, including ligation of the middle colic artery and an ileum–distal transverse colon anastomosis.

CANCER OF THE TRANSVERSE COLON

Transverse colon cancer usually requires an extended resection owing to the technical difficulty of bringing the right and left colon together for creation of an anastomosis. For proximal transverse lesions, an extended right hemicolectomy with resection of the splenic flexure and an ileum-descending colon anastomosis is recommended. For distal transverse lesions, the analogous extended left hemicolectomy makes sense. Some authors recommend removing the greater omentum routinely for any transverse colon cancer. This may not be oncologically required (the principle is to remove involved organs en bloc and to remove organs with a shared blood supply), and to do so loses a potentially valuable ally for healing and infection control, the omentum. Total abdominal colectomy may be considered for transverse lesions, to remove the lymphatic drainage basin completely and eliminate the risk of metachronous polyps or cancer, but there is no evidence suggesting a better prognosis for this. At the opposite extreme, segmental transverse colectomy is probably acceptable when there is a redundant transverse colon and the capability to create a tension-free anastomosis, as long as the dissection is carried down onto the middle colic artery and adequate mesentery is resected to include at least 10 lymph nodes.

CANCER OF THE LEFT COLON

Cancer arising from the splenic flexure can be treated with either a left hemicolectomy with ligation of the left colic artery and creation of a transverse-descending anastomosis or an extended right hemicolectomy and an ileo-descending colon anastomosis. A descending colon cancer mandates a left hemicolectomy, with ligation of the left colic or inferior mesenteric artery and resection of the splenic flexure. Whether the sigmoid colon needs to be resected is debatable. The transverse colon is anastomosed to either the sigmoid or upper rectum. Mobilization of the splenic flexure may be easy or technically challenging, and traction on the splenocolic ligament can result in splenic injury, usually in the form of a capsular tear. When this occurs, the injured spleen can be salvaged with topical hemostatic agents, direct pressure, argon-beam coagulation, omental buttressing, or even partial splenectomy. Such measures should, however, be tempered by the knowledge that the risk of postsplenectomy sepsis in a mature adult is extremely low, and blood transfusion has its own risks (detailed below). In some cases it may be better for the patient to accept the complication of splenectomy than to spend excessive time (and blood) trying to salvage a persistently oozing spleen.

Cancer of the Sigmoid Colon

Cancers arising in the sigmoid colon are treated with segmental sigmoid resection, because the arterial supply is from the sigmoidal arteries arising from the inferior mesenteric artery. If the proximal margin of resection is inadequate, however, a formal left hemicolectomy is indicated. What constitutes an adequate margin in colon cancer resection is not uniformly agreed on, and in segmental sigmoid resection one often harks back to the old 5-cm rule (28).

Two Primary Cancers

Synchronous colon cancers are found in 2 to 9% of patients, emphasizing the need for complete preoperative colonoscopy. Left-sided lesions have the highest rate of co-existing cancers. Although patients with synchronous cancers usually present at a more advanced stage than patients with solitary tumors, their 5-year survival is the same as the single-cancer group, with prognosis based on the stage of the more advanced tumor (32). Treatment for two cancers is either two radical resections, each as described above, or total abdominal colectomy. In cases in which the two lesions are widely separated, the two required major resections will leave the patient with only a minimal length of functional colon, and the risk of two anastomoses and the need for continued endoscopic surveillance are usually outweighed by the benefits of total colectomy. Not only does total colectomy adequately treat both cancers in these cases, but the procedure also decreases the risk of metachronous lesions and eliminates the need for colonoscopic surveillance, although routine simple rigid proctoscopy is still required. Furthermore, total abdominal colectomy is often technically easier and more rapidly performed than two sequential cancer resections, and it may confer less operative morbidity. Functional outcome is satisfactory in 84% (probably not significantly different from patients left with only a small length of colon), and most patients return to their original bowel habits by the 6th postoperative month (33). Finally, the appearance of synchronous cancers should be a warning to review the family history and colonoscopic findings, because one may in fact be dealing with an attenuated form of familial adenomatous polyposis (FAP) or hereditary nonpolyposis colorectal cancer (HNPCC; Lynch syndrome). In these cases, a total abdominal colectomy is clearly indicated (and perhaps also a proctectomy in attenuated FAP), with any debate focusing on whether or not to resect the rectum as well.

THE NO-TOUCH TECHNIQUE

Tumor cells can be found in the mesenteric venous blood of the resected segments in patients with colorectal cancer, suggesting that manipulation may scatter tumor cells (34). In 1952, Barnes (35) described a technique of right hemicolectomy in which he ligated the vascular pedicle *before* dividing and mobilizing the colon. Turnbull (36) then popularized the technique of no-touch isolation for colon cancer resection. This operative technique consists of ligating the lymphovascular pedicles first, then dividing the colon, and only then mobilizing the cancer-bearing segment, all the time minimizing tumor manipulation. Turnbull's reported 5-year survival was 50% compared to 34% using the conventional technique. Others have failed to reproduce this outcome differential, reporting local or regional recurrence and survival rates similar to those of conventional operative techniques (37,38). Although the no-touch technique has receded into surgical history, it emphasizes the fact that tumor manipulation *does* mobilize malignant cells into the circulation. This is one of the more common questions informed patients ask about colon cancer surgery. They (and we) should be optimistic that mechanisms of metastatic development are much more complex than simply sloughing malignant cells into the bloodstream; the vast majority of mobilized cells are likely unprepared seeds that fall onto barren soil, and so most likely do not form metastases.

Blood Transfusion and Cancer Surgery

In the early days of transplantation, it was discovered that pretransplantation blood transfusions resulted in increased allograft survival (39,40). This concept of transfusion-induced immunosuppression also applies to oncologic surgery. From a cellular standpoint, blood transfusions decrease the function of natural killer (NK) cells, which help control metastasis, and decrease the production of interleukin 2 (IL-2), which NK cells require (41). In clinical studies in cancer patients, blood transfusions are associated with increased incidence of metastasis and decreased survival rates (42,43). Interestingly, an increased incidence of wound infection in patients receiving perioperative blood transfusions has not been reported. Based on current information, blood transfusion should be treated like any other medication or intervention associated with major undesirable side-effects in that it should be administered only for specific indications and with significant respect for related risks to patient survival.

Concomitant Oophorectomy

Some authors have recommended bilateral oophorectomy in conjunction with colon cancer resection in perimenopausal or postmenopausal patients. The rationale is both to avoid future ovarian cancer and to eliminate the ovaries as potential sites of colon cancer metastasis. Colon cancer is one of the cancers that most frequently metastasizes to the ovaries (44), and some studies have found ovarian metastases in 3 to 11% of female colon cancer patients at the time of initial bowel operation (45–47). However, isolated ovarian metastases (in the absence of hepatic, peritoneal, or widespread metastasis) are extremely rare; therefore, oophorectomy performed primarily to eliminate this site of potential metastasis is not encouraged. The more logical reason for concomitant oophorectomy is to avoid primary ovarian cancer, which occurs in 1.5% of women > 40 years of age and is lethal in two-thirds of cases (48). The rationale of avoiding ovarian cancer specifically in colon cancer patients has not been subjected to formal, statistical scrutiny, but arguments against incidental removal of healthy organs have been uniformly successful in recent years, most notably in the discussion of incidental appendectomy during elective hysterectomy. Prophylactic oophorectomy should be discussed in this light with perimenopausal and postmenopausal women who harbor colon cancers. We recommend against gratuitous castration, unless the patient specifically requests it for sound medical reasons.

CANCER SURGERY AFTER POLYPECTOMY

Cancer within a polyp that is confined to the mucosa may be managed by endoscopic polypectomy. If the cancer extends into the true bowel wall, is poorly differentiated, has evidence of vascular or lymphatic invasion, or is incompletely excised endoscopically, then resection is indicated. Ideally, the previous polypectomy site should be tattooed as soon as possible via a follow-up colonoscopy. If the site is not tattooed, intraoperative colonoscopy may reveal the scar, and the site can then be marked from inside the abdomen. If the scar cannot be found, a measured resection is necessary.

OBSTRUCTING COLON CANCER

The reported incidence of obstruction in patients with colon cancer is 8 to 21%, although it is probably lower and decreasing annually as people become more medically savvy and cancer detection programs proliferate. Each obstructing cancer represents a double failure of health maintenance, both of the cancer screening program and of the patient's primary care program, because most lesions that obstruct are within reach of a flexible sigmoidoscope, and virtually all will have at least recently been symptomatic. More than half of obstructed patients are incurable on presentation owing to distant metastases (49,50). Attempted curative resection, however, still yields a 5-year survival rate of 23% (51).

Most patients will have undergone an abdominal x-ray and either a contrast study or endoscopy to prove obstruction. Preoperative care includes nasogastric decompression and correction of hypovolemia, electrolyte deficiencies, and anemia. Some obstructing colon cancers can be converted to partially obstructing lesions with bowel rest, nasogastric decompression, colonic stents and enemas; and a slow, gentle bowel preparation with polyethylene glycol is possible. Thus the goal of the brief preoperative period is to convert the impending operation into a one-stage procedure by allowing for a mechanical bowel preparation. Antibiotics to cover enteric gram-negative and anaerobic bacteria should be started on admission, because bacteria both proliferate in and translocate from the obstructed colon. If the bowel preparation is successful, the operation proceeds identically to the elective operations as previously described.

If there is complete obstruction, there are four options: partial colectomy with anastomosis (with or without on-table lavage), three-stage resection, two-stage resection, and total abdominal colectomy with ileorectal anastomosis. A right colon lesion can probably be resected with the safe performance of a primary anastomosis, because the bacterial count in the region is relatively low, the stool is liquid, and the size mismatch at the anastomosis is not so dramatic. The usual situation of a left-sided cancer presents a more difficult problem.

Historically, for an obstructing left colon lesion, a three-stage operation was performed, with initial proximal stomal decompression, delayed tumor resection, and finally anastomosis. Two-stage operations with immediate resection along with diversion (such as Hartmann's operation) gained favor when they were shown to have equal operative mortality and better 5-year survival rates than the three-stage approach. One-stage options include left colectomy with on-table lavage and primary anastomosis, left colectomy without lavage, and total abdominal colectomy with ilcorectal anastomosis. The rationale for on-table lavage is that the major reason that anastomotic leaks are more common when obstructed colon is used to create the anastomosis is the proximal stool load. When segmental colectomy with lavage was compared to subtotal colectomy without lavage, the anastomotic leak and death rates were equal (52). Working against the proximal fecal loading concept is the increasing evidence from the trauma literature that bowel preparation makes little difference in postoperative morbidity. The real test of on-table lavage, a randomized trial of segmental resection with and without lavage for obstructing sigmoid cancers, remains to be performed; and on-table lavage enjoys only limited popularity in the United States. Certainly the literature on on-table lavage has opened the question of one-stage operations for obstructing cancers; and in the future, surgeons may be more willing to select favorable patients for such one-stage procedures.

The main reason for the shift toward the apparently riskier one-stage operative approach is that it spares the patient a second procedure, itself a major, morbid operation by any measure. Attention has recently focused on the hidden morbidity of Hartmann's procedure: Not only is the second stage beset by complications, but at least 30% of "temporary" stomas for large bowel obstructions are never taken down (53).

POSTOPERATIVE CARE

Care after all colon operations is fairly standard, and it is amenable to further standardization through clinical pathways that have the potential to save resources and decrease morbidity. Clearly postoperative care must be individualized, but some guidelines are appropriate. Postoperative antibiotics should not be given. Recent studies confirm that routine use of nasogastric suction is unnecessary, and that early postoperative feeding is safe, does not prolong postoperative ileus, and has no higher rate of anastomotic leak or aspiration pneumonia (54,55). Thus after resection of nonobstructing colon cancers, routine nasogastric suction is unnecessary. The patient's diet is advanced by stages, usually starting with liquids on the 1st postoperative day and advancing to a regular diet as tolerated. Most of the length-of-stay decreases reported for laparoscopic colectomy appear to relate to these management changes rather than to the use of the laparoscopic technique itself. All surgeons owe a debt to the laparoscopic enthusiasts for identifying ways to make conventional surgical postoperative care more efficient and more comfortable for the patient.

The patient may be discharged when able to walk, take solid food, and have good pain control on an oral agent. This usually occurs between postoperative days 3 and 6. There is no need to wait for the first bowel movement, which may be a long time in coming because of the effects of ileus and narcotics on an already cleansed colon. There is also no need to hasten bowel movements through meddlesome measures such as laxatives or cathartics.

There may be disturbances in bowel function after colon resection, depending on the length and location of the segment removed. Diarrhea after colon resection may be the result of removal of the major absorptive surfaces, particularly the right and transverse colon, or of resection of the ileocecal valve. Without the ileocecal valve, there is reflux of colonic contents into the distal ileum, resulting in bacterial degradation of bile salts and consequent diarrhea. Antidiarrheal agents may be necessary in the short term, and fiber supplementation should continue over the long term. In one study, 87% of patients had satisfactory function, even after extensive colon resection (33).

ADJUVANT TREATMENT

Although this topic is fully addressed in chapter 9, suffice it to say that patients with stage III colon cancer are candidates for adjuvant chemotherapy. So probably are all stage II patients with T4 lesions and some with T3N0 lesions. Further risk stratification by genetic defects at sites such as K-*ras*, DCC, or p53 may add further detail to future recommendations for postoperative chemotherapy, but at present these are research tools only. Postoperative radiation therapy to the colon has not been as well defined as it has for rectal cancers. There is a subset of colon cancer patients that may benefit from local or regional radiation therapy in controlling local disease and improving survival compared to surgery alone. The patients who benefit are those at high risk for local failure, T4N0–2M0, or T4N0 with perforation or fistula, and those with residual disease (56,57).

PATIENT FOLLOW-UP

Follow-up for colon cancer patients is discussed fully in chapter 10 but is touched on here. There are two types of colon cancer follow-up: recurrence detection and polyp detection. Although most of the time and resources are spent on recurrence detection, it is reasonable to be skeptical, even somewhat nihilistic, about the true benefits of aggressive follow-up for recurrent disease in terms of patient survival and even quality of life. There is no place for nihilism in regard to polyp detection, however. The rate of metachronous cancers (second primary lesions) can and should be reduced to zero through colonoscopic surveillance and polypectomy, and the only question is how often the endoscopy should be performed. Thus we come full circle to the idea that each colon adenocarcinoma was once an adenomatous polyp that could have been detected and removed endoscopically, and the disease thereby eradicated.

REFERENCES

1. Landis SH, Murray T, Bolden S, Wingo PA. Cancer statistics, 1998. CA Cancer J Clin 1998;48:6–29.

2. August DA, Ottow RT, Sugarbaker PH. Clinical perspective of human colorectal cancer metastases. Cancer Metastasis Rev 1984;3:303–324.

3. Fabre JM, Rouanet P, Ele N, et al. Colorectal carcinoma in patients aged 75 years and more: factors influencing short and long-term operative mortality. Int Surg 1993;78:200–203.

4. Fitzgerald SD, Longo WE, Daniel GL, Vernava AM 3rd. Advanced colorectal neoplasia in the high-risk elderly patient: is surgical resection justified? Dis Colon Rectum 1993;36:161–166.

5. Hobler KE. Colon surgery for cancer in the very elderly. Cost and 3-year survival. Ann Surg 1986;203:129–131

6. Staab HJ, Anderer FA, Brümmendorf T. Prognostic value of preoperative serum CEA level compared to clinical staging. I. Colorectal carcinoma. Br J Cancer 1981;44:652–662.

7. Wanebo HJ, Rao B, Pinsky CM, et al. Preoperative carcinoembryonic antigen level as a prognostic indicator in colorectal cancer. N Engl J Med 1978;299:448–451.

8. Langevin JM, Nivatvongs S. The true incidence of synchronous cancer of the large bowel. A prospective study. Am J Surg 1984;147:330–333.

9. Wagner HE, Barbier PA, Luder PJ, Niederhäuser U. Prognosis in synchronous colorectal carcinomas. Z Gastroenterol 1988;26:117–120.

10. Shida H, Yamamoto T, Hiraiwa M, et al. Colorectal cancer and synchronous adenomatous or malignant polyps—factors influencing its incidence. Gan No Rinsho 1987;33:929–935.

11. Sause WT, Pajak TF, Noyes RD, et al. Evaluation of preoperative radiation therapy in operable cancer. Ann Surg 1994;220:668–675.

12. Willis AT, Ferguson IR, Phillips KD, et al. Metronidazole in prevention and treatment of bacteroides infections in elective colonic surgery. Br Med J 1977;1:607–610.

13. Norwegian Study Group for Colorectal Surgery. Should antimicrobial prophylaxis in colorectal surgery include agents effective against both anaerobic and aerobic microorganisms? A double-blind, multicenter study. Surgery 1985;97:402–408.

14. Beck DE, Fazio VW, Jagelman DG. Comparison of oral lavage methods for preoperative colonic cleansing. Dis Colon Rectum 1986;29:699–703.

15. Weaver M, Burdon DW, Youngs DJ, Keighley MR, et al. Oral neomycin and erythromycin compared with single-dose systemic metronidazole and ceftriaxone prophylaxis in elective colorectal surgery. Am J Surg 1986;151:437–442.

16. Lau WY, Chu KW, Poon GP, Ho KK. Prophylactic antibiotics in elective colorectal surgery. Br J Surg 1988;75:782–785.

17. Nichols RL, Broido P, Condon RE, et al. Effect of preoperative neomycin-erythromycin intestinal preparation on the incidence of infectious complications following colon surgery. Ann Surg 1973;178:453–462.

18. Solla JA, Rothenberger DA. Preoperative bowel preparation. A survey of colon and rectal surgeons. Dis Colon Rectum 1990;33:154–159.

19. Adachi Y, Mori M, Matsushima T, et al. The distribution of lymph node metastases in right-sided colon cancer. J Clin Gastroenterol 1994;19:210–213.

20. Machi J, Sigel B. Operative ultrasound in general surgery. Am J Surg 1996;172:15–20.

21. Kane RA, Hughes LA, Cua EJ, et al. The impact of intraoperative ultrasonography on surgery for liver neoplasms. J Ultrasound Med 1994;13:1–6.

22. Martin EW Jr, Mojzisik CM, Hinkle GH Jr, et al. Radioimmunoguided surgery using monoclonal antibody. Am J Surg 1988;156:386–392.

23. Nieroda CA, Mojzisik C, Sardi A, et al. The impact of radioimmuno-guided surgery (RIGS) on surgical decision-making in colorectal cancer. Dis Colon Rectum 1989;32:927–932.

24. Kuhn JA, Corbisiero RM, Buras RR, et al. Intraoperative gamma detection probe with presurgical antibody imaging in colon cancer. Arch Surg 1991;126:1398–1403.

25. Cohen AM, Martin EW Jr, Lavery I, et al. Radioimmunoguided surgery using iodine 125 B72.3 in patients with colorectal cancer. Arch Surg 1991;126:349–352.

26. Sickle-Santanello BJ, O'Dwyer PJ, Mojzisik C, et al. Radioimmunoguided surgery using the monoclonal antibody B72.3 in colorectal tumors. Dis Colon Rectum 1987;30:761–764.

27. Manayan RC, Hart MJ, Friend WG. Radioimmunoguided surgery for colorectal cancer. Am J Surg 1997;173:386–389.

28. Grinnell RS. Distal intramucosal spread of carcinoma of the rectum and rectosigmoid. Surg Gynecol Obstet 1954;99:421–430.

29. Weese JL, O'Grady MG, Ottery FD. How long is the five centimeter margin? Surg Gynecol Obstet 1986;163:101–103.

30. Hunter JA, Ryan JA Jr, Schultz P. En bloc resection of colon cancer adherent to other organs. Am J Surg 1987;154:67–71.

31. MacRae HM, McLeod RS. Handsewn vs. stapled anastomoses in colon and rectal surgery: a meta-analysis. Dis Colon Rectum 1998;41:180–189.

32. Passman MA, Pommier RF, Vetto JT. Synchronous colon primaries have the same prognosis as solitary colon cancers. Dis Colon Rectum 1996;39:329–334.

33. Walsh RM, Aranha GV, Freeark RJ. Mortality and quality of life after total abdominal colectomy. Arch Surg 1990;125:1564–1566.

34. Fisher ER, Turnbull RB Jr. The cytologic demonstration and significance of tumor cells in the mesenteric venous blood in patients with colorectal carcinoma. Surg Gynecol Obstet 1955;100:102–108.

35. Barnes JP. Physiologic resection of the right colon. Surg Gynecol Obstet 1952;94:722–726.

36. Turnbull RB Jr, Kyle K, Watson FR, Spratt J. Cancer of the colon: the influence of the no-touch isolation technic on survival rates. Arch Surg 1967;166:420–427.

37. Wiggers T, Jeekel J, Arends JW, et al. No-touch isolation technique in colon cancer: a controlled prospective trial. Br J Surg 1988;75:409–415.

38. Stearns MR Jr, Schottenfeld D. Techniques for the surgical management of colon cancer. Cancer 1971;28:165–169.

39. Halasz NA, Orloff MJ, Hirose F. Increased survival of renal homografts in dogs after injection of graft donor blood. Transplantation 1964;2:453–463.

40. Opelz G, Sengar DP, Mickey MR, Terasaki PI. Effect of blood transfusions on subsequent kidney transplants. Transplant Proc 1973;5:253–259.

41. Waymack JP, Fernandes G, Yurt RW, et al. Effect of blood transfusions on immune function. Part VI. Effect on immunologic response to tumor. Surgery 1990;108:172–177.

42. Burrows L, Tartter P. Effect of blood transfusions on colonic malignancy recurrence rate. Lancet 1982;2:662.

43. Voogt PJ, van de Velde CJ, Brand A, et al. Perioperative blood transfusion and cancer prognosis. Different effects of blood transfusion on prognosis of colon and breast cancer patients. Cancer 1987;59:836–843.

44. Webb MJ, Decker DG, Mussey E. Cancer metastatic to the ovary: factors influencing survival. Obstet Gynecol 1975;45:391–396.

45. MacKeigan JM, Ferguson JA. Prophylactic oophorectomy and colorectal cancer in premenopausal patients. Dis Colon Rectum 1979;22:401–405.

46. Blamey S, McDermott FT, Pihl E, et al. Ovarian involvement in adenocarcinoma of the colon and rectum. Surg Gynecol Obstet 1981;153:42–44.

47. Graffner HO, Alm PO, Oscarson JE. Prophylactic oophorectomy in colorectal carcinoma. Am J Surg 1983;146:233–235.

48. Yancik R. Ovarian cancer. Age contrasts in incidence, histology, disease stage at diagnosis, and mortality. Cancer 1993;71:517–523.

49. Welch JP, Donaldson GA. Management of severe obstruction of the large bowel due to malignant disease. Am J Surg 1974 127:492–499.

50. Kelley WE Jr, Brown PW, Lawrence W Jr, Terz JJ. Penetrating, obstructing, and perforating carcinomas of the colon and rectum. Arch Surg 1981;116:381–384.

51. Kasperk R, Braun J, Schumpelick V. Obstructive colorectal carcinoma. Principles and technique in 134 cases. Zentralbl Chir 1992;117:67–71.

52. Phillips RK, Hittinger R, Fry JS, Fielding LP. Malignant large bowel obstruction. Br J Surg 1985;72:296–302.

53. Isbister WH, Prasad J: The management of left-sided large bowel obstruction: an audit. Aust NZ J Surg 1996;66:602–604.

54. Petrelli NJ, Stulc JP, Rodriguez-Bigas M, Blumenson L. Nasogastric decompression following elective colorectal surgery: a prospective randomized study. Am Surg 1993;50:632–635.

55. Reissman P, Teoh TA, Cohen SM, et al. Is early oral feeding safe after elective colorectal surgery? A prospective randomized trial. Ann Surg 1995;222:73–77.

56. Willett CG, Fung CY, Kaufman DS, et al. Postoperative radiation therapy for high-risk colon carcinoma. J Clin Oncol 1993;11:1112–1117.

57. Duttenhaver JR, Hoskins RB, Gunderson LL, Tepper JE. Adjuvant post-operative radiation therapy in the management of adenocarcinoma of the colon. Cancer 1986;57:955–963.

CHAPTER

9

Adjuvant Therapy for Colon Cancer: Management and Current Concepts

May C. Chen, M.D., and James M. Ford, M.D.

Colorectal cancer ranks third in overall incidence of cancers in the United States population and remains the second leading cause of cancer-related deaths (1). Successful prevention and treatment depends on the detection of colonic polyps and tumors at early stages. Surgery remains the primary treatment and the only successful means of cure for early disease. The role of adjuvant radiotherapy is limited to attempted local control of disease when the risk of local failure is considered to be high (> 10%), as in many rectal cancer patients, but is not clearly defined for colon cancers (2). This chapter focuses primarily on the role of adjuvant chemotherapy for colorectal cancer for surgically resectable disease. The treatment of recurrent and metastatic colorectal cancer is discussed in separate chapters.

Colon and Rectal Cancer, Edited by Peter S. Edelstein, M.D.
ISBN 0-471-35145-8

PROGNOSTIC FACTORS

Substantial progress has been made in recent years in the treatment of colorectal cancer. Improvements in the radiographic detection of tumors, a better understanding of the molecular biology of colon lesions, and recent advances in drug development have affected survival. Numerous studies have documented the importance of prognostic markers in predicting overall survival or recurrence (3). Predictors of poor outcome include location of primary tumors (right-sided tumors have a slightly better prognosis than rectal tumors) (3–5); elevated preoperative carcinoembryonic antigen (CEA) (6–9); age > 50 years (3); high histologic grade (poorly differentiated) (10,11); the presence of signet ring histopathology (12); initial presentation with an obstructive or perforating tumor (13); DNA aneuploidy (14–16); allelic loss of chromosome 18q (17–19); increased S-phase fraction (20,21); and the presence of certain genetic alterations, most notably mutations in the *p53* tumor-suppressor gene (22–26) and loss of the deleted in colon cancer (DCC) gene (27).

Tumor staging has been shown to be the most important predictor of survival (Table 9.1) (3,28,29). The original Dukes' classification system developed in 1932 used depth of tumor penetration into bowel wall and nodal involvement to predict survival (30). The Aster-Coller system was developed in an attempt to subdivide patients with nodal metastases into two groups based on tumor penetration into (C1) or beyond (C2) the muscularis propria. A 5-year survival difference of 42.8 versus 22.4%, respectively, was found between these two groups (31). More recently, the TNM system, developed by the Union Internationale Contre le Cancer (UICC), and subsequently adopted by the American Joint Committee on Cancer (AJCC), uses characteristics of the tumor (T) and nodal status (N) to determine stages I to IV and prognosis (Table 9.1) (28). Using this staging system, current best estimates for 5-year survival for stage I colorectal tumors range from 85 to 100%. Stage II

TABLE 9.1. COLORECTAL CANCER STAGING AND SURVIVAL

TNM Staging	
Tx	Primary tumor not assessable
Tis	Carcinoma in situ
T1	Tumor invades into submucosa
T2	Tumor invades into but not through muscularis propria
T3	Tumor invades through the muscularis propria into the subserosa or into nonperitoneal pericolic or perirectal tissues
T4	Tumor perforates the visceral peritoneum or directly invades other organs or structures
Nx	Lymph node status not assessable
N0	No nodal metastases
N1	One to three pericolic or perirectal nodes involved
N2	Four or more pericolic or perirectal nodes involved
N3	Involvement of any regional node along a named vascular trunk
Mx	Metastatic status not assessable
M0	No distant metastases
M1	Distant metastases found

TNM Stage		Modified Aster-Coller	5 year survival, %
I	T1N0M0	A	> 80
	T2N0M0	B1	> 80
II	T3N0M0	B2	75
	T4N0M0	B3	75
III	T1–2N1–3M0	C1	50–75
	T3N1–3M0	C2	30–50
	T4N1–3M0	C3	30–50
IV	any T any N M1	D	< 5

patients (no nodal involvement) have an estimated 5-year survival of 62 to 70%, but survival decreases to 60% in stage III patients with N1 disease (one to three involved pericolic lymph nodes) and drops to 30% with N2 (four or more involved pericolic nodes) or N3 (involved nodes along a major named vessel) disease. The 5-year survival for stage IV (metastatic) disease is dismal at $< 5\%$.

ADJUVANT THERAPY

A major goal in the management of colorectal cancer has been to identify therapies, in addition to surgical resection, that might improve the chances for long-term survival in high-risk patients (adjuvant treatment). It is now recognized that certain groups of patients clearly benefit from the use of postoperative adjuvant systemic chemotherapy. Most patients with stage I colorectal cancer are cured by surgical resection alone. Presently the standard of care for patients with stage II (T3–4N0) lesions is surgical resection alone, although a proportion will ultimately relapse; therefore, the presence of poor prognostic markers often influences the decision to offer adjuvant therapy. Thus stage II patients with poor prognostic factors (histopathology, genetic, etc.) are frequently offered adjuvant chemotherapy. In particular, stage II patients with T4 lesions (direct invasion by tumor into an adjacent organ) have been shown to have 5-year survival rates only slightly better than or similar to N1 stage III patients (32). This has led some investigators to evaluate other features of stage II patients that may predict a poorer outcome, suggesting a rational argument for the administration of adjuvant chemotherapy for those at greater risk of relapse. Changes in gene expression, such as overexpression of mutant *p53*, have been shown to predict poorer outcome (6,22–26). In addition, patients whose tumors demonstrate chromosomal deletions 17q (including the *p53* gene locus) or 18q (including the DCC gene locus) are more likely to develop metastasis (27,33–37). One current intergroup study by the Cancer and Leukemia Group B (CALGB) and the Eastern Cooperative Oncology Group (ECOG) is analyzing the predictive value of the 18q deletion and DNA ploidy status as a measure of risk of recurrence in patients with Dukes' B2 colorectal cancers (CALGB 9581). Recently, Liefers et al. (38) in the Netherlands used polymerase chain reaction (PCR) based molecular diagnostic techniques to demonstrate that the presence of microscopic metastases in patients with histologically negative lymph nodes after resection predicted a poorer outcome. The 5-year observed survival rate for the patients harboring micrometastases was 36% compared to 75% for patients without micrometastases (P = .03). This again suggests that a subpopulation of patients with stage II disease and micrometastases within lymph nodes may benefit from systemic adjuvant therapy.

Presently, standard treatment for patients with stage III (N1–3) colorectal cancer after surgical resection is adjuvant systemic chemotherapy; 6 months of 5-fluorouracil/leucovorin is considered the standard of care after surgery. Data to support these findings come from several randomized trials that demonstrate statistically significant improvement in both overall survival and disease-free survival in selected stage III patients treated postoperatively with adjuvant systemic chemotherapy (39–43).

5-FLUOROURACIL

For more than 30 years, 5-fluorouracil (5-FU) has been considered the most active single agent available for the treatment of colorectal cancer. 5-FU is a metabolite that interferes with the function of thymidylate synthase, a key enzyme involved in DNA synthesis. 5-FU is enzymatically converted to 5-fluoro-2′-deoxyuridine (floxuridine, FudR) and subsequently to 5-fluoro-2′-deoxyuridine monophosphate (FdUMP). FdUMP is the active metabolite that, in the presence of the reduced folate cofactor 5,10-methylenetetrahydrofolate, forms a stable complex with thymidylate synthase, leading to the inhibition of DNA synthesis and repair (44). Clinical response rates of 15 to 20% have generally been reported for the use of 5-FU as a single agent in advanced colorectal cancer (45,46). The first trials of adjuvant systemic chemotherapy for resected colorectal cancer were initiated in the 1950s and involved various combinations of agents such as nitrogen mustard, thiotepa, and 5-FU (47,48). The activity of 5-FU as a single agent for adjuvant treatment has been extensively studied in randomized controlled trials, dating to the early 1970s, and compared surgery alone to surgery plus 5-FU; no overall statistically significant survival advantage was shown with adjuvant 5-FU (49–55) (Table 9.2). However, a meta-analysis of all trials using adjuvant 5-FU, involving 25 randomized trials and nearly 10,000 patients, did demonstrate a marginal benefit in overall survival in those receiving adjuvant chemotherapy (56). The studies included in the analysis used heterogeneous patient populations with differing drug administration schedules and suboptimal dosing (by today's standards). Buyse et al. (56) concluded that future trials should use a larger sample population to detect small differences in patient subpopulations.

TABLE 9.2. ADJUVANT SINGLE AGENT 5-FU CHEMOTHERAPY: EARLY RANDOMIZED, CONTROLLED TRIALS[a]

Trial	Patients, *n*	Drug	Duration	Survival Advantage[b]	Reference
VASAG	548	FUDR	7 weeks	No	49
VASAG	308	5-FU	6 weeks	No	51
VASAG	522	5-FU	18 months	No	52
Grossi et al.	487	5-FU	2 days	No	50
Lawrence et al.	156	5-FU	10 months	No	54
COG	233	5-FU	12 months	No	55

[a] Adapted from Ref. 46
[b] Statistically significant survival advantage in treatment versus control group.
VASAG, Veterans Administration Surgical Adjuvant Group; *COG*, Central Oncology Group.

The use of 5-FU in combination with other chemotherapeutic agents in the adjuvant setting has also been extensively studied and includes a series of trials beginning in 1975 involving Dukes' stage B2 or C colon cancer patients treated with 5-FU in various combinations with semustine, bacillus Calmette-Guerin (BCG), or methanol extraction residue (57–62) (Table 9.3). No survival advantage was

TABLE 9.3. ADJUVANT 5-FU/SEMUSTINE COMBINATION CHEMOTHERAPY: EARLY RANDOMIZED, CONTROLLED TRIALS[a]

Trial	Patients, *n*	Treatment Regimen	Survival Advantage[b]	Reference
VASOG	645	Observation vs.		57
		5-FU/semustine	No	
GITSG	572	Observation vs.		61
		MER of BCG		
		5-FU/semustine vs.		
		5-FU/semustine/ MER of BCG	No	
SWOG	279	Observation vs.		59
		5-FU/semustine		
		5-FU/semustine/BCG	No	
Cross Cancer Center	253	Observation		58
		BCG		
		5-FU/semustine/BCG	No	
ECOG	162	5-FU vs. 5-FU/semustine	No	62
NSABP	1116	Observation vs.		60
		BCG	[c]	
		MOF	No	

[a] Adapted from Ref. 46.
[b] Statistically significant survival advantage for treatment versus control group (or versus 5-FU for ECOG study).
[c] Fewer noncancer-related deaths in BCG arms; no survival advantage when noncancer deaths were excluded.
VASOG, Veterans Administration Surgical Oncology Group; *GITSG*, Gastrointestinal Tumor Study Group; *SWOG*, Southwest Oncology Group; *NSABP*, National Surgical Adjuvant Breast and Bowel Program; *MER*, methanol extraction residue; *MOF*, semustine (methyl-CCNU), vincristine, and 5-FU.

observed among patients treated with any of these combinations. Subsequent review of patients treated with combinations including semustine demonstrated a disproportionate number of secondary leukemias, leading to the discontinuation of the drug's use (63).

Subsequently, attempts have been made to modulate the activity of 5-FU to improve patient survival. The use of agents (e.g., leucovorin, methotrexate, allopurinol, hydroxyurea, and recombinant interferon α) to biochemically modulate 5-FU activity has improved objective response rates and, in some cases, overall survival. In particular, the use of levamisole, an antihelminthic agent that is known to enhance delayed hypersensitivity reactions in immunosuppressed patients has been shown to potentiate the effect of 5-FU. The exact mechanism of levamisole's effect on 5-FU is not known but has been attributed to levamisole's ability to act as an immunomodulator (64). As a single agent, however, levamisole has not been shown to affect disease-free or overall survival (65). The side effects of levamisole include myalgias, arthralgias, and taste abnormalities. The primary toxicities of the combination of 5-FU and levamisole include those seen with 5-FU alone: nausea, vomiting, diarrhea, stomatitis, dermatitis, and leukopenia. Hepatic toxicity, which is not seen with either agent alone, is a side effect of the drug combination (66). A potentially more troubling but rare reported side effect involves sporadic cases of multifocal inflammatory leukoencephalopathy with the 5-FU/levamisole combination (67). Patients present with symptoms of ataxia and progressive decline in mental status. Fortunately, these symptoms have been shown to be reversible with discontinuation of chemotherapy and a short course of steroid therapy (67).

The possible benefit of levamisole in combination with other chemotherapeutic agents was initially suggested by animal models, which showed a benefit in survival (64). The results of several studies in human patients with advanced colorectal cancer have been inconclusive, although one widely quoted study did show a statistically significant benefit in overall survival (64,68). The results of a trial initiated in 1974 by Verhaegen et al. (69) in which patients with resected Dukes' A, B, or C colorectal cancer plus adjuvant chemotherapy including levamisole were compared to control patients with resection alone showed an improved 5-year survival in the adjuvant group, particularly in patients with stage B2 or C cancers. Although several follow-up studies failed to redemonstrate this advantage, subsequent studies conducted at the Mayo Clinic and elsewhere have shown an increase in disease-free survival when levamisole has been part of an adjuvant approach, particularly among patients with nodal involvement (65,70–72) (Table 9.4). This led to more definitive studies in the 1980s aimed at precisely answering the question, "Which adjuvant therapy confers any survival benefit and to which patients?"

Two subsequent studies, the North Central Cancer Treatment Group (NCCTG) and Mayo Clinic, which enrolled 401 patients, and the Intergroup Trial, which enrolled 1296 (929 evaluable) patients, were aimed at patients with Dukes' stage B2 or C colorectal cancer (72,73) (Table 9.5). NCCTG randomized patients after surgical resection to observation, levamisole alone, or 5-FU/levamisole. In a subset of patients with Dukes' C disease, treatment with 5-FU/levamisole resulted in a statistically significant advantage in 5-year disease-free survival and borderline statistical improvement in overall survival. The Intergroup Trial randomized patients with Dukes' C colorectal cancer who had undergone resection to observation, levamisole alone, or 5-FU/levamisole and grouped patients with resected Dukes' B2 disease to 5-FU/levamisole or observation alone. With an initial median follow-up of 36 months, both disease-free and overall survival were enhanced by the combination 5-FU/levamisole regimen in patients with Dukes' C disease; this benefit was not observed in the Dukes' B2 patient group. Among Dukes' C patients, a reduction of 41% in the relative rate of recurrence and a reduction of 33% in the relative risk of death were observed in the combination group compared to the observation alone group. No statistically significant advantage in overall

TABLE 9.4. ADJUVANT CHEMOTHERAPY FOR STAGE B2 AND C COLORECTAL CANCER: RANDOMIZED CONTROLLED TRIALS COMPARING 5-FU/LEVAMISOLE WITH OBSERVATION ALONE[a]

Trials/Group	Patients, *n*	Treatment Regimens	Disease-free Survival Advantage	Overall Survival Advantage[b]	Reference
Verhaegen et al.	60	Observation vs.			69
		Levamisole	Not reported	Yes[c]	
Western Cancer Study Group	78	Placebo vs.			70
		Levamisole	Not reported	No	
EORTC	287	Placebo vs.			
		Levamisole	No	No	65
Windle et al.	141	Observation vs.			71
		5-FU (PO)	Not reported	No	
		5-FU (PO)/levamisole	Not reported	Yes	
NCCTG	408	Observation vs.			72
		Levamisole	Yes	No	
		5-FU/levamisole	Yes	No	

[a] Adapted from Ref. 46.
[b] Statistically significant survival for treatment versus control group.
[c] Trial not randomized.
EORTC, European Organization for Research and Treatment of Cancer; *NCCTG*, North Central Cancer Treatment Group.

TABLE 9.5. ADJUVANT CHEMOTHERAPY IN NODE-POSITIVE COLORECTAL CANCER: RANDOMIZED CONTROLLED TRIALS

Trial	Patients, *n*	Treatment Regimen	5-year Disease-free Survival	5-year Overall Survival	Reference
NCCTG	262	Observation vs.	38%	45%	72
		Levamisole	50%[a]	50%[a]	
		5-FU/levamisole	50%[a]	54%[a]	
Intergroup	929	Observation vs.	45%	54%	43
		Levamisole	45%[a]	54%[a]	
		5-FU/levamisole	63%	65%	

[a] Statistically significant survival advantage in treatment versus control group.

TABLE 9.6. ADJUVANT CHEMOTHERAPY IN NODE-NEGATIVE COLORECTAL CANCER: 7-YEAR RESULTS FROM THE INTERGROUP STUDY[a]

Patients, *n*	Treatment Regimen[b]	7-year Disease-Free Survival	7-Year Overall Survival
159	Observation	71%	72%
159	5-FU/levamisole	79%[c]	72%[d]

[a] Intergroup study 0035 (75).
[b] Both groups of patients had undergone surgery.
[c] P = .10.
[d] Not statistically significant.

survival was noted for patients treated with levamisole alone (73). These results were subsequently upheld when extended to a 7-year follow-up analysis (43). This led to subsequent National Cancer Institute (NCI) guidelines in 1989 adopting adjuvant systemic therapy with 5-FU/levamisole administered for 1 year as standard therapy for Dukes' stage C colorectal cancer (74).

Studies of patients with stage II (Dukes' B2, node-negative) colorectal cancer involving adjuvant 5-FU/levamisole have not shown a survival advantage for the combination chemotherapy. With a 7-year median follow-up, results of the Intergroup INT-0035 study conducted on 318 patients with resected stage II colorectal cancer showed a decrease in recurrence of 31%, which did not approach statistical significance in terms of overall survival (75) (Table 9.6). However, there may be as yet unidentified subsets of stage II patients who would indeed benefit from such adjuvant treatment, based on previously mentioned prognostic factors.

The next generation of trials for adjuvant treatment of colorectal cancer has used biochemical modulators such a leucovorin to enhance the cytotoxic effects of 5-FU. Initial evidence for the effect of leucovorin was suggested in laboratory studies that showed enhanced biologic activity when 5-FU was used in combination with reduced folates (76–79). Leucovorin may enhance 5-FU activity by increasing the intracellular store of 5,10-methylenetetrahydrofolate, thus increasing the duration of thymidylate synthase activity (76,80). This has been supported by clinical studies that demonstrate increased antitumor activity of 5-FU with leucovorin in patients with advanced colorectal cancer, though this improvement in response did not result in improved survival in patients with metastatic disease (81). Subsequent trials to assess the efficacy of the combination 5-FU/leucovorin compared to the standard 5-FU/levamisole treatment have been conducted in patients with high-risk stage II and III colorectal cancer.

Results from the IMPACT International Multicenter Pooled Analysis of Colon Cancer Trials study published in 1995 showed that patients with resected Dukes' B or C colorectal cancer had improved survival when treated with 6 months of adjuvant 5-FU and high-dose leucovorin, suggesting that 5-FU/leucovorin may be comparable to 5-FU/levamisole (82). The IMPACT study included three independently randomized trials and showed that 5-FU/leucovorin improved both 3-year event-free survival (62 to 71%) and overall survival (78 to 83%). The tolerability and efficacy of the 6-month 5-FU/leucovorin regimen led to subsequent studies comparing 5-FU/leucovorin with 5-FU/levamisole.

The Intergroup Trial INT-0089 accrued 3759 patients with high-risk stage II or III colorectal cancer and randomized them to one of four treatment arms (five planned treatment comparisons; Table 9.7), either 7 to 8 months of 5-FU plus high-dose leucovorin at 500 mg/m^2 daily, 7 to 8 months of 5-FU plus low-dose leucovorin at 20 mg/m^2 daily, 7 to 8 months of 5-FU plus low-dose leucovorin with levamisole (standard levamisole regimen combined with 5-FU/low-dose leucovorin), or the standard 12 months of 5-FU plus levamisole (83,86). With a median follow-up of 5 years and all planned treatment comparisons mature, the only significant treatment benefit noted was that of overall survival in the subset of stage III patients favoring 5-FU/low-dose leucovorin/levamisole over 5-FU/levamisole (overall survival 63% versus 60% among stage III patients; $P = .0054$). In addition, no statistically significant survival

TABLE 9.7. Adjuvant Trials of 5-FU with Biochemical Modulators: Randomized Controlled Trials in Stage II and III Colorectal Cancers

Trial	Patients, *n*	Treatment regimens	Disease-Free Survival, % (Significance/Advantage)	Overall Survival, % (Significance/Advantage)	Reference
INT-0089	3759	5-FU/LDLV vs.	60[a] (P = .68)	66[a] (P = .56)	83
		5-FU/HDLV	59 (No)	65 (No)	
		5-FU/LDLV vs.	59 (P = .16)	66 (P = .09)	
		5-FU/LEV	56 (No)	63 (No)	
		5-FU/HDLV vs.	60 (P = .18)	65 (P = .20)	
		5-FU/LEV	56 (No)	63 (No)	
		5-FU/LDLV vs.	59 (P = .24)	66 (P = .24)	
		5-FU/LDLV/LEV	60 (No)	67 (No)	
		5-FU/LEV vs.	56 (P = .014)	63 (P = .0074)	
		5-FU/LDLV/LEV	60 (Yes)	67 (Yes)	
NSABP C-04	2151	5-FU/LEV	60	69	84
		5-FU/HDLV vs.	64 (P = .12)	74 (P = .14)	
		5-FU/HDLV/LEV	64 (No)	72 (No)	
NSABP C-05	2129	5-FU/HDLV vs.	69[b] (P = .35)	80[b] (P = .41)	85
		5-FU/HDLV/IFN-α	70 (No)	81 (No)	

[a] Reflects 5-year disease-free and overall survival data.
[b] Reflects 4-year disease-free and overall survival data.
LDLV, low-dose leucovorin; *HDLV*, high-dose leucovorin; *LEV*, levamisole; $IFN - \alpha$, interferon α.

advantage was observed in any of the treatment comparisons for stage II patients, which represented approximately 20% of the study population (83). The results of INT-0089 established the comparable efficacy of 6 months of 5-FU/leucovorin with 12 months of 5-FU/levamisole. Similarly, the NSABP C-04 study randomized patients with resected stage II or III colorectal cancer to 5-FU/levamisole, or 5-FU/high-dose leucovorin versus 5-FU/high dose leucovorin plus levamisole and found no statistically significant difference in overall survival (Table 9.7) (84). Based on these two large randomized studies, most experts now recommend 6 months of therapy with 5-FU plus low-dose leucovorin as the standard adjuvant treatment for patients with resected stage III (Dukes C) colorectal cancer.

5-FU ADMINISTRATION Subsequent studies have been aimed at improving on the results of adjuvant therapy using knowledge of drug pharmacokinetics and various dosing schedules in the treatment of colon cancer. The use of continuous-infusional 5-FU therapy has been evaluated as an alternative to bolus treatment, primarily among patients with advanced colorectal cancer (87,88). 5-FU given by continuous infusion has theoretical advantages over bolus 5-FU in that a greater dose intensity of the drug can be delivered via continuous infusion without the degree of myelosuppression commonly seen with bolus treatments (88–90). In addition, it has been suggested that bolus administration inhibits RNA synthesis, whereas continuous infusion selectively targets thymidylate synthase (91). The Intergroup INT-0153 study initiated March 1995 was a phase III randomized trial aimed at addressing the effectiveness of bolus 5 FU/leucovorin/levomisole versus continuous infusional 5 FU/levamisole as adjuvant therapy for patients with stage B2, C1, or C2 colorectal cancer. At its first interim analysis in August 1999, at which time 1078 patients had been accrued, no statistically significant difference was observed in the two arms. Moreover, while a greater number of patients in the bolus arm experienced grade 4 toxicity, twice as many patients in the continuous infusion arm discontinued therapy early. The study committee recommended early closure of the study. The final recommendations to practicing oncologists are that either bolus or infusional 5 FU can be utilized depending on physician and patient preference (91a). The Intergroup INT-0136 study is currently accruing patients to study the role of perioperative 7-day infusional 5-FU followed by 5-FU/levamisole beginning in the 4th postoperative week versus 5-FU/levamisole without infusion in the 4th postoperative week. Although results have yet to be reported, such studies suggest other intriguing possibilities for the management of resectable colorectal cancer.

The next generation of trials will continue to optimize duration of adjuvant therapy while incorporating newer agents such as CDT-II, oxolipatin, and oral-fluoropyrimidines.

High-Risk Stage II (Node-Negative) Colorectal Cancer

Presently the standard of care for patients with stage II (T3–4N0) lesions is surgical resection alone. Although a majority of patients will be cured with resection, a significant minority will ultimately relapse, suggesting the need to identify patients who may benefit from adjuvant therapy. Current guidelines for adjuvant therapy of high-risk stage II colorectal cancer are not well established. Results from the INT-0035 study, a 7-year median follow-up study of 318 patients with resected stage II colorectal cancer, demonstrated a decrease in recurrence of 31% in patients treated with adjuvant 5-FU/levamisole compared to observation alone. Although suggestive, these results did not reach statistical significance and did not demonstrate an overall survival advantage (75). Several tumor features have been identified as prognostic markers for poor patient outcome or metastatic recurrence. These include growth rate markers such as DNA ploidy and proliferation, genetic markers such as *p53* mutations and DCC (18q) deletions, elevation of serum

CEA, CA19-9, and lipid-associated sialic acid (LASA), and *ras* oncogene overexpression (6). Use of such markers may aid in the decision to offer adjuvant therapy for high-risk stage II colon cancer patients. The American Society of Clinical Oncology has recently published guidelines on the use of tumor markers in patients with colon cancer (Table 9.8) (6).

Patients who present with obstructing or perforating node-negative colorectal cancers are known to have survival rates comparable to nonobstructed and nonperforated patients with node-positive disease. Data from several randomized trials of 5-FU/levamisole comparing the subset of stage II patients with perforating tumors suggests a significantly decreased 5-year disease-free and overall survival. Five-year relapse-free survival in stage II patients with perforated tumors was 43% in the intergroup trial INT-0035, comparable to that of patients with nodal involvement (75). As such, stage II patients with perforating or obstructing tumors are considered high risk, and it is now widely accepted that such patients should receive adjuvant therapy with 6 months of 5-FU/leucovorin.

ADJUVANT THERAPY IN THE ELDERLY PATIENT POPULATION

As for all decisions regarding chemotherapy, the benefits of treatment should be weighed against the potential toxicities, particularly among elderly patients who may have difficulty completing a full course of chemotherapy. One recent population-based study of elderly patients receiving adjuvant chemotherapy reported a drop-out rate of > 50% among patients > 70 years who were scheduled for 1 year of treatment with adjuvant 5-FU/levamisole (92). However, a recent intention-to-treat meta-analysis of 3351 patients (aged > 50, 50–60, 60–70, > 70) from 7 trials showed significant positive effect of overall survival and disease-free survival. The

TABLE 9.8. SUMMARY OF CLINICAL PRACTICE GUIDELINES FOR THE USE OF TUMOR MARKERS IN COLORECTAL CANCER[a]

Carcinoembryonic Antigen

Role in screening: not recommended

Role in initial staging: may be ordered preoperatively in patients to assist in staging and surgical treatment planning, because elevated preoperative CEA (> 5 mg/mL) may correlate with poorer prognosis; insufficient data to support the use of CEA to determine treatment of patients with adjuvant therapy

Role in surveillance: if resection of identified liver metastases would be tolerated, postoperative serum CEA testing may be performed every 2–3 months in patients with stage II or II disease for ≥ 2 years after diagnosis; further evaluation of metastatic disease is warranted for elevated CEA but does not justify the use of adjuvant therapy for presumed metastatic disease

Role in monitoring treatment: insufficient data to recommend routine use of CEA alone; if no other simple test (such as CT scan) is available, CEA should be measured at the start of treatment for metastatic disease and then every 2–3 months during active treatment; two values above baseline are adequate to document progressive disease even in absence of supporting radiographs

LASA, CA19-9, *p53* expression or mutation, and *Ras* oncogene

Role in screening: not recommended

Role in diagnosis: not recommended

Role in staging: not recommended

Role in surveillance: not recommended

Role in monitoring treatment: not recommended

DNA Ploidy, DNA Proliferation (%S phase and related indices)

Insufficient data to recommend routine use in management of colorectal cancers

[a] Adopted from Ref. 6.

study concluded that elderly patients benefit from 5-FU based adjuvant therapy without significant increase in toxicity (92a).

IMMUNOMODULATION

An immunomodulatory role for interferon (IFN) has been suggested in tumor models showing synergy between 5-FU and IFN (93,94). In particular, IFN-α and IFN-β, which belong to the type I interferons, have been shown to biochemically enhance the activity of 5-FU in vitro by increasing the intracellular levels of FdUMP and increasing binding to the target enzyme thymidylate synthase (94–96). IFN-β has 30% amino acid homology to IFN-α and a higher receptor binding specificity (97,98). Although previous phase II studies of 5-FU and IFN-α have reported increased response rates compared to 5-FU alone (99–103), more recent phase III studies of 5-FU and IFN-α have not shown survival benefit in advanced colorectal cancer (104,105). Based on the results of the NSABP C-04 study and on the observation that IFN-α2a when combined with 5-FU/leucovorin (5-FU/LV) shows some improved objective response in patients with advanced colorectal cancer, additional studies have been undertaken in patients with resectable colorectal cancer to evaluate the benefits of interferon as a modulator of adjuvant 5-FU/LV. NSABP C-05 enrolled 2129 stage II and III patients into two treatment arms: 5-FU/LV versus 5-FU/LV plus IFN-α2a. At a median follow-up of approximately 54 months, initial results indicate no significant difference in disease-free or overall survival (85). Patients receiving 5-FU/LV with IFN experience a higher incidence of grade 4 and 5 toxicities, resulting in higher rates of discontinuation of therapy. Clinical trials using 5-FU with IFN-β in advanced colorectal cancer are currently under way (106,107). IFN-γ, the third class of interferons, has shown no benefit in phase II studies of advanced colorectal cancer (108).

ACTIVE-SPECIFIC IMMUNOTHERAPY

While the results of IFN-α2a have been less than encouraging, much interest has been generated in recent years in the area of immunotherapy. The concept of active-specific immunotherapy (ASI) originated in the 1960s when animal models stimulated with killed tumor cells demonstrated delayed tumor growth, suggesting that proteins expressed by tumor cells might elicit a host immune response that could destroy tumors but spare the host (109). One of the first ASI studies of adjuvant immunotherapy in colorectal cancer involved the use of BCG. In the NSABP C-01 study, patients with resected Dukes' B2 or C colorectal cancer were randomized to receive either observation alone or chemotherapy with semustine, vincristine, and 5-FU (MOF) or intradermal BCG (110). Although a slight benefit was noted in patients receiving BCG over surgery alone, there was no overall statistical significance in survival. The authors concluded that BCG's further study was no longer warranted given the lack of this agent's benefit in preventing recurrence.

Subsequently, more specific targets of immunotherapy have been studied using tumor vaccines. The results of a phase III randomized trial of adjuvant tumor vaccine therapy were reported in 1993 (111). With a 6.5-year median follow-up, patients with high-risk colon or rectal cancers (Dukes' B2 to C2) were randomized to receive either adjuvant autologous tumor cell-BCG vaccine or surgery alone. Patients receiving adjuvant vaccine therapy demonstrated a slight benefit in disease-free and overall survival; these benefits were statistically significant only in patients with colon primaries. The small size and heterogeneous study population led to skepticism regarding the vaccine's efficacy. A larger trial initiated by ECOG in 1986 compared adjuvant tumor vaccine to surgery alone in patients with high-risk stage II and III colorectal cancer but was prematurely terminated after publication of data on adjuvant 5-FU/levamisole in 1989. The study was subsequently revised in 1990 to include stage III patients who received either adjuvant therapy with 5-FU/levamisole or 5-FU/levamisole plus tumor vaccine (42,111). Results of the ECOG study E5283 comparing the efficacy of surgical resection with ASI versus surgery alone in stage II and III colon cancer patients showed no statistically significant difference in disease free survival, overall survival, or time to relapse in all randomized patients after a 7.5 year median follow-up (111a).

MONOCLONAL ANTIBODIES

Another area under intensive investigation involves the use of monoclonal antibodies. The high degree of specificity of monoclonal antibodies offers a promising alternative to conventional generalized chemotherapies. A number of monoclonal antibodies directed against tumor-specific antigens present on colorectal cancer cells have been identified, although their exact mechanism of antitumor activity remains speculative. Monoclonal antibody stimulation of antibody-dependent cellular cytotoxicity involving monocytes, macrophages, and natural killer cells appears to play a role in tumor cell destruction. The monoclonal antibody 17-1A is the best characterized of the single agent antibodies. It is an IgG2a that recognizes the cell surface glycoprotein CO17-1A, present on 90% of colorectal carcinoma cells (112–114). Use of the murine monoclonal antibody 17-1A has demonstrated only sporadic efficacy in advanced colorectal cancer, but results are encouraging in patients with resected Dukes' C colorectal cancer (114–116). The results of a multicenter randomized study of 189 Dukes' cancer C colorectal patients comparing postoperative observation alone versus monoclonal antibody treatment were published in 1994. With a 5-year median follow-up, patients receiving adjuvant monoclonal antibody treatment had up to a 30% reduction in mortality ($P = .09$) and a 27% reduction in recurrence rate ($P = .03$). Side effects of the treatment were minimal and far less toxic than with the 5-FU-based regimens and included mild gastrointestinal symptoms, chills, fever, transient flushing, and occasional transient allergic or anaphylactic reactions (controlled with intravenous steroids). These results were provocative enough to warrant larger monoclonal antibody trials, which are currently under way. The phase III study—initiated by the CALGB and activated in August 1997—is a randomized comparison of adjuvant monoclonal antibody 17-1A versus observation in resected stage II (Dukes B2) colorectal cancer. Another phase III trial comparing adjuvant 5-FU/levamisole with 5-FU/levamisole plus 17-1A in patients with resected stage III colorectal cancer is also under way.

HEPATIC INFUSIONAL THERAPIES

The use of hepatic-specific adjuvant therapy for colorectal cancer has been actively investigated. The theoretical advantage of hepatic infusional therapy lies in the prevention of hepatic recurrences, which are known to be the most common site of metastases in colorectal cancer patients (117–119). In addition, the high rate of extraction of 5-FU administered directly to the liver would potentially reduce the toxicities associated with systemic therapy. Adjuvant therapy can be administered through the portal vein, a common site of tumor embolization (120). The results of several randomized trials of adjuvant perioperative portal vein infusion versus surgery alone have suggested a small but statistically significant benefit in disease-free and overall survival with portal vein infusion. The first controlled trial of adjuvant portal vein chemotherapy randomized 244 patients to either no further treatment after curative bowel resection or to 1 g of 5-FU with 5000 U heparin administered each day for 7 successive days via the portal vein. This study demonstrated a reduction in the number of hepatic metastases and a statistically significant reduction in the number of deaths in the treatment group (121) (Table 9.9). In a study of 370 patients randomized to observation, urokinase, or 5-FU/heparin, Wereldsma et al. (122) demonstrated a statistically significant reduc-

TABLE 9.9. ADJUVANT PORTAL VEIN THERAPY: RANDOMIZED CONTROLLED TRIALS IN STAGE II AND III COLORECTAL CANCER[a]

Trial	Patients, *n*	Treatment Regimen(s)	Reduction in Liver Metastases	Benefit in Overall Survival[b]	Reference
Taylor et al.	244	Observation vs.			121
		5-FU/heparin	No	Yes	
Wereldsma et al.	370	Observation vs.			122
		Urokinase	No	No	
		5-FU/heparin	Yes	No	
NCCTG	224	Observation vs.			123
		5-FU/heparin	No	No	
SAKK	469	Observation vs.			124
		5-FU/mitomycin C/heparin	No	Yes	
NSABP C-02	1158	Observation vs.			125
		5-FU/heparin	No	Yes	
Fielding et al.	398	Observation vs.			126
		Heparin	No	No	
		5-FU/heparin	No	No	

[a] Adapted from Ref. 46.
[b] Statistically significant survival advantage in treatment versus control group.
SAKK, Swiss Group for Clinical Cancer Research.

tion in hepatic metastasis (23% in controls versus 7% in the 5-FU/heparin arm) but no significant difference in overall survival (122). Subsequent studies have failed to show a consistent reduction in hepatic metastasis or benefit in overall survival (123,124). A larger study was conducted, the NSABP C-02, which randomized 1158 patients with Dukes' A, B, or C colorectal cancer to resection alone or perioperative portal vein 5-FU infusion (125). Recently updated results after a 7-year median follow-up showed sustained and continued improvement in overall and disease-free survival among those treated with perioperative infusion (126). A recent meta-analysis of nine randomized trials of adjuvant infusional portal vein therapy involving > 4000 patients has confirmed the survival advantage of portal vein infusion (127). Interestingly, the incidence of hepatic metastasis has not been shown to be consistently reduced after portal vein infusional therapy, suggesting that the timing of adjuvant chemotherapy may be as much a factor in reducing the incidence of recurrence as the loco-regional delivery of 5-FU. Presently the use of portal vein infusion therapies continues to be limited to large institutional studies.

CPT-11 in the Adjuvant Setting

CPT-11 (or irinotecan) is a newly approved cytotoxic agent that has demonstrated promising activity in advanced colorectal cancer patients in several large, randomized trials (128–133). The mechanism of action appears to involve inhibition of topoisomerase I, which is one of a family of nuclear enzymes responsible for spatial and topologic control of DNA during transcription and replication (134). Both topoisomerase I and II mediate ligation and religation interactions in the DNA-enzymes complex, and inhibition results in DNA strand breaks and subsequent cell death. Currently the use of CPT-11 is limited to the treatment of patients with recurrent or metastatic colorectal cancer (135). A randomized phase II trial was initiated in August 1997 to address the issue of CPT-11 in the adjuvant setting.

Patients with resected stage III colorectal cancer are randomized to sequential versus concurrent administration of 5-FU/leucovorin plus CPT-11. The current NSABP C-07 is studying adjuvant therapy with 5 FU+LV with or without oxoliplatin. A randomized intergroup study planned by the Mayo Clinic is also preparing to begin accrual.

ROLE OF ADJUVANT RADIATION THERAPY

Traditionally, the role of radiation therapy in the treatment of colorectal cancer has been reserved for cases in which a high rate of local failure (> 10%) is likely and when adequate doses can be safely delivered to a limited field (2,136,137). Because of the high incidence of local recurrence in rectal cancers, adjuvant radiation treatment of locally advanced rectal cancer is well established (136).

Colon cancers differ from rectal cancers in their natural history in that the most likely site of local recurrence after curative colon cancer resection is extrapelvic (intra-abdominal). As such, the role of adjuvant radiotherapy after resection of colon cancer is less clearly defined. The most comprehensive study of adjuvant radiotherapy involved 203 patients with Aster-Coller stage B2, B3, C2, and C3 colon tumors (138). After resection, patients were randomized to receive postoperative radiation therapy with and without concurrent 5-FU. The 173 patients treated with adjuvant radiation therapy were compared with a historical control group of 395 patients treated with surgery only. Results showed a selective benefit in local control and recurrence-free survival with postoperative radiation therapy in selective patient groups. Patients with stage B3 and C3 lesions, tumors associated with abscess or fistula formation, and with residual disease after resection appeared to benefit from high-dose radiation therapy, which served as a salvage after resection. This supports the growing body of evidence that certain high-risk features predict for recurrence and that each patient's treatment should be individualized. A phase III Intergroup trial, INT-0130, is currently under way to randomize high-risk stage T4N1–2M0 and selected T3N1–2M0 tumors (gross penetration into the retroperitoneum) to 5-FU/levamisole versus 5-FU/levamisole with concurrent 45-Gy local or regional radiation therapy.

In summary, the use of local or regional radiation therapy for adjuvant treatment of resected colon cancer is less clearly defined than for rectal cancer. Treatment should be reserved for cases in which there is a high risk of local recurrence, those patients presenting with bulky node-negative or positive lesions, patients with associated malignant abscess or fistula formation, and patients with residual disease after resection. As with all treatment plans, therapy should be individualized to the patient.

ISOLATED HEPATIC METASTASES

The liver is the most frequent site of tumor recurrence after curative surgery for colorectal cancer (139–141). After resection, approximately 50% of patients will develop metastases isolated to the liver. At the time of recurrence, only 5 to 10% of these patients will have potentially resectable disease. Median survival after the occurrence of liver metastasis ranges from 6 to 22 months. In a retrospective historical analysis, the median survival of patients with unresectable solitary and multiple unilobar lesions was 21 and 15 months, respectively, although 20% of patients with solitary residual liver lesions survived 3 or more years (142). For patients with resectable hepatic disease, surgery offers the greatest hope for possible cure and long-term survival. The 5-year survival of hepatic metastases without resection from colorectal cancer is approximately 25% (142). Generally, patients with three or fewer resectable liver metastases are considered candidates for operation, although this is not a firm rule. Relative contraindications to surgical resection include four or more metastases (highly variable between institutions), concurrent metastases to the common bile duct or celiac lymph nodes, and anatomic inability to obtain adequate resection margins (142).

Adjuvant therapy after resection of hepatic metastases has not been shown to benefit patient survival in randomized clinical trials (143–145). However, several small single-institution trials have suggested benefit in median survival time using postoperative adjuvant hepatic arterial chemotherapy. Recently, two large randomized, prospective trials incorporating hepatic arterial infusion (HAI) after resection of hepatic metastases have reported preliminary results favoring hepatic arterial infusion in both disease-free survival and overall survival (146,147). Preliminary results from the Memorial Sloan-Kettering Cancer Center (MSKCC) study involving 156 patients randomized to receive either HAI and systemic chemotherapy or chemotherapy alone showed a statistically significant difference favoring the HAI/systemic chemotherapy arm in both hepatic disease-free survival and overall survival at 2 years (146). Interim analysis of the intergroup study INT-0103 involved patients with one to three isolated hepatic metastases who were assigned to observation or to a combination of postoperative arterial FudR and intravenous 5-FU. A significantly improved 3-year recurrence-free rate was noted in patients given HAI and systemic chemotherapy with a trend toward increased survival benefit in the HAI/chemotherapy group (147). At the present time, adjuvant therapy after complete resection of the isolated liver shows promise in terms of both disease-free and overall survival.

ROLE OF CEA AND TUMOR MARKERS IN MANAGEMENT OF COLORECTAL CANCER

The role of tumor markers as predictors of poor outcome has been studied extensively, though mainly in retrospective analyses. The use of markers such as CEA, DCC, DNA ploidy, and proliferation have been used in the clinical setting as adjuncts to decision-making concerning further treatments. Guidelines for the use of markers in patients with colon cancer have recently been reviewed (Table 9.10)

(6). Presently, the use of tumor markers is recommended only as an adjunct to decision making in terms of prognosis and cannot be advocated as independent predictors of outcome. Current National Comprehensive Cancer Network (NCCN) practice guidelines advocate the inclusion of CEA as part of the preliminary laboratory evaluation in patients newly diagnosed with colorectal cancer. An elevated postoperative CEA is an adverse prognostic indicator. If elevated, the CEA should be repeated postoperatively every 6 months for approximately 2 years and then annually for an additional 3 years. More frequent monitoring of CEA in hopes of identifying early recurrence has not been shown to be cost-effective or to affect survival in the absence of measurable disease (148–151). Although several studies do not advocate the routine monitoring of CEA to detect recurrence, it has been recognized that an elevated CEA detects resectable disease earlier than no screening and that a minute subset of patients with single, resectable hepatic metastases might benefit from treatment after such aggressive CEA monitoring (152–156). Therefore, current guidelines from the ASCO panel recommend the routine monitoring of CEA only in patients medically qualified to undergo hepatic resection should early, resectable metastatic disease be identified (6). Current trials such as the INT-0135 will address the issue of tumor markers, particularly in the setting of high-risk stage II disease, to better clarify their importance in predicting outcomes. Routine use of other tumor markers such as CA19-9, LASA, DNA index, DNA flow cytometric proliferation, *p53*

TABLE 9.10. Ongoing Trials of Adjuvant 5-FU with Biochemical Modulators: Randomized Controlled Trials in Stage II and III Colorectal Cancer

INT-0136	Perioperative 5-FU infusion vs. surgery alone→ 5-FU/LEV
INT-0153	5-FU/LDLV/LEV vs. PVI 5-FU/LEV*

LEV, levamisole; *LDLV,* low-dose leucovorin; *PVI,* protracted venous infusion.
*Study closed at first interim analysis 8/1999; See Ref. 91a.

tumor-suppressor gene, and *ras* oncogene is not generally recommended for diagnosis, screening, staging, or monitoring after treatment of colorectal cancers in clinical practice (Table 9.10) (6).

UNRESECTABLE METASTATIC COLORECTAL CANCER

The treatment of metastatic colorectal cancer has seen encouraging advances in recent years with the discovery and development of more precise targets of biological therapy. For more than 30 years, 5-FU has been the primary chemotherapeutic treatment for colorectal cancer and the only agent to show significant activity against this relatively refractory malignancy. Although response rates with bolus 5-FU alone have been low, encouraging results both in tumor response and toxicity profile have been reported with 5-FU delivered by continuous infusion (157–160). In particular, the activity and toxicity profile of 5-FU differ significantly when given as a continuous infusion, allowing the delivery of more drug and changing the dose-limiting toxicity from myelosuppression to stomatitis and hand-foot syndrome. A recent meta-analysis, involving 1219 patients with advanced colorectal cancer in six randomized trials comparing continuous infusion versus bolus 5-FU, showed improved tumor response rates (22%, continuous infusion vs. 14% bolus) and a slight increase in overall survival in patients treated with infusional 5-FU (160). Myelosuppression was far less significant in the continuous infusion group, though more hand-foot syndrome was observed (160).

More recently a number of new agents have been developed that target specific pathways of cancer development. One of the most promising agents recently approved for the treatment of recurrent or metastatic colorectal cancer is irinotecan (CPT-11), a topoisomerase I inhibitor that has been shown to have moderate activity against colorectal cancer. Based on recent phase II trials, which demonstrated a modest (13%) response in patients refractory to 5-FU-based chemotherapy, CPT-11 was approved as a single agent for the treatment of recurrent colorectal cancer (129–134,161). Since then, two phase III studies comparing CPT-11 after fluorouracil failure with best supportive care or infusional 5-FU have reported significant improvements in progression-free and overall survival among patients treated with CPT-11 (162,163). In patients randomized to CPT-11 versus best supportive care, quality of life was significantly improved among patients receiving CPT-11, despite the side effects and toxicities of treatment (163). Toxicities are significant and include up to a 31% incidence of grade 3 or 4 diarrhea, requiring dose reduction or withdrawal of therapy (161).

Other agents include folate-based thymidylate synthase inhibitors, some of which are in various phase I to III clinical trials, including raltitrexad (Tomudex), nolatrexad, LY231514 (MTA), and ZD931 (164–170). Oral fluorinated pyrimidines (UFT, S-1, capcitabine and eniluracil) have been widely studied and used as adjuvant treatment in Japan and are currently under study in the U.S. in phase II and III trials comparing these oral agents to intravenous 5-FU (170). Oxaliplatin is a platinum derivative with single-agent activity against previously treated and untreated advanced colorectal tumors (171–174).

More recently, based on promising animal studies, much attention has been focused in the media on the use of angiogenesis inhibitors to treat tumors. Early clinical trials are currently under way for several drugs that are known to inhibit new vessel formation in vitro. Recently a monoclonal antibody against the vascular endothelial growth factor (VEGF) has been synthesized for use in phase II and III clinical trials in colorectal as well as breast, lung, and prostate cancers (175). Because of their mechanism of action in preventing tumor growth without actually killing tumor cells, angiogenesis inhibitors may be useful in combination with other cytotoxic agents. Current trials are investigating several different angiogenesis inhibitors in combination with other cytotoxic chemotherapeutic agents.

SUMMARY

The management of colorectal cancer involves a multimodality approach, with surgery being the primary treatment modality in limited-stage disease. 5-FU-based chemotherapy remains the standard adjuvant treatment for stage III disease and a subset of high-risk stage II patients. New agents targeting the molecular mechanisms of colorectal cancer biology are encouraging in their potential for the treatment of this common but relatively refractory cancer.

REFERENCES

1. U.S. Surveillance, Epidemiology and End Results Study (SEER). Cancer Incidence in the U.S. 1973–1991.
2. Gunderson LL, Sosin H. Areas of failure found at reoperation following "curative surgery" for adenocarcinoma of the rectum. Clinicopathological correlation and implications for adjuvant therapy. Cancer 1974;34:1278–1292.
3. Lev R, Lee M. Colorectal Carcinoma. Pathology In: Rustgi AK, ed. Gastrointestinal cancers, biology, diagnosis, and therapy. Philadelphia: Lippincott-Raven; 1995:379–398.
4. Pihl E, Hughes ESR, McDermott FT, et al. Clinicopathologic correlation of lymph node enlargement, tumor spread and survival in 1505 colorectal cancer patients treated with curative resection. Am J Proctol Gastroenterol Colon Rectal Surg 1983;34:5–27.
5. Shepherd NA, Sarga EP, Love SB, Jass JR. Prognostic factors in colonic cancer. Histopathology 1989;14:613–620.
6. American Society of Clinical Oncology. Clinical practice guidelines for the use of tumor markers in breast and colorectal cancer. J Clin Oncol 1996;14:2843–2877.
7. Costanza ME, Das S, Nathanson L, et al. Carcinoembryonic antigen: report of a screening study. Cancer 1974;33:583–590.
8. Wanebo HJ, Rao B, Pinsky CM, et al. The use of the preoperative

carcinoembryonic antigen level as a prognostic indicator to complement pathologic staging. N Engl J Med (1978);299:448–451.

9. Ng IOL, Ho J, Pritchett CJ, et al. A tissue staining in colorectal cancer patients—correlation with plasma CEA, histology and staging. Pathology 1993;25:219–222.
10. Henson DE. The histological grading of neoplasms. Arch Pathol Lab Med 1988;112:1091–1096.
11. Halvorsen TB, Sein E. Degree of differentiation in colorectal adenocarcinomas: a multivariate analysis of the influence on survival. J Clin Pathol 1988;41:532–537.
12. Kirkham N. Colorectal signet ring cell carcinoma in young people. J Pathol 1988;155:93–94.
13. Willett C, Tepper JE, Cohen A, et al. Obstructive and perforative colonic carcinoma: patterns of failure. J Clin Oncol 1985;3:379–384.
14. Scott NA, Wieand HS, Moertel CG, et al. Colorectal cancer: Dukes' stage, tumor site, preoperative plasma CEA level and patient prognosis related to tumor DNA ploidy pattern. Arch Surg 1987;122:1375–1379.
15. Kokal WA, Gardine RL, Sheibani K, et al. Tumor DNA content in resectable, primary colorectal carcinoma. Ann Surg 1989;209:188–193.
16. Albe X, Vassilakos P, Helfer-guarnori K, et al. Independent prognostic value of ploidy in colorectal cancer. A prospective study using image cytometry. Cancer 1990;66:1168–1175.
17. Jen J, Kim H, Piantadosie S, et al. Allelic loss of chromosome 18q and prognosis in colorectal cancer. N Engl J Med 1994;331:213–221.
18. Lanza G, Matteuzzi M, Gafa, et al. Int J Cancer 1998;79:390–395.
19. Ogunbiyi OA, Goodfellow PJ, Herfarth K, et al. Confirmation that chromosome 18q allelic loss in colon cancer is a prognostic indicator. J Clin Oncol 1998;16:427–433.
20. Witzig TE, Loprinzi CL, Gonchoroff NJ, et al. DNA ploidy and cell kinetic measurements as predictors of recurrence and survival in stages B2 and C colorectal adenocarcinoma. Cancer 1991;68:879–888.
21. Schutte B, Reynder MMJ, Wigger T, et al. Retrospective analysis of the prognostic significance of DNA content and proliferative activity in large bowel carcinoma. Cancer Res 1987;47:5494–5496.
22. Ahnen DJ, Feigl P, Quan G, et al. *Ki-ras* mutation and *p53* overexpression predict the clinical behavior of colorectal cancer: a Southwest Oncology Group study. Cancer Res 1998;58:1149–1158.
23. Bell SM, Scott N, Cross D, et al. Prognostic value of *p53* overexpression

and *c-Ki-ras* gene mutations in colorectal cancer. Gastroenterology 1993;104:57–64.

24. Hamelin R, Laurent-Puig P, Olschwang S, et al. Association of *p53* mutations with short survival in colorectal cancer. Gastroenterology 1994;106:42–48.
25. Yamaguchi A, Kurosaka Y, Fushia S, et al. Expression of *p53* protein in colorectal cancer and its relationship to short-term prognosis. Cancer 1992;70:2778–2784.
26. Remvikos Y, Tominaga O, Hammel P, et al. Increased *p53* protein content of colorectal tumours correlates with poor survival. Br J Cancer 1992;66:758–764.
27. Shibata D, Reale, MA, Lavin P, et al. The DCC protein and prognosis in colorectal cancer. N Engl J Med 1996;335:1727–1732.
28. American Joint Committee on Cancer. Manual for staging of cancer. 4th ed. Philadelphia: Lippincott, 1992.
29. Hutter RVP, Sobin LH. A universal staging system for cancer of the colon and rectum: let there be light. Arch Pathol Lab Med 1986;110:367–368.
30. Dukes CE. The classification of cancer of the rectum. J Pathol 1983;35:323–332.
31. Aster VB, Coller FA. The prognostic significance of direct extension of the colon and rectum. Ann Surg 1954;139:846–851.
32. Hermanek P. pTNM and residual tumor classifications: problems of assessment and prognostic significance. World J Surg 1995;19:184–190.
33. Kern SE Fearon ER, Tersemette KWF, et al. Clinical and pathological associations with allelic loss in colorectal carcinoma. JAMA 1989;261:3099–3103. (Erratum, JAMA 1989;262:1952).
34. Goldberg DM, Diamandis EP. Models of neoplasia and their diagnostic implications: a historical perspective. Clin Chem 1993;39:2360–2374.
35. Hedrick L, Cho KR, Fearon ER, et al. The DCC product in cellular differentiation and colorectal tumorigenesis. Genes Dev 1994;8:1174–1183.
36. Froggatt NJ, Levenson SH, Garner RC. Low frequency and late occurrence of *p53* and DCC alterations in colorectal tumors. J Clin Res Clin Onc 1995;121:7–15.
37. Meling GI, Lothe RA, Borreson AL, et al. The *TP53* suppressor gene in colorectal carcinomas, II. Relation to DNA ploidy pattern and clinicopathologic variable. Br J Cancer 1993;67:93–98.
38. Liefers GJ, Cleton-Jansen AM, Van de Velde CJH, et al. Micrometas-

tases and survival in stage II colorectal cancer. N Engl J Med 1998;339:223–228.

39. NIH Consensus Conference: adjuvant therapy for patients with colon and rectal cancer. JAMA 1990;264:1444–1450.
40. Diaz-Canton EA, Pazdur R. Adjuvant medical therapy for colorectal cancer. Surg Clin North Am 1997;77:211–228.
41. NIH Consensus Development Conference. Adjuvant therapy for patients with colon and rectum cancer. NIH Consensus Dev Conf Consensus Statement 1990;8:16–18.
42. Vaughn DJ, Haller DG. Adjuvant therapy for colorectal cancer: past accomplishments, future directions. Cancer Invest 1997;15:435–447.
43. Moertel CG, Fleming TR, MacDonald JS, et al. Fluorouracil plus levamisole as effective adjuvant therapy after resection of stage III colon carcinoma: a final report. Ann Intern Med 1995;122:321–326.
44. Allegra CJ, Grem JL. Antimetabolites In: DeVita VT, Hellman S, Rosenberg SA, eds. Cancer. Principles and practice of oncology. Vol. 1. 5th ed. Philadelphia: Lippincott-Raven 1997:436–440.
45. Carter SK. Correlation of chemotherapy in advanced disease with adjuvant results. In: Salmon SE, ed. Adjuvant chemotherapy of cancer. Amsterdam: Elsevier/North Holland 1977:589–595.
46. Fuchs C, Mayer RJ. Colorectal cancer chemotherapy. In: Rustgi AK, ed. Gastrointestinal cancers, biology, diagnosis, and therapy. Philadelphia: Lippincott-Raven; 1995:423–442.
47. Mrazek R, Economou S, McDonald GO, et al. Prophylactic and adjuvant use of nitrogen mustard in the surgical treatment of cancer. Ann Surg 1959;150:745–754.
48. Dixon WJ, Longmire WP, Holden WD. Use of triethylenethiophosphoramide as an adjunct to the surgical treatment of gastric and colorectal carcinoma. Ann Surg 1971;172:26–39.
49. Dwight RW, Humphrey EW, Higgins GA, Keehn RJ. FUDR as a adjuvant to surgery in cancer of the large bowel. J Surg Oncol 1973;5:243–249.
50. Grossi CE, Wolff WI, Nealon TF Jr, et al. Intraluminal fluorouracil chemotherapy adjunct to surgical procedures for resectable carcinoma of the colon and rectum. Surg Gynecol Obstet 1977;145:549–554.
51. Higgins GA, Dwight RW, Smith JV, Keehn RJ. Fluorouracil as an adjuvant to surgery in carcinoma of the colon. Arch Surg 1971;102:339–343.
52. Higgins G, Humphrey E, Juler G, et al. Adjuvant chemotherapy in the surgical treatment of large bowel cancer. Cancer 1976;38:1461–1467.

53. Higgins GA, Donaldson RC, Humphrey EW, et al. Adjuvant therapy for large bowel cancer. Update of Veterans Administration Surgical Oncology Group trials. Surg Clin North Am 1981;6:1311–1320.

54. Lawrence W Jr, Terez JJ, Horsley S, et al. Chemotherapy as an adjuvant to surgery for colorectal cancer. A follow-up report. Arch Surg 1978;113:164–168.

55. Grage TB, Moss SE. Adjuvant chemotherapy in cancer of the colon and rectum: demonstration of effectiveness of prolonged 5-FU chemotherapy in prospectively controlled, randomized trial. Surg Clin North Am 1981;61:1321–1329.

56. Buyse M, Zeleniuch-Jacquotte A, Chalmer TC. Adjuvant therapy of colorectal cancer. Why we still don't know. JAMA 1988;259:3571–3578.

57. Higgins GA, Amadeo JH, Mcelhinney J, et al. Efficacy of prolonged intermittent therapy with combined 5-fluorouracil and methyl-CCNU following resection of carcinoma of the large bowel. Cancer 1984;53:1–8.

58. Adbi E, Harbora D, Hanson J, et al. Adjuvant chemoimmunotherapy and immunotherapy in stage B2 and C colorectal cancer [Abstract]. Proc Am Soc Clin Oncol 1987;6:93.

59. Panettiere FJ, Goodman PJ, Costanzi JJ, et al. Adjuvant therapy in large bowel adenocarcinoma: long term results of a Southwest Oncology Group study. J Clin Oncol 1988;6:947–954.

60. Wolmark N, Wickerham DL, Fisher B, et al. Postoperative adjuvant therapy for Dukes' B And C adenocarcinoma: NSABP protocols C-01, C-03, C-04. In: Hamilton JM, Elliot JM, eds. NIH Consensus Development Conference: adjuvant therapy for patients with colon and rectum cancer. Bethesda, Md.: National Institutes of Health, 1990;45–46.

61. Mayer RJ, Stablein DM. Adjuvant colon cancer trials of the Gastrointestinal Tumor Study Group. In: Hamilton JM, Elliot JM, eds. NIH Consensus Development Conference: adjuvant therapy for patients with colon and rectum cancer. Bethesda, Md.: National Institutes of Health, 1990;25–30.

62. Mansour E, Ryan L, Lerner H, et al. Lack of effectiveness of 5-FU and methyl-CCNU as compared to 5-FU for adjuvant therapy in colon cancer: a randomized trial of the Eastern Cooperative Oncology Group (EST 2276) [Abstract]. Proc Am Soc Clin Oncol 1989;8:115.

63. Boice JD, Greene MN, Killen JY, et al. Leukemia and preleukemia after adjuvant treatment of gastrointestinal cancer with semustine. N Engl J Med 1983;309:1079–1084.

64. Stevenson HC, Green I , Hamilton JM, et al. Levamisole: known effects on the immune system, clinical results and future applications to the treatment of cancer. J Clin Oncol 1991;9:2052–2066.

65. Arnaud JP, Buyse M, Nordlinger B, et al. Adjuvant therapy of poor prognosis colon cancer with levamisole: results of an EORTC double-blind randomized clinical trial. Br J Surg 1989;76:284–289.

66. Moertel CG, Fleming TR, Macdonald JS, et al. Hepatic toxicity associated with fluorouracil plus levamisole adjuvant therapy. J Clin Oncol 1993;11:2386–2390.

67. Hook CC, Kimmel DW, Kvols LK, et al. Multifocal inflammatory leukoencephalopathy with 5-fluorouracil and levamisole. Ann Neurol 1992;31:262–267.

68. Borden EC, Davdis TE, Crowley JJ, et al. Interim analysis of a trial of levamisole and 5-fluorouracil in metastatic colorectal carcinoma. In: Terry W, Rosenberg S, eds. Immunotherapy of human cancer. New York: Elsevier, 1982:225–229.

69. Verhaegen H, Decree J, Decock W. Levamisole therapy in patients with colorectal cancer In: Terry W, Rosenberg S, eds. Immunotherapy of human cancer. New York: Elsevier, 1982:225–229.

70. Chlebowski RT, Nystrom S, Reynold R, et al. Long-term survival following levamisole or placebo adjuvant treatment of colorectal cancer: a Western Cancer Study Group trial. Oncology 1988;45:141–143.

71. Windle R, Bell PRF, Shaw D. Five year results of a randomized trial of adjuvant 5-fluorouracil and levamisole in colorectal cancer. Br J Surg 1987;74:569–572.

72. Laurie JA, Moertel CG, Fleming TR, et al. Surgical adjuvant therapy of large-bowel carcinoma: an evaluation of levamisole and the combination of levamisole and fluorouracil. J Clin Oncol 1989;7:1447–1456.

73. Moertel CG, Fleming TR, Macdonald JS, et al. Levamisole and fluorouracil for adjuvant therapy of resected colon carcinoma. N Engl J Med 1990;322:352–358.

74. National Cancer Institute. The efficacy of the group C status of levamisole and 5-FU for patients with Dukes' C colon cancer. NCI, Oct. 1989.

75. Moertel CG, Fleming TR, Macdonald JS, et al. Intergroup study of fluorouracil plus levamisole as adjuvant therapy for stage II/Dukes' B2 colon cancer. J Clin Oncol 1995;13:2936–2943.

76. Rustum YM. Modulation of fluoropyrimidines by leucovorin: rationale and status. J Surg Oncol 1991;2(suppl):116–123.

77. Kemeny N, Lokich JJ, Anderson N, et al. Recent advances in the treatment of advanced colorectal cancer. Cancer 1993;71:9–18.

78. Fuchs CS, Mayer RJ. Adjuvant chemotherapy for colon and rectal cancer. Semin Oncol 1995;22:472–487.

79. Mini E, Trave F, Rustum YM, et al. Enhancement of the antitumor effects of 5-fluorouracil by folinic acid. Pharmacol Ther 1990;47:1–19.

80. Zaniboni A. Adjuvant chemotherapy in colorectal cancer with high dose leucovorin and fluorouracil: impact on disease-free survival and overall survival. J Clin Oncol 1997;15:2432–2441.

81. Piedbois P, Buyse M Rustum Y, et al. Modulation of fluorouracil by leucovorin in patients with advanced colorectal cancer: evidence in terms of response rates. J Clin Oncol 1992;10:896–903.

82. Labianca R, Marsoni S, Pancera G, et al. Efficacy of adjuvant fluorouracil and folinic acid in colon cancer. Lancet 1995;345:939–944.

83. Haller DG, Catalano PJ, Macdonald JS, Mayer RJ. Fluorouracil, leucovorin and levamisole adjuvant therapy for colon cancer: five year final report of INT-0089 [Abstract]. Proc Am Soc Clin Oncol 1998; 17:256.

84. Wolmark N, Rockette H, Mamounas EP, et al. The relative efficacy of 5-FU-leucovorin-levamisole in patients with Dukes' B and C carcinoma of the colon: First report of NSABP C-04 [Abstract]. Proc Am Soc Clin Oncol 1996;15:205.

85. Wolmark N, Bryant J, Hyams DM, et al. The relative efficacy of 5-FU + leucovorin and 5-FU-leucovorin+ interferon alfa-2a in patients with Dukes' B and C carcinoma of the colon: the first report of NSABP C-05 [Abstract]. Proc Am Soc Clin Oncol 1998;17:255.

86. Haller DG, Catalano PJ, Macdonald JS, et al. Fluorouracil (FU), leucovorin (LV) and levamisole (LEV) adjuvant therapy for colon cancer: preliminary results of INT-0089 [Abstract]. Proc Am Soc Clin Oncol 1996;15:211.

87. DeGramont A, Bosset JF, Milan C, et al. Randomized trial comparing monthly low-dose leucovorin and fluorouracil bolus with bimonthly high-dose leucovorin and fluorouracil bolus plus continuous infusion for advanced colorectal cancer: a French Intergroup study. J Clin Oncol 1997;15:808–815.

88. Piedbois P, Rougier P, Buyse M, et al. Efficacy of intravenous continuous infusion of fluorouracil compared with bolus administration in advanced colorectal cancer. J Clin Oncol 1998;16:301–308.

89. Fraile RJ, Baker LH, Buroker TR, et al. Pharmacokinetics of 5-fluorouracil administered orally by rapid intravenous and by slow infusion. Cancer Res 1980;52:1855–1864.

90. Carlson R. Continuous intravenous infusion chemotherapy In: Perry MC, ed. The Chemotherapy Source book. Baltimore, MD, Williams and Wilkins, 1996:225–251.

91. Aschele C, Sobrero A, Faderan MA, et al. Novel mechanism(s) of resistance to 5-fluorouracil in human colon cancer (HCT-8) cell lines following exposure to two different clinically relevant dose schedules. Cancer Res 1992;52:1855–1864.

91a. Poplin E, Benedetti J, Estes N, et al. Phase III randomized trial of bolus 5FU/leucovorin/leuarricule versus 5-FU continuous infusion/ leuarrisole as adjuvant therapy for high risk colon cancer (SWDG 9415/INT 0153) [Abstract] Proc Am Soc Clin Oncol 2000;19:240.

92. Ratain MJ. New agents for colon cancer: topoisomerase I inhibitors. In: Perry MC, ed. American Society of Clinical Oncology/Educational Book, Philadelphia: Saunders, 1998:311–315.

92a. Sargent D, Goldberg R, MacDonald J, et al. Adjuvant chemotherapy for colon cancer is beneficial without significantly increased toxicity in elderly patients: results from a 3351 pt metoanlysis. [Abstract] Proc Am Soc 2000;19:241.

93. Wadler S, Wersto R, Weinberg V, et al. Interaction of fluorouracil and interferon in human colon cancer cell lines: Cytotoxic and cytokinetic effects. Cancer Res 1990;50:5735–5739.

94. Schwartz EL, Hoffman M, O'Connor CJ, et al. Stimulation of 5-fluorouracil metabolic activation by interferon alpha in human colon carcinoma cells. Biochem Biophys Res Commun 1992;182:1232–1239.

95. Elias L, Sandoval JM. Interferon effects upon fluorouracil metabolism by HL-60 cells. Biochem Biophys Res Commun 1989;163:867–874.

96. Hoffman MA, Wadler S. Mechanisms by which interferon potentiates chemotherapy. Cancer Invest 1993;11:310–313.

97. Taniguchi T, Mantei N, Schwarzstein M. Human leukocyte and fibroblast interferons are structurally related. Nature 1980;285:547–549.

98. Ruzicka FJ, Jach ME, Barton EC. Binding of recombinant-produced interferon-beta-ser to human lymphoblastoid cells. J Biol Chem 1987;262:16142–16149.

99. Wadler S, Wierniek PH. Clinical update on the role of fluorouracil and recombinant interferon alpha-2a in the treatment of colorectal carcinoma. Semin Oncol 1990;17(suppl 1):16–21.

100. Huberman M, Bering H Tessitore J, et al. 5-fluorouracil plus recombinant alpha interferon in advanced colorectal cancer [Abstract]. Proc Am Soc Clin Oncol 1990;9:116.

101. Pazdur R, Abbruzzese J, Faintuch J, et al. Phase II study of recombinant interferon alpha and 5-flurouracil in patients with advanced colorectal carcinoma [Abstract]. Proc Am Soc Clin Oncol 1990;9:117.

102. Kemeny N, Kelsen D, Derby S, et al. Combination 5-fluorouracil and recombinant alpha-interferon in advanced colorectal carcinoma: activity but significant toxicity [Abstract]. Proc Am Soc Clin Oncol 1990;9:109.

103. Wadler, S. The role of immunotherapy in colorectal cancer. Sem Oncol 1991;18(suppl 1):27–38.

104. Greco FA Figlin R, York M, et al. Phase III randomized study to compare interferon alfa-2a in combination with fluorouracil versus fluorouracil alone in patients with advanced colorectal cancer. J Clin Oncol 1996;14:2674–2681.

105. Hill M, Norman A, Cunningham D, et al. Royal Marsden phase III trial of fluorouracil with or without interferon alfa-2b in advanced colorectal cancer. J Clin Oncol 1995;13:1297–1302.

106. Wadler S, Haynes H, Tenteromano L, et al. Results of sequential phase II clinical trials of 5-fluorouracil and interferon-beta-ser in patients with advanced colorectal carcinoma [Abstract]. Proc Am Soc Clin Oncol 1995;14:205.

107. Joffe JK, Bradley C, Selby PJ, et al. A phase II study of recombinant interferon-beta in combination with 5-fluorouracil in the treatment of patients with advanced colorectal carcinoma. Abstract presented at the BACR meetings, 1995.

108. Pavlidis N, Nicolaides C, Athanassiadis A, et al. Phase II study of 5-fluorouracil and interferon-gamma in patients with metastatic colorectal cancer. Oncology 1996;53:159–162.

109. Hanna MG Jr, Hoover HC Jr, Peter LC, et al. Fundamental applied aspects of successful active specific immunotherapy of cancer. In: Oldham RK ed. Principles of cancer biotherapy. New York: Raven, 1987:195–221.

110. Wolmark N, Fisher B, Rockett H, et al. Postoperative adjuvant chemotherapy or BCG for colon cancer: results from NSABP protocol C-01. J Natl Cancer Inst 1988;80:30–36.

111. Hoover HC, Brandhorst JS, Peters LC, et al. Adjuvant active specific immunotherapy for human colorectal cancer: 6.5 median follow-up of a phase III prospectively randomized trial. J Clin Oncol 1993;11:390–399.

111a. Ryan L, Hoover H, Stuart R, et al. Delayed cutaneous hypersensitivity

(DCH) as a measure of effectiveness for adjuvant active specific immunotherapy (ASI) in surgically resected Stage II and Stage II colon cancer: ECOG 5283. [Abstract] Proc Am Soc Oriol 1999;18:438.

112. Gottlinger HG, Funke I, Johnson JP, et al. The epithelial cell surface antigen 17-1A, a target for antibody mediated tumor therapy: its biochemical nature, tissue distribution and recognition by different monoclonal antibodies. Int J Cancer 1986;38:47–53.
113. Maxwell-Armstrong CA, Durrant LG, Scholefield JH. Colorectal cancer vaccines. Br J Surg 1998;85:149–154.
114. Zbar AP, Lemoine NR, Wadhwa M, et al. Biological therapy: approaches to colorectal cancer. Strategies to enhanced carcinoembryonic antigen (CEA) as an immunogenic target. Br J Cancer 1998;77:683–693.
115. Mellstedt H, Frodine JE, Masucci G, et al. The therapeutic use of monoclonal antibodies in colorectal carcinoma. Semin Oncol 1991;2:462–477.
116. Riethmuller G, Schneider-Gadicke E, Schlimok G, et al. Randomized trial of monoclonal antibody for adjuvant therapy of resected Dukes' C colorectal carcinoma. Lancet 1994;343:1177–1183.
117. Olson RM, Perencevich NP, Malcolm AW, et al. Patterns of recurrence following curative resection of adenocarcinoma of the colon and rectum. Cancer 1980;45:2969–2974.
118. Bergmark S, Hafstrom L. The natural history of primary and secondary tumors of the liver, I. The prognosis for patients with hepatic metastases from colonic and rectal carcinoma by laparotomy. Cancer 1969;23:198–202.
119. Welch JP, Donaldson GA. The clinical correlation of an autopsy study of recurrent colorectal cancer. Ann Surg 1979;189:496–502.
120. Nitto D, Wills J, Shammed T, et al. Final results of a phase III clinical trial on adjuvant intraportal infusion with heparin and 5-fluorouracil in resectable colon cancer (EORTC GITCCG 1983-1987). Eur J Cancer 1997;33:1209–1215.
121. Taylor I, Rowling J, West C. Adjuvant cytotoxic liver perfusion for colorectal cancer. Br J Surg 1979;66:833–837.
122. Wereldsma JCJ, Bruggink ERM, Meijer WS, et al. Adjuvant portal liver infusion in colorectal cancer with 5-fluorouracil/heparin versus urokinase versus control: results of a prospective randomized clinical trial (colorectal adenocarcinoma trial I). Cancer 1990;65:425–432.
123. Beart RW, Moertel CG, Wieand HS, et al. Adjuvant therapy for resectable colorectal carcinoma with fluorouracil administered by portal vein infusion. Arch Surg 1990;125:879–901.
124. Metzger U, Laffer U, Aerberhard P, et al. Randomized multicenter trial

of adjuvant intraportal chemotherapy for colorectal cancer 40/811: an interim report. Acta Chir Scand 1990;156:467–474.

125. Wolmark N, Rockette H, Wickerham DL, et al. Adjuvant therapy of Dukes' A, B, and C adenocarcinoma of the colon with portal-vein fluorouracil hepatic infusion: preliminary results of national surgical adjuvant breast and bowel project protocol C-02. J Clin Oncol 1990;8:1466–1475.

126. Fielding, L, Hittinger R, Grace R, et al. Randomized controlled trial of adjuvant chemotherapy by portal vein perfusion after curative resection for colorectal adenocarcinoma. Lancet 1992;340:502–506.

127. Wolmark N, Rockette H, Petrelli N, et al. Long-term results of the efficacy of perioperative portal vein infusion of 5-FU for treatment of colon cancer: NSABP C-02 [Abstract]. Proc Am Soc Clin Oncol 1994;13:194.

128. Piedbois P, Buyse M, Gray R, et al. Portal vein infusion is an effective adjuvant treatment for patients with colorectal cancer [Abstract]. Proc Am Soc Clin Oncol 1995;14:192.

129. Rothenberg ML. Topoisomerase I inhibitors: Review and update. Ann Oncol 1997;8:837–855.

130. Shimada Y, Yoshino M, Wakui A, et al. Phase II study of CPT-11, a new camptothecin derivative, in metastatic colorectal cancer. J Clin Oncol 1993;11:909–913.

131. Conti JA, Kemeny NE, Saltz LB, et al. Irinotecan is an active agent in untreated patients with metastatic colorectal cancer. J Clin Oncol 1996;14:709–715.

132. Rothenberg ML, Eckardt JR, Kuhn JG, et al. Phase II trial of irinotecan in patients with progressive or rapidly recurrent colorectal cancer. J Clin Oncol 1996;14:1128–1135.

133. Rougier P, Bugat R, Douillard JY, et al. Phase II study of irinotecan in the treatment of advanced colorectal cancer in chemotherapy naïve patients and patients pretreated with fluorouracil-based chemotherapy. J Clin Oncol 1997;15:251–260.

134. Pitot HC, Wender DB, O'Connell JM, et al. Phase II trial of irinotecan in patients with metastatic colorectal carcinoma. J Clin Oncol 1997;15:2910–2919.

135. Chen AY, Liu LF. DNA topoisomerases: essential enzymes and lethal targets. Ann Rev Pharmacol Toxicol 1994;34:191–218.

136. Brower M, Asbury R, Kramer K, et al. Adjuvant chemotherapy for colorectal cancer in the elderly: population-based experience (Abstract). Proc Am Soc Clin Oncol 1993;12:195.

137. Minsky BD. The role of adjuvant radiation therapy in the treatment of colorectal cancer. Hematol Oncol Clin North Am 1997;11:679–697.

138. Rich T, Gunderson LL, Lew R, et al. Patterns of recurrence of rectal cancer after potentially curative surgery. Cancer 1983;52:1317–1329.

139. Willett CG, Fung CY, Kaufman DS, et al. Postoperative radiation therapy for high risk colon carcinoma. J Clin Oncol 1993;11:1112–1117.

140. Scheele J, Stangle R, Altendorf-Hofman A. Hepatic metastases from colorectal carcinoma: impact of surgical resection on natural history. Br J Surg 1990;77:1241–1246.

141. Adson MA. Resection of liver metastases: when is it worthwhile? World J Surg 1987;11:511–520.

142. Wagner JS, Adson MA, Van Heerden JA, et al. The natural history of hepatic metastases from colorectal cancer. Ann Surg 1984;199:502–507.

143. Hughes KS, Simons R, Songhorabodi S, et al. Resection of the liver for colorectal carcinoma metastases: a multi-institutional study of indications for resection. Surgery 1988;103:278–288.

144. Gastrointestinal Tumor Study Group. Adjuvant therapy of colon cancer: results of a prospectively randomized trial. N Engl J Med 1984;310:737–743.

145. O'Connell MJ, Adson MA, Schutt AJ, et al. Clinical trial of adjuvant chemotherapy after surgical resection of colorectal cancer metastatic to the liver. Mayo Clin Proc 1985;60:517–520.

146. Kemeny O, Cohen A, Huang Y, et al. Randomized study of hepatic arterial infusion (HAI) and systemic chemotherapy (SYS) alone as adjuvant therapy after resection of hepatic metastases from colorectal cancer [Abstract]. Proc Am Soc Clin Oncol 1999;18:263.

147. Kemeny MM, Adak S, Lipsitz B, et al. Results of the Intergroup (Eastern Cooperative Oncology Group (ECOG) and Southwest Oncology Group (SWOG)) prospective randomized study of surgery alone versus continuous hepatic artery infusion of FUDR and continuous systemic infusion of 5-FU after hepatic resection for colorectal liver metastases [Abstract]. Proc Am Soc Clin Oncol 1999;18:264.

148. Wagman LD, Kemeny MM, Leon L, et al. A prospective randomized evaluation of the treatment of colorectal cancer metastatic to the liver. J Clin Oncol 1990;8:1885–1893.

149. Kievit J, van de Velde CJH. Utility and cost of carcinoembryonic antigen monitoring in colon cancer follow-up evaluation: a Markov analysis. Cancer 1990;65:2580–2587.

150. Moertel CG, Gelming TR, Macdonald JS, et al. An evaluation of the carcinoembryonic antigen (CEA) test for monitoring patients with resected colon cancer. JAMA 1993;270:943–947.

151. Minton JP, Hoehn JL, Gerbe DM. Results of a 400 patient carcinoembryonic antigen second-look colorectal cancer study. Cancer 1985;55:1284–1290.

152. Makela JT, Laitinen SO, Kairaluoma MI. Five year follow-up after radical surgery for colorectal cancer results of a prospective randomized trial. Arch Surg 1995;130:1062–1067.

153. Arnaud JP, Bergamaschi R, Casa C, et al. The rationale for CEA dosage in the follow-up of patients operated for colorectal cancer. A prospective study on 800 cases. Spec Int Col Mtg Surg Oncol; 25 (1992).

154. Tartter PL, Slater G, Gelernt I, et al. Screening for liver metastases from colorectal cancer with carcinoembryonic antigen and alkaline phosphatase. Ann Surg 1981;193:357–360.

155. Bruinvels DJ, Stiggelbout AM, Kievit J, et al. Follow-up of patients with colorectal cancer. Ann Surg 1994;219:174–182.

156. McCall J, Black R, Rich C. The value of serum carcinoembryonic antigen in predicting recurrent disease following curative resection of colorectal cancer. Dis Colon Rectum 1994;37:875–881.

157. Lokich JJ, Bothe A, Fine, et al. Phase I study of protracted venous infusion of 5-fluorouracil. Cancer 1981;48:2565–2568.

158. Leichman L, Leichman CG, Kinzie J, et al. Long-term low dose 5-fluorouracil in advanced measurable colon cancer: No correlation between toxicity and efficacy [Abstract]. Proc Am Soc Clin Oncol 1985;4:333.

159. Belt RJ, Davidner JL, Myron MC, et al. Continuous low dose 5-fluorouracil for adenocarcinoma: confirmation of activity [Abstract]. Proc Am Soc Clin Oncol 1985;4:349.

160. Wolmark N, Piedbois P, Buyse M, et al. Efficacy of intravenous continuous infusion of fluorouracil compared with bolus administration in advanced colorectal cancer. J Clin Oncol 1998;16:301–308.

161. Von Hoff DD, Rothenberg ML, Pitot HC, et al. Irinotecan (CPT-11) therapy for patients with previously treated metastatic colorectal cancer: overall results of FDA-reviewed pivotal US clinical trials [Abstract]. Proc Am Soc Clin Oncol 1997;16:228.

162. Rougier P, Cutsem EV, Bajetta E, et al. Randomised trial of irinotecan versus fluorouracil by continuous infusion after fluorouracil failure in patients with metastatic colorectal cancer. Lancet 1998;352:1407–1412.

163. Cunningham D, Pyrhonen S, James RD, et al. Randomised trial of

irinotecan plus supportive care versus supportive care alone after fluorouracil failure for patients with metastatic colorectal cancer. Lancet 1998;352:1413–1418.

164. Zalcberg JR, Cunningham D, Van Cutsem E, et al. ZD1694: a novel thymidylate synthase inhibitor with substantial activity in the treatment of patients with advanced colorectal cancer. J Clin Oncol 1996;14:716–721.

165. Kerr DJ. Clinical efficacy of Tomudex (raltitrexed) in advanced colorectal cancer. Anticancer Drugs 1997;8(suppl 2):S11–S15.

166. Rafi I, Taylor GA, Calotte JA, et al. A phase I clinical study of the novel antifolate AG337 given by a 5 day continuous infusion [Abstract]. Proc Am Assoc Cancer Res 1995;36:240.

167. Rinaldi DA, Burris HA, Dorr FA, et al. A phase I evaluation of LY231514, a novel multitargeted antifolate, administered every 21 day [Abstract]. Proc Am Soc Clin Oncol 1996;15:489.

168. Cripps MC, Burnell M, Jolivet J, et al. Phase II study of a multi-targeted antifolate (LY231514) as first-line therapy in patients with locally advanced or metastatic colorectal cancer [Abstract]. Proc Am Soc Clin Oncol 1997;16:949.

169. John W, Clark J, Burris H, et al. A phase II trial of LY231514 in patients with metastatic colorectal cancer [Abstract]. Proc Am Soc Clin Oncol 1997;16:1038.

170. Jackman AL, Kimbell R, Brown M, et al. The antitumor activity of ZD9331, a non-polyglutamatable quinazoline thymidylate synthase inhibitor. Adv Exp Med Biol 1995;370:185–188.

171. Pazdur R. New agents for colorectal cancers: oral fluorinated pyrimidines and oxaliplatin In: Perry MC, ed. American Society of Clinical Oncology educational book. Philadelphia: Saunders, 1998:300–310.

172. De Gramant A, Vignaud J, Tournigand C, et al. Oxaliplatin with high dose leucovorin and 5-fluorouracil 48 hour continuous infusion in pretreated metastatic colorectal cancer. Eur J Cancer 1997;33:214–219.

173. Extra JM, Espie M, Calvo J, et al. Phase I study of oxaliplatin in patients with advanced cancer. Cancer Chemother Pharmacol 1990;25:299–303.

174. Becouarn Y, Ychou M, Ducruex M, et al. Oxaliplatin (L-OHP) as first-line chemotherapy I metastatic colorectal cancer (MCRC) patients: preliminary activity/toxicity report [Abstract]. Proc Am Soc Clin Oncol 1997;16:229.

175. Nelson NJ. Inhibitors of angiogenesis enter phase III testing. J Natl Cancer Inst 1998;90:960–963.

CHAPTER

10

FOLLOW-UP AFTER TREATMENT OF COLON CANCER

WAYNE DE VOS M.D., PH.D.

After curative resection of colon cancer, 30 to 40% of patients will develop a recurrence (1,2), the majority of which will occur in the first 2 postoperative years. The most common locations where cancer is found after curative resection are the liver, lungs, remaining colon, and previous site of resection; thus these areas are the most commonly surveyed in any given follow-up program. The argument for surveillance after curative resection of colon cancer is based on the supposition that timely discovery of asymptomatic recurrent cancer significantly improves survival. Two important points in this statement bear clarification. First, to truly benefit from surveillance, the patient must be asymptomatic at the time of discovery. Timely discovery of symptomatic cancer is not a benefit of scheduled follow-up, because this group of patients will identify themselves without any surveillance efforts. Second, the end point of measuring success of any surveillance method is survival: not the number of patients found to have recurrent cancer or the number of patients taken back to the operating room for a second, "curative" operation,

Colon and Rectal Cancer, Edited by Peter S. Edelstein, M.D.
ISBN 0-471-35145-8

but rather the number of patients who live a significant length of time beyond what would be expected without surveillance.

Unfortunately, when these basic criteria are applied to the literature, and compared to the results of either no follow-up or follow-up based on symptomatic recurrence, essentially no study has proven that postoperative surveillance for asymptomatic recurrence of colon cancer has anything other than an anecdotal effect on survival (1,3–5). The reason for this is not clear: It may relate to the studies themselves, most of which are hampered by small size, retrospective approach, lack of control groups, and short follow-up, or it may relate to a lack of understanding of the biology of adenocarcinoma of the colon, particularly with respect to mechanisms of metastasis. Nonetheless, despite the inability of researchers to prove that any one method of surveillance significantly improves survival, what is shown in the many publications is reasonable proof that some method of follow-up is appropriate for most patients, and that a nihilistic approach is not necessary or acceptable for the majority of potentially cured patients.

In addition, what is rarely mentioned in print, but what is most likely very important to the individual patient, is not only the quantity of life but also the quality of life after resection. The quality of life in a patient with recurrent and incurable disease may be significantly improved by the "act of follow-up"—that is, awareness in the patient that he or she is in the care of a professional trained to find recurrence at the earliest possible instance (of course, return visits may also serve negatively to remind the patient of his or her diagnosis)—and by timely and palliative, though not lifespan-extending, surgery or interventions. Also, while medicolegal concerns should not be the sole motivation for a particular method of care, establishment of some pattern of postoperative follow-up may be important to avoid possible feelings of abandonment, particularly in patients who develop recurrence.

Balanced against these arguments supporting follow-up is the tremendous cost of postoperative surveillance, ever an increasing concern in today's health care arena, and the cost (both financial and in terms of patient risk) of more advanced diagnostic studies and procedures that are used to further evaluate false-positive basic surveillance tests. Simply put, for postoperative surveillance of colon cancer to be reasonably implemented, it must show a significant benefit to the population at a reasonable cost and with acceptable risk to the patient.

METHODS OF POSTOPERATIVE SURVEILLANCE

The techniques and tools potentially available for postoperative surveillance include interval history and physical examination, endoscopy, chest radiography, laboratory analyses, and CT. Additional testing implemented when recurrence is suspected includes immunoscintigraphy and PET scanning. Each may play a small or a more expanded role in an individual patient's care, depending on the original operation, the stage of the tumor, and the health of the patient.

HISTORY AND PHYSICAL EXAMINATION

After curative resection of a colon cancer, the median length of time to recurrence is 22 months, with 60 to 80% of recurrences being found in the first 2 years, and 90% occurring within 4 years after initial resection (6,7). Optimal frequency of follow-up has been evaluated in numerous studies; unfortunately, more frequent follow-up has not been shown to have a significant effect on survival (1,5). Although frequent scheduled patient visits have been shown to detect recurrent cancer earlier than patient visits based solely on the development of symptoms, frequent scheduled visits have never been shown to increase resectability or patient survival. Also, although intense follow-up has been shown to increase the odds of a second, attempted curative excision, this has not been shown to translate into increased survival. Nonetheless, follow-up in the office is reasonable for the following reasons. (1) Between 1 and 2% of the patients in the surveyed group will ultimately have their life prolonged significantly after resection of a recurrent tumor. (2) The majority of patients can be reasonably assured during these physician interactions that they do not have recurrent cancer. (3) In the event of unresectable recurrence, palliation may be more successfully achieved with earlier onset of therapy. (4) The office visits provide a framework around which other components of postoperative surveillance can be managed, such as laboratory testing, radiologic studies, and endoscopic examinations. (5) Finally, some studies have supported an increase in the incidence of other neoplasms in patients with a history of colon cancer, such as breast, endometrial, ovarian, and intestinal tract other than colon or rectum (8). The increased contact with medical staff during scheduled follow-up visits may increase early discovery of these neoplasms.

Because the majority of recurrences are found in the first two postoperative years, early follow-up should be more intense than later follow-up (9). A common schedule of office visits after the patient has recovered from surgery is quarterly for 2 years, then every 6 months for 3 years, followed by yearly visits for the rest of the patient's life. During each office visit, an interval history should be taken and should include information about changes in bowel habits, new symptoms, and changes in constitution. During the physical examination, particular attention should be directed toward the abdominal examination, including a careful palpation of the liver and inspection of the incision. If the anastomosis is located at or below the rectosigmoid junction, rigid proctosigmoidoscopy should be performed regularly at these visits, with careful inspection of the anastomosis.

ROUTINE LABORATORY STUDIES

Elevation of liver function tests (LFTs) has been shown to correlate with growth of metastatic tumor within the liver. However, although

LFTs are often included in postoperative surveillance programs, they do not greatly add to the results of simple clinical evaluation, because significant LFT elevation generally occurs only in the presence of unresectable malignant replacement of the liver parenchyma (10). In addition, specificity of LFT elevation is poor, potentially leading to unnecessary further testing. This is also true for CBC: although a patient with postoperative anemia should certainly be followed until normal counts return, recurrent anemia is rarely an indicator of recurrent or metachronous cancer in the absence of other clinical or laboratory findings. Thus the routine evaluation of simple blood count and liver chemistry levels is not indicated in the follow-up of colon cancer.

CARCINOEMBRYONIC ANTIGEN

Carcinoembryonic antigen (CEA) was first described as a possible marker for gastrointestinal malignancies by Gold and Freedman (11) in 1965. CEA, however, was also found to be elevated in a variety of common benign conditions and in smokers and to be only inconsistently increased in the presence of cancer. Thus CEA is unfit for use as a screening tool. Nevertheless, other characteristics of CEA levels with colon cancer have supported its use in postoperative surveillance. For example, many publications have shown a clear relationship between preoperatively elevated CEA levels and risk of recurrence (12). In patients with an elevated preoperative CEA, postoperative return to normal is a reasonable assurance that a curative resection has been performed. Furthermore, a significant persistent increase in CEA after curative resection has been demonstrated to be significantly correlated with recurrence, and an increase in CEA levels usually precedes clinical symptoms by 5 to 7 months (13,14).

Unfortunately, the utility of following postoperative CEA levels is at best not clear, and although some studies have shown a significant increase in the odds of reoperation for attempted cure when serial CEA levels are monitored (13,15), translation into actual improved survival when compared to clinically directed reoperation for cure has not been demonstrated (15–17). In addition, a significant percentage of patients may have false-positive test results, leading to unnecessary testing, attempted biopsy, and even reoperation (18–20). And although the cost of following CEA levels in any one individual is small, the actual cost per asymptomatic recurrence discovered and re-resected for cure may rise into the millions of dollars, making the cost-effectiveness of regular CEA testing unclear.

No other readily available, inexpensive test is available that detects recurrences earlier or with a higher rate of resectability for cure than CEA analysis. And although the number of patients actually helped by following serial CEA levels is extremely small, long-term survival is possible in this very limited patient population. The most common pattern of CEA determination involves preoperative testing and then postoperative testing at 3-month intervals for the first 2 years, 6-month intervals for the next 2 years, and then yearly thereafter. Any increase in the value is followed by a repeat CEA test 1 month later. An increase in the CEA level on two consecutive dates warrants further evaluation to rule out recurrence. Unfortunately, in patients whose CEA is not elevated preoperatively, the role of postoperative CEA surveillance is even less clear.

Chest X-Ray

Approximately 10% of all patients with colorectal adenocarcinoma will develop isolated lung metastases (4,20), and of these patients, approximately 10% will have isolated lesions amenable to attempted curative resection. Because thoracotomy for limited pulmonary metastatic lesions is well tolerated and can lead to 5-year survival rates of 30 to 35%, an annual chest x-ray is believed by many clinicians to be appropriate for detecting the few patients who may have isolated spread to the lungs (6,7). However, it is again important to emphasize that only 1% of all colorectal cancer patients will develop pulmonary metastases that are resectable for cure; of these patients, at best 35% will actually be cured. Thus the cost-benefit ratio of an annual chest x-ray is questionable.

COLONOSCOPY

Anastomotic recurrence is more common after resection in rectal cancer patients than in colon cancer patients. For colon cancer, it is a rare finding on follow-up endoscopy. When discovered, it most often represents local ingrowth of recurrent disease external to the bowel rather than a true anastomotic origin and thus is a poor prognostic indicator. Therefore, postoperative colonoscopy for colon cancer patients is completed primarily for the detection of synchronous and metachronous precancerous and invasive lesions.

Significant support for the use of polyp clearance in the prevention of colorectal cancer was provided by Winawer et al. (21), indirectly supporting the theory that clearance of polyps postresection will also decrease the risk of recurrent colon cancer (new lesions). The development of adenomatous polyps has been found to occur in 10 to 56% of patients treated for adenocarcinoma (7,22,23). Khoury et al. (24) in their follow-up of 389 patients with colon cancer found that the risk for finding polyps on initial postoperative colonoscopy was 18.3%; subsequently, after a negative colonoscopy, the risk fell to 10.4%, but after a positive colonoscopy, the risk for finding polyps at a subsequent examination rose to 43%, with a risk of 70.4% if multiple polyps were found. Therefore, the presence of multiple synchronous polyps warrants repeat colonoscopy at an early postoperative interval, such as within 3 to 6 months. Also, the presence of synchronous adenomatous polyps at the time of cancer resection has been shown to be a strong predictor of metachronous polyps (7); therefore, detection of polyps on colonoscopy in the 1st postoperative year is an important initiator of surveillance for metachronous polyps. If polyps are found, repeat endoscopy should be completed 1 to 2 years later. The subsequent schedule should be determined by the pathology present in the particular patient: If polyps < 1 cm or few in number are found, the interval can be lengthened to every 3 to 5 years; however, the discovery of multiple or large (> 1 cm) polyps at any endoscopic procedure warrants repeat colonoscopy at an earlier interval, such as within 6 months to 2 years, depending on the ability of the endoscopist to remove all of the polyps.

Generally, the risk for synchronous invasive lesions, as shown by discovery of a second carcinoma in the first 1 to 2 years, is thought to be 2 to 8% (23,25). Therefore, if endoscopic evaluation cannot be completed before the initial planned resection, colonoscopy should follow segmental colon resection for malignancy within 3 to 6 months. If complete colonoscopy is possible preoperatively, a repeat examination should be scheduled approximately 1 year postoperatively to rule out missed precancerous or invasive lesions.

Multiple studies have demonstrated an increased risk for metachronous invasive lesions after colon cancer resection. Based on a retrospective study of > 5400 patients, Cali et al. (26) calculated the annual risk of a second primary adenocarcinoma of the colon to be 0.35%, with a cumulative risk of 6.3% at 18 years. An overall risk of 2 to 4.5% in the 20 years after resection found in other studies supports this estimate (6,27–29). Nonetheless, in spite of this identified increased risk, demonstration of improved survival with close surveillance by endoscopy has been difficult, as demonstrated by a study showing that yearly postoperative surveillance by colonoscopy, liver CT, and chest radiography did not alter 5-year survival in patients with colorectal cancer (20). However, that study, like most others that emanate from single institutions, is limited by small numbers: For instance, in the 5-year follow-up of 325 patients, only eight metachronous colon lesions were found on colonoscopy, only one of which was found by scheduled screening endoscopy in the absence of symptoms or clinical abnormalities. Also, long-term follow-up is lacking in most studies, and the efficacy of polypectomy during postresection surveillance is not addressed. Therefore, although definitive proof either supporting or disproving the use of postoperative colonoscopy in improving survival is not available, basing practice on what is acceptable for patients with a moderately increased risk of colon cancer would seem reasonable: colonoscopy every 1 to 3 years in the presence of recurrent polyps, and every 5 years after repeat examination shows durable clearance (30).

COMPUTERIZED TOMOGRAPHY

As a surveillance tool, CT scan of the abdomen with special attention to the liver and lymphatics has been found to have poor utility in screening for metastases. In a study by Sugarbaker et al. (18), only 2 of 33 recurrences were demonstrated initially on CT scan in the absence of other symptoms or signs of recurrence, and a high false-positive rate of 45% was found. Shoemaker et al. (20) found that, although annual CT scans did increase detection of asymptomatic liver metastases, resection rate was not significantly different when compared to a group in which CT scan was performed only in the presence of suspected disease (symptoms or abnormal screening tests).

A more appropriate role for CT scan of the abdomen and pelvis after curative resection of colon cancer is that of a secondary evaluation test following the onset of new symptoms or the detection of abnormal screening tests, such as persistently elevated CEA levels, that suggest metastatic disease. In this context, significant information regarding resectability may be obtained. Also, CT-guided fine-needle aspiration may often be performed to confirm malignancy in equivocal radiographic lesions.

SECOND-LOOK OPERATION

In 1949, Wangensteen et al. (31) introduced the concept of blind re-exploration at a specific interval after curative colorectal cancer resection in an attempt to decrease the incidence of disease recurrence. However, the procedure did not gain popularity because operative mortality was significant, 50% of patients had negative laparotomies, and long-term survival was poor (6.2% at 5 years). More recently, with the identification of the biologic marker CEA, this approach has regained attention (13,15,32). Using progressive elevation of CEA levels as an indicator of recurrent disease, negative exploration is significantly reduced and long-term survival in the subgroup of patients re-resected for attempted cure is significantly increased compared to patients with unresectable disease. For example, in the study by Hida et al. (32), a negative laparotomy occurred in only 1 of 72 patients re-explored, and 5-year survival for the resectable and unresectable recurrence groups was 41.3 and 5.2%, respectively. Unfortunately, however, even in this carefully selected group (50% of patients with suspected recurrence did not go to surgery secondary to determination of unresectable disease preoperatively), almost half of re-explored patients were found to have unresectable disease. New methods of preoperative determination of resectability (see below) will possibly allow better screening of patients and a decrease in reoperation for unresectable disease.

SECONDARY TESTING

Following determination of abnormal screening tests or the onset of suspicious symptoms, identification of colon cancer recurrence may elude clinical examination and standard testing modalities. Furthermore, the identification of recurrence and the decision regarding reoperation may be stalled in a given patient secondary to concern regarding unidentified malignant disease that would make any reoperation for cure futile and, therefore, unnecessary. In this context, further evaluation with one or more of the following testing modalities may be appropriate.

COMPUTERIZED TOMOGRAPHY

After the appearance of a new, solid lesion on chest x-ray, a chest CT should be completed to better characterize the abnormality and the remainder of the lung parenchyma. If indicated, CT-guided biopsy can be completed to assist in the diagnosis. It is important to remember that in up to half of such cases, the newly detected lung lesion is of pulmonary origin.

When suspicion for intra-abdominal recurrence arises, as in the context of a consistently elevated CEA, unexplained weight loss, or abdominal pain, an abdominal and pelvic CT scan should be obtained. Size, number, and location of lesions can be determined in the majority of patients with hepatic metastases. Also, evidence of local recurrence may be obtained, although differentiation from postoperative changes and scar tissue may be difficult.

RADIOIMMUNOSCINTIGRAPHY

The development of monoclonal antibody (MAb) technology has allowed for the application of tumor-specific radiolabeled probes in the investigation of metastatic disease. Three such monoclonal antibodies are CEA-Scan (Immunomedics, Morris Plains, N.J.), Oncoscint (Cytogen Corp., Princeton, N.J.), and HumaSPECT-Tc (Intracel Corp. Rockville, Md.). Radioimmunoscintigraphy (RIS) is more sensitive and specific than CT scanning (33,34). MAb technology is particularly useful in the patient in whom recurrence is suspected but cannot be detected using conventional techniques (e.g., the patient with rising CEA but a negative CT scan), recurrence is not suspected but examination detects abnormalities (e.g., the patient with thickening and scarring in the region of the previous resection but otherwise normal screening studies), and apparently resectable recurrence is identified but there is suspicion that nonresectable metastatic disease also exists (e.g., the patient with resectable liver metastasis but also with bulky retroperitoneal lymphadenopathy). Wolf et al. (34) compared HumaSPECT-Tc, a totally human MAb, with CT scanning in the evaluation of 219 patients with recurrent or metastatic disease. In patients with identified disease, they found that HumaSPECT-Tc was significantly more accurate in predicting nonresectability than CT scan (60 vs. 29%), although CT and HumaSPECT-Tc were essentially equivalent in predicting resectability in this group (98 vs. 91%). In patients with occult disease, HumaSPECT-Tc was significantly better at predicting resectability or nonresectability than CT scan (68 vs. 24%). Unfortunately, a relatively high false-negative rate limits the current clinical applicability of this test, particularly when compared to PET. However, it is more widely available than PET, and its current clinical indication is in two groups of patients: for patients with recurrent, apparently resectable disease, RIS will help identify the significant subset of patients with occult, nonresectable disease (up to half of whom would otherwise return to the operating room for attempted curative reoperation) and for patients with rising CEA levels but with unidentifiable disease based on conventional studies.

Positron Emission Tomography

PET is a method of imaging that takes advantage of the increased metabolism of tumor cells by using a positron-emitting isotope-labeled compound that is incorporated into a biochemical process within the body. Flanagan et al. (35) analyzed the utility of PET in the evaluation of 22 patients with rising CEA levels but unidentified disease using conventional techniques (including CT scan). They found a positive predictive value of 89% (15 of 17 patients) and a negative predictive value of 100% (5 of 5 patients) for PET. Several other studies have supported this high accuracy in determining unresectability and differentiating recurrent tumor from benign tissue (36). The best role for this expensive and time-consuming study is not yet clear, and further studies comparing PET to monoclonal antibody techniques are required to answer this question. Nonetheless, at this time, similar to RIS, PET may be useful to rule out the presence of nonresectable metastasis before exploration when radical reoperation is anticipated for identified disease and to identify suspected recurrent disease not demonstrable by conventional studies.

CONCLUSION

Unfortunately, current methods of postoperative surveillance for recurrent or metachronous malignancy after curative resection benefit only 1 to 2% of colon cancer patients and may lead to unnecessary testing and procedures in patients either without true recurrence or with incurable disease. New technologies currently under investigation may help identify patients who will most benefit from more aggressive care. In addition, more evaluation is needed to determine whether selective surveillance for patients at higher risk of recurrence can be more cost-effective without the sacrifice of quality patient care. It is likely that the best approach to determining which techniques will be beneficial in the follow-up of colon cancer patients will be enrollment in clinical trials.

REFERENCES

1. Bruinvels DL, Stiggelbout AM, Kievet J, et al. Follow-up of patients with colorectal cancer: a meta-analysis. Ann Surg 1994;219:174–182.
2. Richard CS, McLeod RS. Follow-up of patients after resection of colorectal cancer. A position paper of the Canadian Society of Surgical Oncology and Canadian Society of Colon and Rectal Surgeons. Can J Surg 1997;40:90–100.
3. Tornqvist A, Ekeland G, Leandoer L. The value of intensive follow-up after curative resection for colorectal carcinoma. Br J Surg 1982;69:725–728.
4. Safi F, Link KH, Begar HG. Is follow-up of colorectal cancer patients worthwhile? Dis Colon Rectum 1993;36:636–644.

5. Kjeldsen BJ, Kronberg O, Fenger C, Jorgensen OD. A prospective randomized study of follow-up after radical surgery for colorectal cancer. Br J Surg 1997;84:666–669.
6. Gordon PH and Nivatvongs S. Principles and practice of surgery for the colon, rectum and anus. Quality Medical Publishing, 2nd ed. 1999.
7. Chen F, Stuart M. Colonoscopic follow-up of colorectal carcinoma. Dis Colon Rectum 1994;37:568–572.
8. Enblad P, Adami H-O, Glimelius B, et al. The risk of subsequent primary malignant diseases after cancers of the colon and rectum. Cancer 1990;65:2091–2100.
9. Steele G Jr. Follow-up plans after treatment of primary colon and rectal cancer. World J Surg 1991;15:583–588.
10. Nicholls RJ, Dozois RR. Surgery of the colon and rectum. XX: Churchill Livingstone, 1997.
11. Gold P, Freedman SO. Demonstration of tumor specific antigens in human colonic carcinomata by immunological tolerance and absorption techniques. J Exp Med 1965;121:439–462.
12. Wang JY, Tang R, Chiang JM. Value of carcinoembryonic antigen in the management of colorectal cancer. Dis Colon Rectum 1994;37:272–277.
13. Martin EW, Cooperman M, Carey LC, Minton JP. Sixty second-look procedures indicated primarily by rise in serial carcinoembryonic antigen. J Surg Res 1980;28:389–394.
14. Hine KR, Dykes PW. Serum CEA testing in the post-operative surveillance of colorectal carcinoma. Br J Cancer 1984;49:689–693.
15. Minton JP, Hoehn JL, Gerber DM, et al. Results of a 400-patient carcinoembryonic antigen second-look colorectal cancer study. Cancer 1985;55:1284–1290.
16. Beart RW, O'Connell MJ. Postoperative follow-up of patients with carcinoma of the colon. Mayo Clin Proc 1983;58:361–363.
17. Moertel CG, Fleming TR, MacDonald JS, et al. An evaluation of the carcinoembryonic antigen (CEA) test for monitoring patients with resected colon cancer. JAMA 1993;270:943--947.
18. Sugarbaker PH, Gianola FJ, Dwyer A, Neuman NR. A simplified plan for follow-up of patients with colon and rectal cancer supported by prospective studies of laboratory and radiologic test results. Surgery 1987;102:79–87.
19. DeVesa JM, Morales V, Enriquez JM, et al. Colorectal cancer: the bases for a comprehensive follow-up. Dis Colon Rectum 1988;31:636–652.

20. Schoemaker D, Black R, Giles L, Toouli J. Yearly colonoscopy, liver CT, and chest radiography do not influence 5-year survival of colorectal cancer patients. Gastroenterology 1998;14:7–14.

21. Winawer SJ, Zauber AG, Ho MH, et al. Prevention of colorectal cancer by colonoscopic polypectomy. N Engl J Med 1993;329:1977–1981.

22. Koppel M, Bailar JC, Waekley FL, Shimkin MB. Incidence of cancer in the colon and rectum among polyp-free patients. Dis Colon Rectum 1962;5:439–455.

23. Barlow AP, Thompson MH. Colonoscopic follow-up after resection for colorectal cancer: a selective policy. Br J Surg 1993;80:781–784.

24. Khoury DA, Opelka FG, Beck DE, et al. Colon surveillance after colorectal cancer surgery. Dis Colon Rectum 1996;39:252–256.

25. Cunliffe WJ, Hasleton PS, Tweedle DE, Schofield PF. Incidence of synchronous and metachronous colorectal carcinoma. Br J Surg 1984;71:941–943.

26. Cali RL, Pitsch RM, Thorson AG, et al. Cumulative incidence of metachronous colorectal cancer. Dis Colon Rectum 1993;36:388–353.

27. Luchtefeld MA, Ross DS, Zander JD, Folse JR. Late development of metachronous colorectal cancer. Dis Colon Rectum 1987;30:180–184.

28. Heald RJ, Bussey HJR. Clinical experience at St. Mark's Hospital with multiple synchronous cancers of the colon and rectum. Dis Colon Rectum 1975;18:6–10.

29. Lautenbach E, Forde KA, Neugut AN. Benefits of colonoscopic surveillance after curative resection of colorectal cancer. Ann Surg 1994;220:206–211.

30. Simmang CL, Senatore P, Lowry A, et al. Practice parameters for detection of colorectal neoplasms. Dis Colon Rectum 1999;42:1123–1129.

31. Wangensteen OH, Lewis FJ, Tongen LA. The "second-look" in cancer surgery. Lancet 1951;71:303–307.

32. Hida J, Yasutomi M, Shindoa K, et al. Second-look operation for recurrent colorectal cancer based on carcinoembryonic antigen and imaging techniques. Dis Colon Rectum 1996;39:74–79.

33. Lange MK, Martin EW. Monoclonal antibodies in imaging and therapy of colorectal cancer. World J Surg 1991;15:617–622.

34. Wolf BG, Bolton J, Baum R, et al. Radioimmunoscintigraphy of recurrent, metastatic or occult colorectal cancer with technetium Tc 99m 88BV59H21-2V67-66 (HumaSPECT-Tc), a totally human monoclonal antibody. Patient management benefit from a phase III multicenter study. Dis Colon Rectum 1998;41:953–962.

35. Flanagan FL, Dehdashti F, Ogunbiyi OA, et al. Utility of FDG-PET for investigating unexplained plasma CEA elevation in patients with colorectal cancer. Ann Surg 1998;227:319–323.

36. Tempero M, Brand R, Holdeman K, Matamoros A. New imaging techniques in colorectal cancer. Semin Oncol 1995;22:448–471.

PART

III

ADENOCARCINOMA OF THE RECTUM

CHAPTER

11

PATIENT PRESENTATION AND PRETREATMENT EVALUATION OF RECTAL ADENOCARCINOMA

PETER S. EDELSTEIN, M.D.

Although anatomically contiguous, the colon and the rectum give rise to adenocarcinomas with unique and differing natural histories and, as a result, frequently require altogether different treatment strategies. Thus, as discussed in Chapter 7, colon cancer virtually always is initially treated with surgical resection. The use of adjuvant therapy for colon cancer patients depends on the pathologic evaluation of the surgical specimen and usually is in the form of chemotherapy alone. Radiation therapy is reserved for the rare cases of colon cancer in which a locally advanced tumor is present and the surgical margins of resection are in doubt. Local recurrence is an extremely uncommon event after resection of colon cancer, and the majority of cancer-related mortalities are secondary to metastatic disease. Rectal adenocarcinoma is an entirely different entity. By virtue of its location, trapped within the bones of the pelvis, wide excision of anything greater than the rectum and its mesentary is fraught with operative risks and clinical sequellae. Thus at present,

Colon and Rectal Cancer, Edited by Peter S. Edelstein, M.D.
ISBN 0-471-35145-8

total mesorectal excision (TME) with wide lateral margins is the most aggressive initial resection usually performed for rectal cancer. The risk of local recurrence, rarely a concern with colon cancer, is all too frequently encountered in rectal cancer patients and is a source of both patient death and significant symptomatic morbidity.

Another significant difference between colon and rectal cancer concerns the not infrequent need to create a permanent colostomy for patients whose tumors originate very distally within the rectal vault. Even when a low coloanal anastomosis is performed after complete proctectomy, functional outcome is a major concern, especially if the neorectum (the portion of the sigmoid or descending colon that has been anastomosed to the proximal anal canal and acts as a reservoir) is subjected to adjuvant radiation therapy, creating an injured, permanently stiffened neorectal conduit. Such concerns rarely exist after colonic resection, which with the occasional exception of mild diarrhea, usually leads to no significant permanent quality of life issues after recovery.

Thus as is outlined in several chapters within this text, the approach to treatment of rectal cancer has already changed significantly and continues to evolve. For numerous reasons, including the potential for performing sphincter-sparing rectal resection, increased resectability of large tumors, avoidance of radiation injury to the neorectum after resection and reanastomosis, the possibility of decreasing lymphatic and small venous spread of tumor at the time of surgical resection, and the potential for increased tumor toxicity in the presence of undisturbed tumor blood flow, neoadjuvant therapy (the delivery of radiation to the pelvis and possibly limited chemotherapy before surgical resection) has become the mainstay approach to the treatment of stage II and III rectal cancers. Furthermore, some stage I lesions are actually amenable to curative treatment either via transanal excision or using endocavitary (transanal) irradiation.

Yet to identify patients who would benefit from neoadjuvant therapy before surgery or to select those appropriate for local curative treatment approaches, it is vital to accurately stage each patient's disease. Inaccurate staging can be problematic and even disastrous when, for example, patients who do not truly require radiation are overstaged and receive treatment, patients who do require radiation are understaged and then suffer the sequellae of postoperative irradiation, and when understaged patients undergo local treatment when metastatic lymph nodes were not identified. Therefore, unlike colon cancer patients, it is crucial for patients who are diagnosed with adenocarcinoma of the rectum and are, therefore, possible candidates for neoadjuvant therapy or local treatments to be accurately and completely staged before the initiation of any treatment. Although this chapter also discusses the presentation of patients suffering from rectal cancer, it focuses on current methods to achieve this accurate pretreatment disease staging.

PATIENT PRESENTATION

The demographics of patients with colorectal cancer were presented in Chapter 3. Likewise, specific high-risk groups, such as those suffering from inflammatory bowel disease, familial adenomatous polyposis, and hereditary nonpolyposis colorectal cancer (Lynch Syndromes), are discussed elsewhere in this work. This section describes presenting symptoms and signs of sporadic rectal cancer in patients with no known risk factors for the disease.

Unlike colon cancer, in which bowel obstruction is commonly a presenting symptom (especially with left-sided lesions), true complete bowel obstruction rarely occurs secondary to rectal cancer. This is likely owing to several factors, among which is the significant capacity of the rectal vault and the exophytic, noncircumferential growth pattern displayed by most rectal lesions. These and other factors make total bowel obstruction uncommon, at least until a lesion becomes massive enough to obstruct either the rectum itself or, in the case of distal lesions, the anal canal. However, partial obstruction likely plays the major causal role in the second most common presenting complaint of patients suffering from rectal cancer, altered bowel habits. Diarrhea, constipation, and an alternating pattern of the two are frequently associated with this neoplasm. While secretory activity by the neoplasm, especially those with a villous component, may contribute to the genesis of diarrhea, partial mechanical obstruction is likely the major cause of both diarrhea and constipation. Even mild narrowing of stool caliber may indicate the presence of a partially obstructing lesion. The change in habits is often of several weeks or longer duration and may be subtle, given the normal variability of bowel habits within the general population. Unfortunately, even when a patient finally becomes aware and then concerned about such seemingly innocuous bowel habit changes, all too frequently the evaluating physician initially fails to do more than perform a digital examination and then provide reassurance. It is crucial that in any normal-risk patient, and particularly in those aged 50 and older, the physician take such subtle complaints seriously and perform a more extensive large bowel evaluation.

Anyone who cares for rectal cancer patients routinely hears those patients state, "The doctor told me that the bleeding was from hemorrhoids." These words can serve as the battle cry of negligent medical care, because in most cases such physician reassurance is not based on anoscopic identification of bleeding hemorrhoids and, in fact, is often delivered without even the performance of a digital rectal examination. It is all too common to find an obvious distal rectal mass on digital examination in a patient whose bright red rectal bleeding has for months been attributed by a physician to hemorrhoids. Even in the presence of hemorrhoids, the physician must be highly suspicious of a slightly more proximal cause for bright red bleeding, especially if the visualized hemorrhoids do not appear friable. Rectal bleeding is, in fact, the most frequent presenting symptom of rectal cancer, occurring in 35 to 40% of patients. The fact that this symptom is also commonly associated with a variety of benign anorectal diseases should never lessen its potential significance.

Rectal or pelvic pain is an uncommon presenting symptom and often signals extensive growth of the tumor with posterior compression or invasion of the sacrum. Tenesemus, the continuous sensation of the need to strain or defecate, also frequently signals the presence of a larger lesion. Fecal incontinence is an infrequent complaint that is associated with high-grade obstruction or interference with the anal sphincter either by growth through the anal canal or invasion into the musculature. On rare occasions, a rectal cancer will perforate, with the subsequent development of a malignant perirectal abscess or fistula. Thus a fistula that fails to heal and the anatomy of which does not mimic that of a routine benign cryptoglandular fistula should raise physician suspicion and lead to aggressive evaluation, including biopsy. Another malignant fistula, a rectovaginal fistula, is, fortunately, a rare presentation. Weight loss is an unusual presenting symptom in an unobstructed patient and is of concern for the presence of metastatic disease. Finally, some rectal tumors are asymptomatic, discovered only during routine physical examination or screening flexible sigmoidoscopy.

INITIAL EVALUATION

Although many of the most common presenting symptoms of rectal cancer are far from specific for malignant disease (bleeding, constipation, diarrhea), the failure to identify rectal cancer in patients with these nonspecific initial complaints is most frequently the fault of the evaluating physician. First, the physician must always include rectal neoplasia in the differential of such common symptoms, even in relatively young patients. And until an obvious cause is identified to explain the symptoms, the physician must continue to consider cancer as a possibility. Furthermore, many rectal cancers are palpable on adequate digital examination. The fact that such lesions are commonly missed on the initial digital examination underlines the reality that many physicians perform a suboptimal rectal examination, often hastily slipping their fingers in and out of the anal canal, never feeling more proximally or fully evaluating the distal rectum, especially where it falls away posteriorly just above the puborectalis muscle. Such a limited, poorly performed digital examination is unacceptable and has been the source of more than one case of medical litigation.

In some patients, the only evidence of a rectal carcinoma will be an irregular area surrounded by soft, smooth mucosa or an area of mild stenosis. However, in the overwhelming majority of palpable cancers, the tumor is unmistakable, presenting either as a large, exophytic mass or as an area of firm, deep ulceration, often surrounded in a crater-like fashion by a firm, raised edge. Once a lesion is identified, the digital evaluation should include an assessment of the location of the lesion (especially, in the case of exophytic lesions, the base of the growth within the mucosa) relative to the upper sphincter musculature; the prostate or vagina: and the posterior, left, and right rectum. Also, the mobility or fixity of the growth, tenderness with palpation, and if possible, the upper and lateral extent of the mass should be digitally evaluated. In female patients with anterior rectal cancers, a combined digital rectal and posterior vaginal examination may provide valuable information concerning vaginal wall involvement.

It is crucial that flexible endoscopy not be exclusively relied on to determine the location of the tumor relative to the anal verge. Flexible scopes, by definition, bend, and every experienced surgeon has cared for a patient whose tumor was actually located significantly more distally than suggested by flexible endoscopy. Thus it is crucial that early on, a rigid proctoscopy is performed to determine the true location of the lesion relative to the anal verge. The location of the distal extent of the mucosal origin of the cancer, the proximal extent, the circumferential involvement, and the morphologic characteristics of the lesion can be clearly demonstrated with accurate, rigid measurements. Such information is critical for identifying lesions that might be appropriate for local treatments, such as transanal excision or endocavitary irradiation, and for determining the possibility of sphincter salvage with and without neoadjuvant therapy.

SECONDARY EVALUATION

After the palpation or visualization of a rectal cancer, much of the pretreatment patient evaluation is similar to that recommended for patients with colon cancer. A detailed history, including family history of any neoplasia, should be obtained. A review of systems should specifically attempt to elicit cancer-related complaints on which the patient might not be focused, such as fatigue, weight loss, and bone or abdominal pain. A complete physical examination must be performed, again with attention focused on both potential sites of metastases (liver) and on those systems that will be crucial for perioperative recovery (such as cardiovascular and pulmonary). A detailed discussion of the preoperative evaluation of systems other than the gastrointestinal tract was presented in Chapter 7. Those recommendations similarly apply to the pretreatment (especially the preoperative) evaluation of rectal cancer patients if not more so, given the greater morbidity and mortality associated with the surgical and adjuvant treatments of rectal malignancies. Likewise, laboratory evaluation, such as a CBC, liver function tests, and carcinoembryonic antigen (CEA) levels, should be obtained. Chest radiographs are also recommended, but as in the case of colon cancer, these studies are actually more useful for identifying cardiopulmonary abnormalities that may have an effect on perioperative care than for identifying pulmonary metastases, given the actual rarity of isolated pulmonary metastases at the time of initial rectal cancer diagnosis.

Once a rectal cancer is identified, a thorough examination of the large bowel is required only to more fully evaluate the primary growth but also to identify (and possibly treat) any synchronous polyps and, less commonly, synchronous cancers. Colonoscopy is usually the procedure of choice to achieve these goals, although flexible sigmoidoscopy followed by double-contrast barium enema is still an acceptable alternative. Needless to say, if any synchronous lesion is identified on barium enema, the patient must then be subjected to a colonoscopy. Given the frequency of synchronous polyps (as high as 60% for all colorectal malignancies) and even cancers (2 to 5%), most physicians prefer to perform the initial large bowel evaluation with colonoscopy, which allows for immediate therapeutic intervention.

DISEASE STAGING

The greatest difference between the initial evaluation of rectal cancer and colon cancer patients concerns the need for accurate pretreatment staging in these two groups. As discussed in chapter 7, initial treatment of colon cancer patients is invariably surgical regardless of disease stage, given that the vast majority of colon tumors are or will rapidly become symptomatic; and thus even in stage IV disease, bowel resection offers the best form of palliation. Furthermore, intraoperative ultrasonography has repeatedly been demonstrated to be the most accurate means of identifying hepatic metastases. In addition, in my experience with 88 colon cancer patients, preoperative staging with CT scanning had no significant effect on the operation performed. For all of these reasons, in colon cancer patients for whom there is no clinical suspicion of metastatic disease, radiographic staging is unnecessary, because the initial treatment is surgical combined with intraoperative staging via liver ultrasonography.

As alluded to in the introduction to this chapter and as is addressed in several of the rectal cancer chapters, in the majority of rectal cancer cases, surgery is not recommended as the initial treatment. However, to appropriately recommend neoadjuvant therapy before resection, the patient must accurately be identified as having either stage II (T3N0M0 or T4N0M0) or stage III (T1–4N2–3M0) disease. Even in rectal cancer patients who do not require neoadjuvant therapy, accurate staging is vital to determine whether initial (and possibly total) treatment can be in the form of endocavitary irradiation or surgical resection and, if the latter, whether the approach can be transanal or via transanal endoscopic microsurgery or whether an abdominal approach is required. Failure to accurately stage rectal cancer patients can lead to serious consequences. Failure to identify hepatic metastases, for example, will lead to the sequellae of unnecessary pelvic irradiation delivered in a futile attempt to cure a stage IV patient who would most likely benefit from a simpler, less morbid form of palliation, such as local fulguration or resection. Likewise, unnecessarily irradiating the pelvis of a stage I patient owing to overstaging is also unacceptable.

Thus, unlike for colon cancer, with so many possible treatment options facing rectal cancer patients and their physicians, accurate staging in a necessity. The target of rectal cancer metastatic spread is, in the vast majority of patients, the liver. And although intraoperative ultrasonography (IOUS) is more accurate in evaluating the liver than is CT scan imaging, given that some form of metastatic evaluation is necessary before surgery in rectal cancer patients, the sensitivity and specificity of abdominal CT is high enough to use this imaging technique in the pretreatment evaluation of rectal cancer patients. Therefore, unlike in the case of colon cancer patient evaluation in which preoperative CT imaging is recommended only when laboratory or clinical suspicion of liver metastasis exists, pretreatment CT evaluation of the liver for staging is required in all patients suffering from adenocarcinoma of the rectum. The demonstration of hepatic metastases, classifying the disease as stage

IV, shifts the treatment approach from curative to palliative, usually leading to the avoidance of unnecessary preoperative chemoradiation therapy and possibly even the abandonment of major surgery, with the associated morbidities and time commitment. That is to say, why put an incurable patient through 5 to 6 weeks of pelvic irradiation and/or a major operation (possibly with a colostomy) if limited medical and/or surgical intervention will rapidly and adequately palliate the patient's symptoms and improve the quality of remaining life?

Once stage IV disease has been excluded by abdominal CT (and with the preoperative chest X-ray) and in the absence of bone pain or cerebral symptoms requiring bone scan or head MRI, respectively, attention must be turned to accurate staging of the primary lesion (T stage) and of the surrounding perirectal lymph nodes (N stage). Until endorectal ultrasonography (ERUS) was developed and refined, the CT scan was the best technique available for evaluating the extent of pelvic disease. Unfortunately, CT is so mediocre at local pelvic staging of rectal (T and N stage) that basing decisions concerning neoadjuvant therapy, endocavitary irradiation, and local versus standard excision is unacceptable. This is owing to the inability of CT to accurately demonstrate the location of the tumor within the layers of the rectal wall and to correctly identify small lymph nodes harboring metastatic deposits. ERUS represents a dramatic improvement in both of these areas of tumor staging.

To determine the T stage of the primary lesion, the level of tumor invasion within the rectal wall must be ascertained. Pelvic CT imaging routinely achieves this goal with only 70% accuracy. The accuracy of ERUS in determining the specific depth of rectal wall invasion is significantly greater, often reported to exceed 90%. This is owing to the ability of ERUS to identify the separate narrow rectal wall layers (usually five, but seven when circular and longitudinal muscles are demonstrable separately) based on the differing echogenicity of these layers (Fig. 11.1). ERUS uses a hand-held rigid probe (flexible scopes are also used), the caliber of which is narrower than a standard rigid proctoscope. The probe is gently passed into the rectum, and a balloon at the tip of the probe is inflated with water. The ERUS transducer within the center of the filled balloon rotates at one of three frequencies selected by the examiner (depending on the tissue depth at which the examiner wishes to focus). The probe is moved back and forth over the tumor so that all aspects of the lesion are imaged. Magnification and several other technical features allow the experienced examiner to accurately identify and analyze the areas of deepest rectal wall invasion and penetration. Furthermore, the intramural extent of tumor invasion can be demonstrated, as can even minuscule areas of invasion into adjacent prostate or vagina. Tumor overstaging occurs more frequently than understaging, usually when a deep T2 lesion (penetrating deeply but not completely through the muscularis propria) is misinterpreted as T3 (full muscle penetration). Tumor understaging

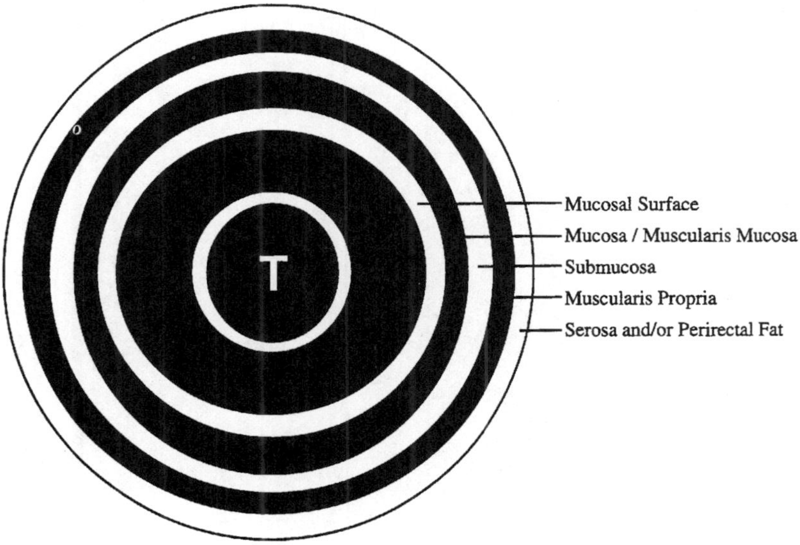

FIGURE 11.1. An ERUS image. *T* is black transducer with white circumference, surrounded by a black, water-filled balloon. Any break in central white submucosal layer indicates invasive disease with metastatic potential. (Reprinted with permission from Ref. 1).

can occur when only a portion of the lesion is evaluated and areas of deeper invasion are never imaged. Figures 11.2 through 11.5 demonstrate primary rectal cancer staging by ERUS.

After staging the primary lesion (designated as uT1, uT2, uT3, or uT4), attention is turned to the evaluation of surrounding perirectal lymph nodes. Whereas pelvic CT imaging is no more accurate at 50% than a coin toss in determining the presence of metastatic perirectal lymph nodes, ERUS routinely has an accuracy of > 75% in determining the status of perirectal lymph nodes. This improvement is based on the ability of ERUS (unlike CT) to identify even tiny nodes, on the order of millimeters in diameter, and on the good fortune of tissue echogenicity. This latter refers to the finding that nonreactive lymph nodes that are free of metastatic disease display an echogenic pattern similar to that of the normal connective tissue and fat surrounding the rectum. Thus on ERUS, uninvolved,

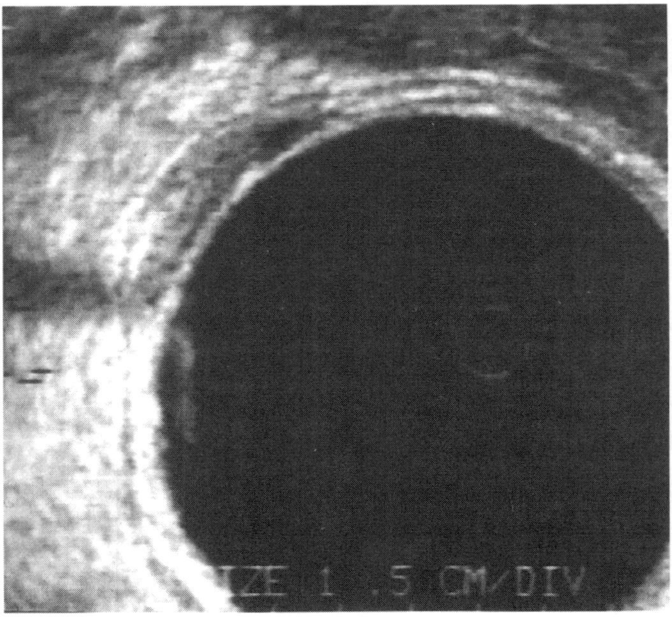

FIGURE 11.2. uT1 rectal cancer (11 o'clock position). Note both the break in the middle white submucosal layer and the normal width of the deeper dark muscularis propria layer.

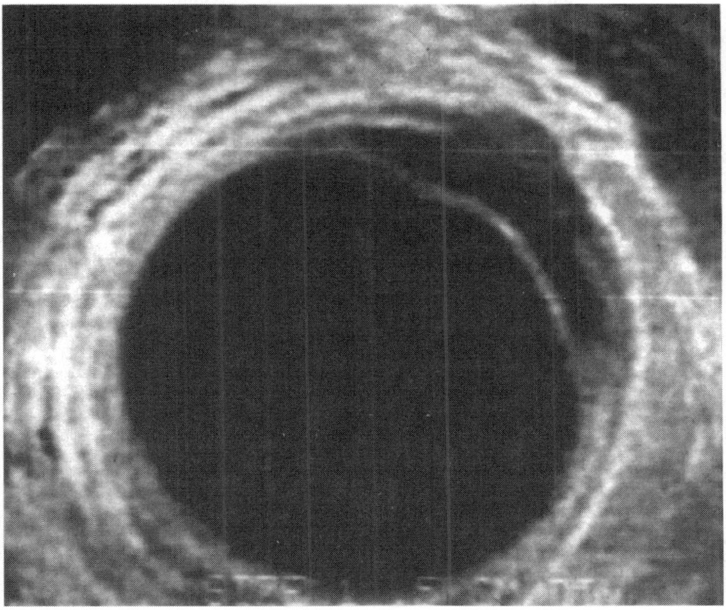

FIGURE 11.3. uT2 rectal cancer (1 o'clock position). Note the break in the middle white submucosal layer, the thickened deeper dark muscularis propria layer but the intact outer white layer, indicating the absence of full-thickness muscular penetration.

nonreactive lymph nodes are usually invisible, blending into the surrounding moderately echogenic perirectal tissues. Lymph nodes harboring metastatic disease, however, are relative hypoechoic and, therefore, are visible as small darker spots within the surrounding lighter background (Fig. 11.6). Although small perirectal vessels also appear hypoechoic, differences in the shape and pattern of echogenecity between metastatic lymph nodes and normal vascular channels can usually be easily detected by the experienced ultrasonographer. Lymph nodes are thus staged as uN0 (no nodal metastases), uN1 (three or less metastatic perirectal lymph nodes), or uN2 (more than three metastatic perirectal lymph nodes).

ERUS is limited by examiner experience (there clearly is a learning curve) and by certain tumor characteristics. Extremely

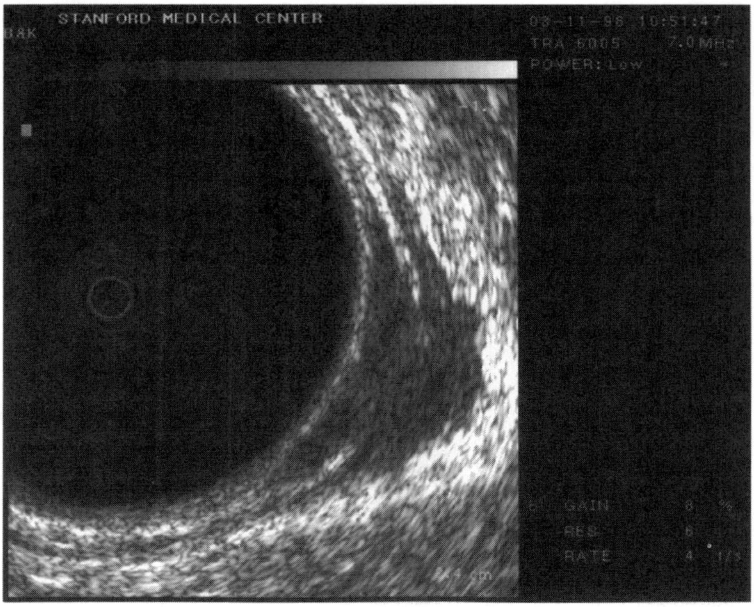

FIGURE 11.4. uT3 rectal cancer, disrupting both the middle white submucosal and outer white layers, indicating full muscular penetration.

large bulky rectal cancers do not allow the probe to pass completely through, thus limiting full evaluation of the lesions. If in such cases, however, either full-thickness rectal wall invasion or lymph node metastasis is identified, the limited examination has adequately achieved its goal of determining the need for neoadjuvant therapy. Furthermore, tumors that are in the proximal rectum, especially those farther than 12 cm above the anal verge, are significantly more difficult to evaluate, even if the probe can successfully negotiate the curves of the middle and distal rectum. Fortunately, rectal lesions higher than this level often lie within the intra-abdominal rectum or more proximally; and such lesions, even when stage II or III, may not require either neoadjuvant or adjuvant radiation if the risk of local pelvic recurrence is deemed minimal based on the tumor's anatomic location relative to the pelvis at the time of operative resection.

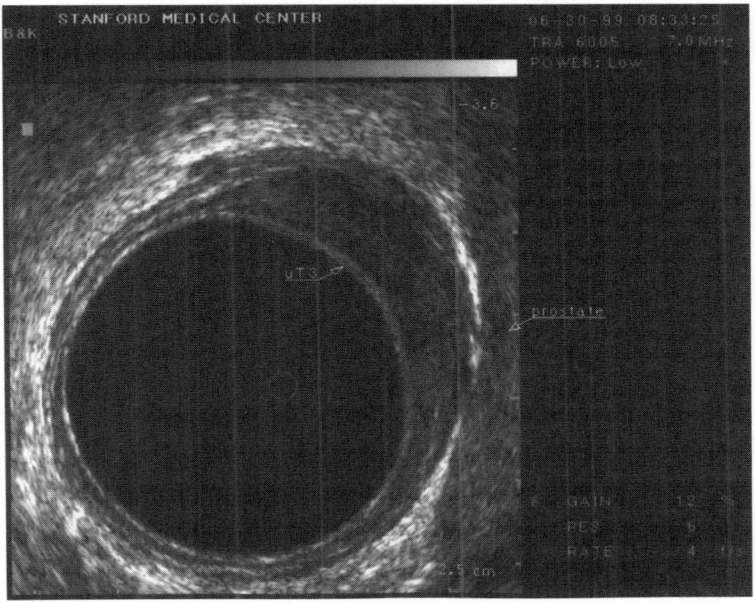

FIGURE 11.5. uT3 rectal cancer. Note the intact white layer of soft tissue between anterior aspect of tumor (1 o'clock position) and prostate gland (3 o'clock position).

SUMMARY

In conclusion, the combination of abdominal CT scan (to evaluate the liver) and ERUS (to evaluate the primary tumor and surrounding lymph nodes) allows for the most accurate pretreatment staging of rectal cancer patients. Although new studies suggest the possibly equivalent staging efficacy of ERUS and MRI using an endorectal coil, the latter technique is more time-consuming, more costly, and less convenient. ERUS is far from perfect for rectal cancer staging, especially in its still limited ability to clearly identify lymphatic metastasis. But as ERUS continues to improve through advances such as three-dimensional imaging and spectral analysis, it is likely that ERUS will further solidify its key role in the pretreatment staging of rectal cancer patients.

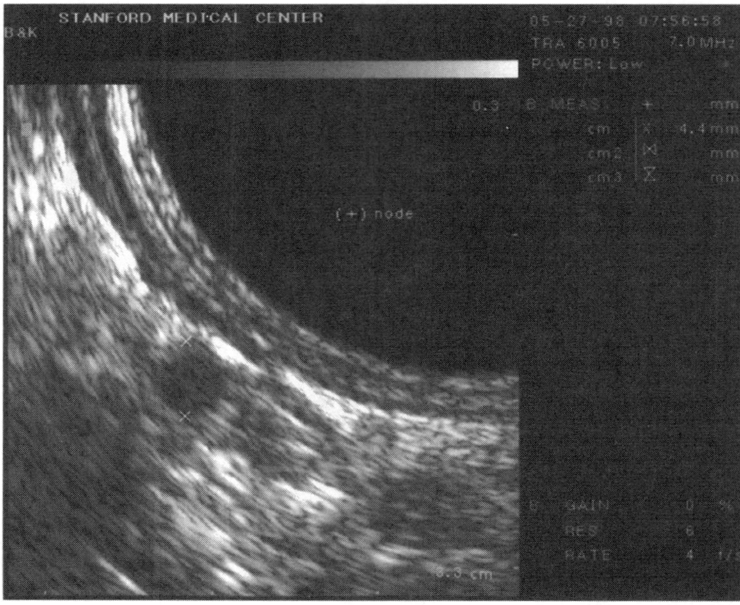

FIGURE 11.6. A 4.4-mm perirectal lymph node harboring metastatic disease. Note the normal rectal wall, with seven layers, is well demonstrated.

References

1. Orrom WJ, Wong WD, Rothenberger DA, et al. Endorectal ultrasound in the preoperative staging of rectal tumors. A learning experience. Dis Colon Rectum 1990;33:654–659.

CHAPTER

12

LOCAL TREATMENT OF RECTAL CANCER

CHARLES O. FINNE III, M.D., FACS, FASCRS, AND JULIO GARCIA-AGUILAR, M.D., PH.D.

Local therapy of rectal cancer may be defined as treatment directed at the primary lesion without regard to regional or distant tissue ablation, i.e., treatment that destroys the tumor with a minimum margin of normal surrounding tissue and with no attempt to remove lymph nodes unless immediately adjacent (or in the paradigm of breast cancer, a lumpectomy). The appeal of such nonradical treatment lies in its low morbidity and mortality and its avoidance of colostomy, analogous to functional and cosmetic concerns experienced by breast cancer patients. Successful local therapy requires that all cancer-bearing tissue be removed or destroyed, hence local treatment is not suitable for any tumor that is large or may have regional spread. Palliative local therapy, eliminating the primary lesion and its attendant symptoms when inoperable metastasis is present, is a different consideration and is often useful. Any modality capable of destroying tissue may be used for local therapy. Local excision by thermal heating (cautery spark, coagulation, laser coagulation, vaporization, or focused microwave heating), freezing, and

Colon and Rectal Cancer, Edited by Peter S. Edelstein, M.D.
ISBN 0-471-35145-8

ionizing radiation have all been used and have advantages and disadvantages.

This chapter focuses on the modalities of local excision (with or without adjuvant therapy) and endocavitary irradiation (Papillon technique), with some consideration of fulguration. Data on local excision are emphasized because partial pathologic staging allows better comparison with radical excision. Local methods of therapy for curative treatment—with one exception (1)—have never been compared to radical surgery of rectal cancer with randomized controlled trials; hence no definitive statement of comparative efficacy can be made. Nevertheless, considerable data suggest that local treatment may be of equivalent efficacy with lower morbidity for selected patients with rectal cancer. Most early cancers are confined to the site of origin and have not established disease beyond that primary site. Finlay et al. (2) demonstrated that mortality from colorectal cancer is related to the presence of metastases too small to be detected at the time of initial treatment of the primary lesion. The metastatic lesions were already established at the time of diagnosis and initial treatment, but became evident and symptomatic only with growth and were responsible for the patients' death. Hence, if it is possible to select patients who have a low likelihood of regional and metastatic disease, it may be possible to use local techniques to treat them with a high degree of success.

HISTOLOGIC CONSIDERATIONS

Three tumor characteristics are powerful predictors of prognosis and stage: depth of invasion into the rectal wall; degree of differentiation or grade; and presence of lymphatic, vascular, or neural invasion. The most important of these features is depth of wall invasion. The incidence of nodal involvement varies somewhat between series, but the general trend is presented in Table 12.1. Without regard to other considerations, 8.4% of patients with involvement confined to the

TABLE 12.1. LYMPH NODE INVOLVEMENT BASED SOLELY ON DEPTH OF INVASION

Depth of invasion	Number with Positive Nodes/total	Reference
T1	2/35 (6%)	3
	3/26 (12%)	4
	0/9	5
	3/46 (6.5%)	6
	5/46 (11%)	7
	6/65 (9%)	8
	4/130 (3%)	9
	3/27 (11%)	10
	0/4	11
	10/78 (13%)	12
	5/28 (18%)	13
	6/65 (9%)	8
	0/6	14
T1 average	47/565 (8.3%)	
T2	21/96 (20%)	3
	28/128 (22%)	4
	14/50 (28%)	5
	(12%)	7
	19/82 (23%)	10
	9/30 (30%)	11
	93/414 (22%)	12
	31/82 (38%)	13
	5/25 (20%)	15
	7/40 (18%)	14
T1 and T2 combined	33/234 (14%)	16
T2 average	250/1131 (22%)	
T3	387/589 (66%)	3
	33/92 (36%)	5
	(58%)	7
	71/126 (56%)	11
	32/69 (46%)	13
	34/51 (67%)	15
	8/13 (62%)	14

(continued)

TABLE 12.1. *(continued)*

Depth of invasion	Number with Positive Nodes/total	Reference
T3 average	565/940 (60%)	
T4	67/85 (79%)	3
	9/17 (53%)	5
	22/25 (88%)	11
	124/210 (59%)	13
T4 average	222/337 (65%)	

submucosal layer (T1) who have standard operations for rectal cancer will have metastases to lymph nodes. If the muscularis propria (T2) is involved this jumps to 22%, and if the perirectal fat (T3) is involved, 60%. Involvement of the serosal surface or adjacent organs (T4) forces this number to 65%. Hermanek and Gall (9) note a difference between tumors that penetrate only the inner muscularis propria and those that penetrate the outer longitudinal muscularis propria. Lesions with favorable histology and that involve only the inner layer are node positive in 9% of cases, those with favorable histology but penetrating the outer layer are node positive in 20%, lesions with high-risk histology and involving only the inner layer are node positive in 40%, and those with high-risk histology and penetrating the outer layer are node positive in 57%.

Histologic grading alone uniformly predicts outcome of treatment, and increasing degrees of dedifferentiation are associated with migration toward advanced stages for both colon and rectal cancer (4,5,7,8,17–24). High-grade tumors treated by local excision are particularly likely to recur. Morson (7) emphasized very early that recurrences after local excision in his series were all in high-grade lesions. These findings are corroborated in all the series that look at histologic grading, and Killingback (14) confirms that even small high-grade lesions recur. The St. Mark's experience with local excision is similar, with only 1 cancer death in 56 low-grade tumors, 8 of 81 (10%) cancer deaths in average-grade lesions, and 5/15 (33%) cancer deaths in patients with high-grade lesions (25).

Combining T stage with differentiation (Tables 12.2 and 12.3) seems to offer useful information, although the numbers are small. Well-differentiated T1 lesions average 4% positive nodes in resected patients, moderately differentiated T1 lesions show 9% positive nodes, and poorly differentiated lesions show about 50% positive nodes. Although the numbers are small for T1 lesions, the literature

TABLE 12.2. INCIDENCE OF NODAL METASTASIS VERSUS DIFFERENTIATION IN T1[a] RECTAL CARCINOMAS SUBJECTED TO RADICAL RESECTION

Differentiation	Number with Positive Nodes/ Total	Reference
Well to moderately differentiated[b]	4/130 (3%)	9
Well differentiated	0/3	4
Well differentiated	0/2	5
Well differentiated	3/44 (7%)	8
Well differentiated average	7/179 (4%)	
Moderately differentiated	0/6	5
Moderately differentiated	2/15 (13%)[c]	4
Moderately differentiated	3/21 (14%)	8
Well to moderately differentiated	0/4	22
Moderately differentiated[d]	2/35 (6%)	3
Moderately differentiated average	7/81 (9%)	
Well to poorly differentiated	5/46 (11%)[e]	7
Poorly differentiated	1/2 (50%)	4
High risk histology	3/20 (15%)	9
Poorly differentiated average	9/68 (13%)	

[a] Into or through the submucosa.
[b] A total of 1.6% poorly differentiated.
[c] Both had vascular or lymphatic invasion.
[d] Includes six well-differentiated cases.
[e] Includes 3 grade IV and 2 grade III lesions; no metastases in low-grade lesions.

TABLE 12.3. INCIDENCE OF NODAL METASTASIS VERSUS DIFFERENTIATION IN T2[a] RECTAL CARCINOMAS SUBJECTED TO RADICAL RESECTION

Differentiation	Number with Positive Nodes/Total	Reference
Well differentiated	0/9	4
Well differentiated	0/2	5
Well differentiated	0/2	22
Well differentiated	3/12 (25%)	15
Well differentiated average	3/25 (12%)	
Moderately differentiated	21/91 (23%)	4
Moderately differentiated	24/41 (58%)	5
Moderately differentiated	25%[b]	22
Moderately differentiated	2/11 (18%)	15
Moderately differentiated[c]	19/96 (20%)	3
Low-risk histology	51/342 (15%)	9
Moderately differentiated average	117/581 (20%)	
High-risk histology	40/84 (48%)	9

[a] Into muscularis propria.
[b] Total not stated.
[c] Includes 11 well-differentiated cases.

is replete with examples showing that poor differentiation is associated with poor outcome (3–5,7,14,15,22). Fortunately, small lesions are infrequently poorly differentiated.

Vascular, lymphatic, and neural invasion have been found to be independent risk factors for metastatic disease and poor outcome (3,5,8,17,19–21,26). Sitzler et al. (3) found that lymphatic invasion was 98% predictive of positive lymph nodes in their series but occurred in <10% of T1 tumors and in approximately 20% of T2 tumors; however, they did not stratify their data in a way to determine if lymphatic invasion occurred exclusively in the node-positive groups within T stage. Saclarides et al. (22) found that perineural invasion had a positive predictive value for nodal metastasis of 86%. Sticca et al. (27) in a selected group of 71 stage I (node-negative T1 and T2) patients found that only 7% had lymphatic invasion and 4% vascular invasion. Special stains to outline blood vessels have been useful for improving yield of angioinvasion (28). Blumberg et al. (19) looked at a similar group of 211 stage I patients and found that only 12% of tumors without angioinvasion recurred, whereas 48% of tumors with angioinvasion recurred. They also found that of patients with two or more unfavorable prognostic factors, 80% with stage I disease died within 3 years.

Few authors have published data substratifying patients in each of the T stage groups according to grade or lymphatic, vascular, and neural invasion. Table 12.4 tabulates what data are available in the literature. Because some studies show a profound adverse effect from these factors, lymphatic, vascular, and neural invasion should be considered contraindications to local therapy alone (3,8).

Mucin production has been viewed as an adverse prognostic factor, but there is no agreement as to what percentage of mucin constitutes mucinous carcinoma. More than 75% mucin confers a slightly decreased survival, whereas signet cell carcinoma is a poorly differentiated variant associated with poor outcome (29). Umpleby et al. (30) believe that 80% mucin content is the cut-off point for

TABLE 12.4. NODAL METASTASIS BASED ON A COMBINATION OF DEPTH OF TUMOR INVASION AND LYMPHATIC, VASCULAR, AND NEURAL INVASION

Depth of Tumor Invasion	Node Positive without Lymphatic, Vascular, or Neural Invasion/Total	Node Positive with Lymphatic, Vascular, or Neural Invasion/Total	Reference
T1	0/15 (0%)	3/9 (33%)	4
T1	0/7 (0%)	0/2 (0%)	5
T2	20/104 (19%)	7/23 (30%)	4
T2	7/28 (25%)	7/22 (32%)	5
T3	10(?)/42 (25%)	20/50 (40%)	5

defining mucinous carcinoma. They found that tumors with 60 to 80% mucin tended to behave as non-mucinous tumors. Poor prognosis was the rule for mucinous carcinoma even though only 25% were poorly differentiated: Only 42% underwent curative operation, and the 5-year survival was 18%. Fortunately, the rectum contained a smaller proportion of high-mucin tumors (24% vs. 43% throughout the rest of the colon), and none of these lesions would have even been considered for local therapy; therefore, mucin-containing tumors that are otherwise suitable for local therapy must be rare. The term *colloid carcinoma* is used to describe mucinous lesions for which poorly differentiated cells float in pools of mucin. Survival and recurrence rates with these lesions are dismal, and they generally are advanced lesions with deep penetration through the bowel wall (4,5,24).

Tumor size alone when corrected for histologic grade and depth of invasion is not an independent risk factor for prognosis (3,4) but does influence the outcome of local therapy. Tumor size >3 cm is associated with more frequent treatment failure by local therapy (14,25,31,33). This has certainly been true in our endocavitary irradiation series, but this factor may relate as much to technical difficulty with margins as to tumor biology (34).

Morphologic descriptions generally divide tumors into two groups: those with an exophytic or protruding growth pattern and those with an endophytic or inward growth pattern. These groups are usually classified as polypoid or ulcerative. Unfortunately, there are no rigid boundaries to this classification and there is a lot of variation in reporting. Killingback (14) makes a distinction between truly ulcerated lesions, in which the ulcer cavitates below the level of the mucosa, and raised lesions with a central ulcer. This does seem to be a valid distinction, but it is not clear whether this is an independent characteristic or whether this may be a morphologic equivalent corresponding to depth of invasion. Montesori and Donald (35) developed an invasion profile, which is a quantitative estimate of the amount of ulceration or invasion by tumor on whole-mount histologic sections. Patients with tumors in which <30% of the bulk of the tumor lays below a line drawn at the level of the mucosa experienced a 90% 5-year survival; survival drops to 27% in patients with tumors in which >30% is below the line.

The literature experience is shown in Table 12.5. In fact, the morphologic pattern may be a predictor of depth of invasion rather than an independent factor, but there is no study that compares ulcerated versus nonulcerated lesions within T stage groups. The data certainly suggest that the search for nodes in the perirectal fat should be vigorous with ulcerated lesions, especially with T2 lesions.

The morphologic characteristics of a tumor (shape and growth pattern) predict treatment success by local excision. Tumors that can be raised into a pseudopolp and excised have a very favorable outcome with local excision alone. Grigg et al. (6) report only one local recurrence (which was successfully salvaged) in 16 tumors excised by tenting up a pseudostalk. Hughes et al. (37) found that 92% of a selected group of patients with polypoid lesions were free of disease, whereas only 33% of the ulcerated group were free of disease after fulguration. Killingback's (14) experience corroborates these data with local excision. One third of the ulcerated tumors in his group treated with local excision recurred, but only 17% of the nonulcerated lesions recurred.

TABLE 12.5. NODAL METASTASIS BASED ON MORPHOLOGIC TUMOR CHARACTERISTICS IN RECTAL CANCER

Number of Nonulcerated Tumors/Total	Number of Ulcerated Tumors/Total	Reference
5/30 (17%)	10/29 (35%)	14
7/30 (23%)	27/69 (39%)	23
1/9 (11%)	21/43 (49%)	36
18/51 (35%)	88/154 (57%)	24

MALIGNANT POLYP

The malignant polyp problem is addressed in chapter 2, mainly with reference to the entire colon and rectum. The classification proposed by Haggett et al. (38) is applicable to rectal lesions, but unless lesions are pedunculated, all T1 rectal lesions are Haggitt level 4 by definition, so the criteria in Table 12.2 apply. Nivatvongs et al. (39) have shown that nodal metastases occur only in the level 4 lesions, whether pedunculated or not, and that all of the primary lesions with metastases had evidence of lymphatic invasion in addition to being level 4. Interestingly, out of 27 poorly differentiated polyps, metastasis occurred only in the level 4 lesions. Each of 3 mucinous carcinomas were level 4 and all had metastases. Any pedunculated polyp that has clear margins and level 3 invasion or less is appropriately treated by polypectomy alone.

PATIENT SELECTION

The data presented up to now strongly suggest that a polypoid lesion <3 or 4 cm in diameter that is well differentiated and confined to the submucosa (T1) carries a risk of nodal metastasis of 3 to 5%, whereas a similar lesion confined superficially to the muscularis propria (superficial T2) carries a risk of 12 to 15%. Such lesions, if found on evaluation with endorectal ultrasound, careful digital examination, and CT scan to have no demonstrable nodes, probably have a risk of <5% and should be considered suitable for local excision even in a patient considered a good risk for major surgery. Lesions confined to the submucosa but moderately differentiated carry a risk of nodal metastasis of 9%, and moderately differentiated lesions within the muscularis propria have a risk of 20%. Negative lymph nodes on ultrasound in these two groups probably cuts the actual risk to between 5 and 10%. The recurrence data from local excision series seem to corroborate these estimates. Poorly differentiated lesions carry a prohibitive risk of nodal metastasis and tend to account for the majority of failures in local excision series, so local treatment alone is contraindicated for poorly differentiated lesions, unless medical circumstances preventing standard treatment prevail. Stretching the criteria for local excision has been associated with increased local, regional, and distant recurrence and poor outcome in all series that have examined for strictness of criteria.

ACCESSIBILITY

The accessibility of a lesion for local removal depends on several factors, including patient body habitus, level of the lesion, whether the lesion will prolapse, whether the lesion is located within intraperitoneal rectum, the skill and experience of the surgeon, availability of special techniques (transanal endoscopic microsurgery, transanal excision, Kraske [posterior proctotomy], York-Mason [division and reconstruction of the sphincter]), and the size of the lesion. Lesions that are marginally approachable should probably undergo anterior resection unless circumstances mitigate against it (in which case the decision then becomes how best to palliate an inoperable lesion, be the reason medical or surgical).

PATIENT EVALUATION

The preoperative evaluation of patients with rectal cancer should include a medical history and general physical examination as well as questions about bowel habits and fecal continence. Digital rectal examination is mandatory to assess location, size, accessibility, and fixity of the tumor, presence of palpable metastatic lymph nodes, and sphincter function. Rigid proctoscopy is the preferred tool to assess distance from the anal verge, relationship to the valves of Houston, size, fixity, and macroscopic appearance. Better biopsy material obtained with the rigid proctoscope is better than the small samples obtained with the flexible scope. Complete colonoscopy should be done to clear the colon of other neoplasms or diseases that might alter the surgical plan. CT scan of the abdomen and pelvis to rule out metastatic disease is mandatory for any patient considered for local therapy because laparotomy will not be performed. The chest should always be evaluated either by chest x-ray or inclusion of the chest on CT. We have had the experience in which several pulmonary lesions found on CT (including a third primary lesion) were not apparent on conventional chest films. Endorectal ultrasound is the single most useful technique for evaluating suitability for local excision, because this study alone can accurately estimate depth of invasion and predict nodal involvement (including areas beyond reach of the finger) with reasonable precision.

TECHNICAL CONSIDERATIONS

Treatment options for local therapy include four varieties of local excision, fulguration, endocavitary irradiation (contact or Papillon technique), brachytherapy with implanted radiation sources, cryotherapy, laser ablation, and other experimental techniques such as microwave thermal ablation and photodynamic therapy. From a practical standpoint, lesions that can be reached with the ultrasound probe are approachable with curative intent. Selected lesions in the upper rectum not accessible to endorectal ultrasound may still be accessible to transanal endoscopic microsurgery.

Posterior proctotomy and sphincter-dividing procedures have seldom been performed in our institution and are associated with an extremely high fistula rate. These operations have been almost abandoned because they are not necessary. Lesions that cannot be resected by exposure through the anus virtually always require formal resection. Thermal ablation (including fulguration, laser ablation, cryotherapy, microwave) has been popular in many institutions but requires the same preoperative preparation and anesthetic as local excision. Ablative procedures do not offer the benefit of histologic evaluation and are often associated with fever and postoperative hemorrhage and are, therefore, less desirable than excision. Contact or endocavitary irradiation, although it produces no specimen, does not burn any bridges by destroying tissue planes, and it is performed with sedation as an outpatient with almost no morbidity.

TRANSANAL EXCISION

With the rare exception of benign anal tumors that can be treated like hemorrhoids, full-thickness rectal excisions require full mechanical bowel preparation with perioperative parenteral antibiotics. The use of oral antibiotics is debatable, but we prefer to use them for reduction of intraluminal bacterial numbers. Bladder catheterization is routine, and general anesthesia is preferable, although regional anesthesia can be used; rarely can lesions be removed with only local anesthesia and sedation. Pudendal or regional local anesthesia may assist in sphincter relaxation. We have come to prefer the prone-jackknife position for all lesions because the lumen of the bowel opens when gravity pulls the sigmoid straight, and exposure is facilitated, even for posterior lesions. In lithotomy position, the lumen of the rectum tends to collapse, interfering with visualization, and bleeding tends to obscure the field rather than flow away from it. Headlights are an essential item. Adequate illumination of the field for a deep transanal procedure is virtually impossible without a good headlight. The anus is partially effaced by taping the buttocks apart, and further effacement and some retraction is achieved with the Lone Star retractor (Houston, Tex.). The Pratt bivalve speculum is used to dilate the anus and expose the lesion and is our instrument of choice, but the Sawyer, Hill-Ferguson, or Ferguson Moon retractors are preferred by others. Occasionally long thin spatulas (like the Wylie renal vein retractors), narrow ribbons, or narrow Deaver retractors are required. The Deaver comes in a "baby" version, which is particularly useful.

A line of resection is marked with the electrocautery striving for a 1-cm margin around the tumor. More proximal lesions can be partially prolapsed by putting one or a series of figure-eight sutures around the lesion and including the sutures within the resection (the parachute technique). The proximal limit of the resection is sometimes difficult to determine when the tumor fills the field, so if there is any difficulty visualizing the proximal line of resection, make the initial distal incision full thickness and then work up to the proximal line of resection from the bottom. Ideally a full-thickness incision is made all around the tumor and then carried across the perirectal fat, leaving a chunk of fat attached to the specimen. Anteriorly, close attention is paid to depth in the rectovaginal septum to avoid vaginal injury in the female and to avoid the urinary tract in the male. Opening into the peritoneal cavity must be recognized and full-thickness anastomosis meticulously carried out to prevent leaks and subsequent peritonitis. We prefer to always close the rectal wall incision using synthetic absorbable suture, even when the injury is entirely retroperitoneal. The ends of the suture are cut long to facilitate identification and exposure in the event of bleeding requiring reoperation. We also believe there is less scarring and that postoperative fever and bleeding are less frequent when the wounds are closed. The rectal lumen can be inadvertently sewn shut; therefore, unless the luminal patency is obvious, postresection proctoscopy should be used liberally to confirm an open lumen and check suture lines.

The specimen is pinned flat on cardboard or corkboard for fixation to facilitate inking margins and serial sectioning.

Postoperative pain is rarely more than minimal because the incisions are above the anus. Urinary retention is not uncommon; and especially in men, catheters are usually left overnight and removed the first postoperative morning. If there is no intraperitoneal injury, a regular diet is started the first day after operation, and patients are usually discharged from the hospital within 24 or 48 h of admission.

Posterior Proctotomy (Transcoccygeal Excision)

Posterior proctotomy for treatment of rectal cancer was introduced by Kraske in 1885 when he removed the coccyx and part of the sacrum to gain access to the rectum, effecting an anastomosis, and leaving the sphincter intact. This procedure is always performed in the prone-jackknife position. The buttocks are taped apart and the operative field prepared with antiseptic solution. Incision may be made either transversely or longitudinally. The midline is opened down to the coccyx, which is removed by incising through the sacrococcygeal joint and dividing the anococcygeal ligament at the coccyx. The levator muscles are retracted laterally, exposing the perirectal fat. Anterior lesions are exposed through a posterior proctotomy, and posterior lesions are digitally palpated within the rectum and are excised with a 1-cm margin over the intraluminal digit. The suture lines are closed in one or two layers according to the surgeon's preference, and the integrity of the suture line is checked by insufflating air into the rectum while submerging the suture line in saline. The remaining incision is closed in layers. Postoperative care is similar to transanal excision. Fecal fistulas have been reported in 5 to 29% of cases, but in the absence of recurrent tumor most will heal, although some require diversion (14,40,41).

In the past complications, including sacral colostomy, were common, and this operation was eventually replaced when Miles introduced his modification of Czerny's combined abdominoperineal operation (APR) in 1908 (42). Fielding and Goldberg (43) have described and illustrated this technique.

York Mason Procedure (Posterior Division of the Sphincter Complex)

Transphincteric resection was introduced by Bevan (44) in 1917 and reintroduced and popularized by York Mason (45) in 1970 for the treatment of tumors of the anterior rectal wall. Patients are placed in the prone-jackknife position. A paracoccygeal incision is made from the lower end of the sacrum down to the anal verge. Each layer of the sphincter complex is sequentially divided and tagged with suture to facilitate reconstruction. The rectal wall incision is extended cephalad sufficient to expose the tumor. Coccygectomy may further extend exposure. The tumor is excised with 1-cm margins as with the other techniques. The excision site is closed transversely with absorbable suture, then the transphincteric access site is closed carefully in layers in a stepwise fashion. Infection and incontinence are common complications, so transphincteric operations are rarely used today (46).

TRANSANAL ENDOSCOPIC MICROSURGERY

Transanal endoscopic microsurgery (TEM) uses a large operating proctoscope with a stereoscopic microscope and a complex set of specially designed instruments, analogous to laparoscopic surgery, to expose and excise rectal tumors. The rectal lumen is held open by CO_2 insufflation. The technique, because of its optics and the construction of its operating instruments, requires careful attention to positioning of the patient. Visualization by this technique is truly superb, but there are some 30 different components to the system, making TEM technically very challenging. TEM requires significant training, including laboratory time with mechanical and animal models. The technique, developed by Buess et al. (47) and introduced for clinical use in Tübingen, Germany, in 1983, was designed for excision of sessile benign tumors in the upper third of the rectum without resorting to laparotomy. TEM has been applied to early rectal cancers as well, and several large series have reported a very favorable experience (Table 12.6). The only prospective randomized trial comparing local excision with traditional radical resection has

TABLE 12.6. LOCAL RECURRENCE RATE (EXCLUDING DISTANT METASTASIS) AFTER TEM EXCISION ALONE

Patients, n	Length of Follow-Up	T1 lesions Local Recurrence	T1 lesions Cancer Deaths	T2 lesions Local Recurrence	T2 lesions Cancer Deaths	T3 lesions Local Recurrence	T3 lesions Cancer Deaths	Reference
69 low risk	Median 29 months	2/52	0	0/13	0	2/4	0	48
46 low risk	Mean 52 months	2/46	1					49
23	Mean 6 months	0/7	0	2/14	0	0/2	0	50
24	Mean 3.4 years	1/24	0					1
31	Mean 17 months	0/6	0	3/17	1	0/5	0	51
54	Not stated	3/30	Not stated	6/15	Not stated	4/6	Not stated	52
30	Median 22 months	1/11	Not stated	3/12[a]	Not stated	1/7[a]	Not stated	53
17 low risk	Mean 29 months	0/17	0					54
294	9/193 (4.6%)	1/193 (< 1%)	14/71 (20%)	1/44 (2%)	7/24 (29%)	0/11		
12 high risk[b]	Mean 43 months	4/12	3					49
5 high risk[b]	Median 29 months	0/3	0			0/2	0	48
29 palliative	Mean 2.5 years	1/6	1	6/14	5	6/9	6	54a
46		5/21 (24%)	4/21 (19%)	6/14 (43%)	5/14 (36%)	6/11 (55%)	6/11 (55%)	

[a] Postoperative radiation therapy given to 13 pathologic T2 and T3 patients (68%).
[b] High risk pathology (poor differentiation; vascular, lymphatic, or neural invasion).

been done with TEM and shows no difference in survival for T1 N0 M0 lesions (1).

THERMAL ABLATION

Thermal ablation techniques employ a variety of different modalities to effect tumor destruction. Electrocautery spark desiccation, laser destruction, freezing, and microwave heating have all been used and all share the difficulty of destruction of the tumor without any retrievable specimen for pathologic examination, rendering some uncertainty in the histologic evaluation of the tumor grade and lymphovascular invasion, and inability to determine actual margins. We regard all of these modalities as similar in their efficacy, but control of the margin of tissue destruction is unique to each and personal experience probably determines their effectiveness. Strauss et al. (55) first reported the use of electrocoagulation alone to treat rectal cancer. Jackman (56) reported on a large series of poor-risk patients treated by fulguration in 1961 with quite favorable results, but the procedure was popularized in this country by Madden and Kandalaft (57), who describe the technique in detail. Their cases require an average of 75 min, some lasting as long as 3 h; more than half of their patients required more than 2 sessions to complete the initial treatment, 20% required 5 to 7 sessions, and 10% from 8 to 13 sessions. This persistence indicates careful attention to complete destruction of the tumor and emphasizes that fulguration is not a casual undertaking. A follow-up report in 1983 detailed 21 years' experience with this technique with 204 patients followed from 5 to 27 years (58). Four sessions were still the average, and nonfatal complications occurred in 24%, including hemorrhage (16%, half of whom required reoperation), rectovaginal fistulas (2%), intraperitoneal perforation (1%), stricture (2.4%), and a variety of others. Of the operable group of patients 62% were alive and free of disease at 5 years. Patients who died of disease averaged 3.4 years of survival, a year longer than patients dying from disease after abdominoperineal resection.

Other large series have been reported by Crile and Turnbull (59), Hughes et al. (37), Salvati et al. (60), and Eisenstat and Oliver (61).

ENDOCAVITARY IRRADIATION

Endocavitary irradiation (ECR; contact radiation) was developed by Papillon and Berard (62) more than 30 years ago and popularized in the United States by Sischy et al. (63). This technique involves placing a 50-kV x-ray source through a special proctoscope in direct proximity to a rectal tumor. Treatments are delivered with the patient in prone-jackknife or left lateral position. Sedation to allow the large proctoscope insertion is achieved with small doses of fentanyl, midazolam, and atropine exactly as for colonoscopy; and patients are discharged within 1 hr of completion of therapy. Typically, treatments are give as three or four fractions of 3000 cGy each, spaced 2 to 4 weeks apart, given through a 2.5- or 3.0-cm aperture. These 50 kV rays have low penetration and are attenuated to 10% of the surface dose at a 2.5-cm depth. This low penetrance allows such a large dose to the tumor surface to be tolerated but limits this form of therapy to use on T2 lesions or less (based on endorectal ultrasound). Hence this form of therapy is limited to small, superficial lesions, which are amenable to local transanal excision as well. Work loss is limited to the period of treatment and recovery from the sedation. There is no sexual or bladder dysfunction, no change in continence, and no acute risk of hemorrhage. Treatments are well tolerated with rare symptomatic side effects related to radiation proctitis in a few patients. Serious complications have not occurred in our series, and minor complications have occurred in one third of patients, including radiation ulcer and radiation proctitis with bleeding. Radiation ulcer spontaneously resolves in most patients; although a few have required topical steroids and oral metronidazole for tenesmus, the majority of these require no treatment and resolve in 2 months to 2 years.

A steel fork filled with iridium sources is used by Papillon to boost the dose to deeper tissue in selected patients. We have not had experience using the fork at our institution because patient selection for its use is not clear to us, but it probably is appropriate for uT2 or deeper lesions or for lesions in which a complete response is not clearly obtained via the proctoscopic approach.

RESULTS OF LOCAL THERAPIES

The results of local treatment are difficult to interpret because the literature is dominated by retrospective analyses from many different institutions whose patients underwent nonstandard treatments for a variety of reasons. The most common reason for a patient to undergo local treatment when a more aggressive approach is warranted is the patient's medical unfitness for major surgery. Few papers contain information on preoperative staging, and most series predate the availability of endorectal ultrasound. Most reports also include patients with poorly differentiated lesions and tumors extending into the perirectal fat; and pathologic comments regarding lymphatic, vascular, and neural invasion are absent. Tumors have been excised by a variety and mixture of techniques, even within series; and compromised margins have been either ignored or approached in a variety of different ways. The intensity and frequency of follow-up and the role of rescue or salvage after failed local treatment is either not discussed or is not clearly related. Despite these limitations, the combined experience of all of these reports still offers some insight into the role of local treatment.

The literature experience with local excision is detailed in tables that examine simple local excision (Table 12.7) and local excision combined with radiation therapy (Table 12.8). Series of patients stratified by depth of invasion and treated by local excision without

TABLE 12.7. MORTALITY AND LOCAL RECURRENCE AFTER LOCAL EXCISION OF RECTAL CANCER

Number	Operative Deaths	Local Recurrence	5-Year Cancer Specific Survival	Reference
54	0	9	92%	64
16	0	0	100%	6
28	0	6	100%	65
59	3	6	96% (at 4 years)	33
60	0	17	73%	14
35	0	0	100%	66
38	0	9	86%	67
63	1	8	92%	68
48	0	3	94%	69
42	0	3	84% (crude, not cancer specific)	16
234[a]	0[b]	49	83%	70
40	0	6	85%	71
29	0	5	93%	72
31	0	3	87%	73
21	0	2	95% (at 40 months)	40
7	0	2	86%	74
24	0	8[c]	100% (6 months to 12 years)	75
36	0	8	89% (at 48 months)	76
20	0	2	95% (minimum 2 years)	77
14	0	2[d]	100% (median 25 months)	78
91	1	3	99%	7
990	*5 (0.5%)*	*149 (15%)*		

[a] This series contains 93 patients with in situ lesions, but the recurrence rate for these is 11%, vs. 27% for invasive lesions, so all are included.
[b] Two unrelated.
[c] Seven local recurrences salvaged with repeat local therapy, one with APR.
[d] Both salvaged by repeat local excision, and both alive and well at 2 and 5 years.

TABLE 12.8. MORTALITY AND LOCAL RECURRENCE AFTER LOCAL EXCISION AND RADIATION THERAPY

Number[a]	Operative Deaths	Local Recurrence	5-Year Cancer Specific Survival	Reference
56 (30)[b]	0	10	72%	79
46[c]	0	8	86% (at 3 years)	80
21	0	3	93%	81
21 (20)	1	4	75%	82
53 (29)	0	3	90%	83
14	0	0	86% (at 2 years)	84
14[b]	0	0	100% (at 2 years)	85
25[d]	0	5	84% (at 40 months)	86
22	0	1	95%	87
86[e]	0	7	94%	32
8 (6)	0	0	100% (at 2 years)	88
22	0	4	68% (at 3 years)	5
26[b]	0	2	92% (at 40 months)	40
16	0	2	94% (minimum 2 years)	77
37 (11)[f]	0	2	100%	89
36 (11)	1	2	97% (at 30 months)	90
47[e]	0	5	96% (median 40 months)	91
16 (15)	0	2	75% (median 33 months)	92
22	0	4	89%	93
45	0	5	88% (minimum 2 years)	94
6	0	2[g]	67%	78
639	*2 (0.3%)*	*71 (11%)*		

[a] Parentheses indicate number receiving radiation if not all patients.
[b] Adjuvant chemotherapy routinely given with radiation.
[c] Adjuvant chemotherapy given to 8 patients.
[d] External beam radiation preoperatively; brachytherapy (irridium implants) postoperatively.
[e] Radiation given preoperative.
[f] Some preoperative, some postoperative radiation.
[g] Both had positive margins.

radiation (Table 12.9) are compared to those in which patients were treated by local excision plus radiation (Table 12.10).

Local excision (with or without radiation) is a remarkably safe operation with mortality of <1% in these combined series despite the fact that a sizable proportion of these patients were treated locally because of medical unfitness for a major operation. The overall addition of radiation appears to have a minimal effect, decreasing local recurrence rates from 15 to 11%. When the data are stratified according to depth of tumor invasion, there is no apparent benefit from the addition of radiation to T1 lesions. The local recurrence rates of 9% and 8% are virtually identical, as are the cancer death rates of 4% and 3%. These are very acceptable results. Local recurrence of T2 lesions, however, appears to be cut in half by the addition of radiation, dropping from 19 to 9%, with a slight beneficial effect on cancer mortality from 13 to 8%. This effect unfortunately seems to disappear for T3 lesions, with the unacceptably high 33% recurrence rate after local excision alone and hovering at 29% after the addition of radiation; cancer mortality actually increased in the T3 patients who received radiation, from 28% to 38%. The patient numbers are small, and, as already mentioned, there is so much variation in the practice among series that the only justifiable conclusion should be that local excision and radiation for T3 lesions is not a viable therapeutic option except under the most dire of circumstances.

The combined results of the three series in which the majority of patients received adjuvant chemotherapy with radiation stand out from the other studies. There were no local recurrences or cancer deaths in 45 T2 patients. The patient numbers are small, but the results support Bleday et al. (40) effort to prospectively study and treat T2 patients with adjuvant chemoradiation (combined therapy) after local excision.

Successful local control even in the presence of distant metastasis should not be considered a treatment failure because palliative results are equivalent to those achieved by major resection. Finlay

TABLE 12.9. LOCAL RECURRENCE RATE (EXCLUDING DISTANT METASTASIS) AFTER LOCAL SURGICAL EXCISION ALONE[a]

Patients, n	Length of Follow-Up	T1 lesions Local Recurrence	T1 lesions Cancer Deaths	T2 lesions Local Recurrence	T2 lesions Cancer Deaths	T3 lesions Local Recurrence	T3 lesions Cancer Deaths	Reference
6	Median 25 months	0/6	0					85
56	Median 36 months (4–162)	2/20	4	1/5	1	3/4	3	95
47	Mean 40 months	2/21	1					40
36	Mean 48 months	4/17	1					76
89	> 5 years	3/36	0	4/15	2	1/3	1	64
119	> 5 years	3/91	1	1/11	1			7
95	Median > 3 years	3/39	0	3/20	2			33

16	> 9 years	1/16	1					6
28	> 4 years	2/16	0	4/9	0			65
31	> 5 years	1/15	1	2/14	2	1/2	1	73
58	> 3 years	0/28	0					66
38	> 4 years	0/17	0	6/14	2			67
63	> 5 years	0/27	0	8/36	5			68
57	> 5 years	1/25	1	6/29	4	1/3	1	69
42	> 5 years			3/42	4			16
29	> 5 years			0/4	0	5/25	2	72
14	> 5 years	2/14[b]	0					78
36	Median 68 months (minimum 24)	0/20	1					77
24	Median probably > 5 years	8/22[b]	0	0/2	0			75
60	> 5 years	7/22	5	7/32	7	3/6	4	14
944		*39/452 (9%)*	*16/452 (4%)*	*45/233 (19%)*	*30/233 (13%)*	*14/43 (33%)*	*12/43 (28%)*	

[a] No chemotherapy or radiation therapy.
[b] All were salvaged.

TABLE 12.10. LOCAL RECURRENCE RATE (EXCLUDING DISTANT METASTASIS) AFTER LOCAL SURGICAL EXCISION OF RECTAL CANCER PLUS RADIATION THERAPY

Patients, *n*	Length of Follow-Up	Percent Receiving Chemotherapy	T1 lesions: Local Recurrence	T1 lesions: Cancer Deaths	T2 lesions: Local Recurrence	T2 lesions: Cancer Deaths	T3 lesions: Local Recurrence	T3 lesions: Cancer Deaths	Reference
14	Median 25 months	87 (5-FU)			0/13	0	0/1	0	85
20	Mean 47 months	70 (5-FU)	0/5	0	0/11	0	0/1	0	96
47	Mean 40 months	100 (5-FU)			0/21	0	2/5[b]	2	40
8 (6)	Median 24 months	12 (5-FU)	0/2	0	0/4	0	0/2	0	88
14[a]	Median 27 months	0	0/8	0	0/3	0	1/3	1	84
19	Median 26 months	27 (5-FU)	1/10	0	2/11	2	2/3	2	95
36 (11)	Mean 30 months	0	2/34	0	0/2	1			90
16 (15)	Median 33 months	0	1/2	0	1/9	1	0/3	3	92
46	Median 36 months	17 (5-FU)	0/16	0	0/15	1	3/15	6	80
22	Median 37 months	9 (5-FU)	0/4	0	3/12	4	2/6	3	5
25	Mean 40 months	0	0/7	0	2/8	1	3/10	3	86

47[c]	Median 40 months	0	3/30	1	0/14	0	2/3	1	91
53 (29)	Median 44 months	0	2/35	1	2/18	1			83
21	Median 54 months	0	1/9	0	2/12	2			81
21 (20)	Median 56 months	0	2/2	2	2/15	2	1/4	1	82
22 (10)	Mean 63 months	20 (5-FU, MMC)	0/13	0	1/6	0	1/3	1	87
4	> 5 years	0			0/4	0			78
22	Median 6 years (minimum 3 years)	0	4/13	2	0/7	0	1/3	1	93
36	Median 68 months (minimum 24)	0			2/16	1			77
37 (11)	Median 155 months	0	1/11	0	1/5	0			89
530			*17/201 (8%)*	*6/201 (3%)*	*18/206 (9%)*	*16/206 (8%)*	18/62 (29%)	*24/62 (39%)*	

[a] Nonoverlapping series.
[b] Both had high risk histology (lymphovascular invasion, positive margin).
[c] Preoperative x-ray and pathologic staging followed radiation therapy.
MMC, .

et al. (2) showed that most metastases have already been established by the time of treatment of the primary cancer; therefore, local or regional control of a tumor is the best that can be achieved by present surgical means.

The TEM data, because the follow-up is short and the pathologic data better stratified, are presented in Table 12.6. The pathologic classifications into "low risk" and "high risk" were developed by Hermanek (97a) based on histologic grading and on the presence of lymphatic or vascular invasion. Tumors with poor differentiation or positive lymphatic or vascular invasion are at high risk for metastasis. The low-risk group experiences a vastly improved prognosis, especially regarding the possible salvage after local treatment failure. The TEM data particularly suffer from short patient follow-up but seem to reflect patterns similar to those of the other local excision data.

THE POSITIVE MARGIN

Clear margins are the goal of every cancer resection. The terrible prognostic implications of a positive margin after major resection are emphasized by Quirke and co-workers' (98a) data, demonstrating local recurrence in 11 of 13 (85%) of patients with pathologically involved margins after resection, but only 1 of 38 (3%) experienced local recurrence with pathologically negative margins. Decosse et al. (69) believe that margins were not important in their patients' outcomes, but our own experience and the literature suggest that clear margins after local excision are indeed important, unless very high doses of postoperative radiation are given (84,93). Tables 12.11 and 12.12 compare the outcome of local excision series in which positive margins were not treated. Clear margins in nonirradiated patients led to a 4% recurrence rate versus 32% for positive margins. Even excluding Morson's (7) data (which include a large number polyps) does not change these figures. Surprisingly, radiation did statistically improve the results, although the patient numbers in the studies are small: Clear margins in the irradiated patients were associated with 13% recurrence vs. 37% for those with positive margins. The data do not support use of adjuvant radiation to

TABLE 12.11. RECURRENCE WITH COMPLETE AND INCOMPLETE SURGICAL MARGINS IN PATIENTS TREATED BY LOCAL EXCISION ALONE

Negative (Clear) Margin	Positive or Doubtful Margin	Reference
No data		64
N/A	N/A	33
N/A	N/A	65
N/A	N/A	66
N/A	N/A	68
N/A	N/A	72
N/A	N/A	76
N/A	N/A	70
N/A	N/A	75
N/A	N/A	74
All clear	—	6
All clear	—	14
All clear	—	67
2/45	3/12	69
3/36	2/6	16
0/25	1/4	71
1/16	3/8	73
1/20	1/1	40
2/33	1/1	77
2/14		78
3/91	7/28	7
0/36[a]	2/10	49
0/7[b]	4/5	49
14/323 (4%)	24/75 (32%)	

[a] Low risk
[b] High risk
N/A, not available.

TABLE 12.12. RECURRENCE WITH COMPLETE AND INCOMPLETE SURGICAL MARGINS IN PATIENTS TREATED BY LOCAL EXCISION PLUS RADIATION THERAPY

Margin Complete	Positive or Doubtful Margin	Reference
N/A	N/A	79
N/A	N/A	80
N/A	N/A	88
N/A	N/A	90
N/A	N/A	91
N/A	N/A	92
N/A	N/A	94
All clear	—	81
All clear	—	85
All clear	—	5
All clear	—	83
All clear	—	77
All clear	—	87
2/17	2/4	82
0/5[a]	1/11[a]	84
2/19	3/6	86
1/26	1/1	40
9/34	3/3	89
0/3	1/6	93
—	2/4	78
14/104 (13%)	*13/35 (37%)*	

[a] Very high dose radiation (average 5300 in complete and 4980 in incomplete group).
N/A, not available.

overcome a compromised margin. There are insufficient data to examine whether conversion of a positive margin to a clear margin with further local excision is as effective as proceeding to major resection, but we believe, if technically feasible, that it probably is, recognizing that further excision should have no effect on the rate of distant metastasis.

RESULTS OF ENDOCAVITARY IRRADIATION

The results of the Papillon technique seem comparable to those of local excision. The literature results are detailed in Table 12.13. Endorectal ultrasound staging is a relatively new entity and has been applied to only a limited number of patients but appears to effectively determine those patients who will do well with this approach. The local recurrence rate of 2 to 17% and the 2 to 10% cancer death rate for T1 lesions are comparable to that achievable by any other modality, and endocavitary radiation has almost no associated morbidity. Endocavity irradiation alone appears to have an unacceptably high recurrence rate for uT2 lesions (41%), but ultimately a good proportion of these recurrences are salvageable, so that the effective cancer death rate of 16% is not much different from that of local excision. The addition of external beam adjuvant radiation to endocavity irradiation appears to be another effective way to elevate results to an acceptable level for selected patients with deeper tumors who are medically unfit for operation (Table 12.14), although the numbers are too small to draw firm conclusions.

FOLLOW-UP

Office follow-up after local excision is usually scheduled for 2 to 4 weeks unless a complication develops. If the margins of resection are clear, then further therapy depends on the histology of the excised specimen. The presence of poor differentiation or lymphatic, vascular, or neural invasion is an ominous finding and should result in reoperation by formal resection, either low anterior or abdominoperineal. If resection is not an option for medical reasons, then adjuvant therapy, preferably combined full-dose chemoradiation, should be delivered, unless compelling factors mitigate against such treatment. The ultimate goal of follow-up is to identify patients who develop recurrences amenable to curative salvage therapy.

TABLE 12.13. RESULTS OF ENDOCAVITARY IRRADIATION ALONE FOR RECTAL CANCER (STAGING BY ENDORECTAL ULTRASOUND)

		uT1 Lesions		uT2 Lesions		uT3 Lesions		
Patients, *n*	Length of Follow-Up	Local Recurrence	Cancer Deaths	Local Recurrence	Cancer Deaths	Local Recurrence	Cancer Deaths	Reference
Series with uT1–uT3								
101	Median 61 months	0/22	0	6/13	1	0/1	0	97b
64	Mean 41 months	1/28	1	7/19	4	6/6	4	34
165		*1/50 (2%)*	*1/50 (2%)*	*13/32 (41%)*	*5/32 (16%)*	*6/7 (86%)*	*4/7 (57%)*	
Series with *clinically staged* T1–3								
1831[a]	>60 months	58/922 (7%)	58/922 (7%)	424/532 (80%)	424/532 (80%)	372/377 (99%)	372/377 (99%)	98b
Series with *no staging needed*								
312	>60	33/312	26					62
72	0–16 years[b]	16/72	5					99
244[c]	>60 months	22/244	6/144					100
20	Mean 55 months	3/20	2					101
62	Mean 31 months	15/62	6					102
32	Mean 43 months	12/32	8					103
126	Mean 52 months	37/126	24					104
38	Median 39 months	8/38	2					105
13	>24 months	8/13	5					106
919		*154/919 (17%)*	84/819 (10%)					

[a] Staged clinically, without use of endorectal ultrasound.
[b] Mean unknown.
[c] Series includes 144 patients followed > 5 years, but recurrence data are based on 244 patients with ≤ 5 year follow-up.

TABLE 12.14. RESULTS OF ENDOCAVITARY IRRADIATION PLUS ADJUVANT EXTERNAL BEAM THERAPY

Patients, *n*	Follow-Up	Recurrence	Cancer Deaths	Reference
67 clinical T2 and T3 lesions	>60 months	9/67	8/67	62
48 palliative	>60 months	18/48	16/48	100
28 ideal cases	>24 months	7/28	5/28[a]	106
15 non-ideal cases	>24 months	2/15	2/15[a]	106
158 total		*36/158 (23%)*	*31/158 (20%)*	

[a] Patients with persistent disease (unclear whether patients have died).

The role of follow-up in colorectal cancer is controversial at best. Only two controlled trials, neither of which was truly randomized, have been published, and neither study separated rectal cancers from colon cancers (107,108). Orvaska et al. (108) did demonstrate a trend, which was not statistically significant, in favor of the patient group that received follow-up. Conventionally followed patients who underwent rectal cancer resection experienced local recurrence rates between 6 (109) and 20% (110), and the number of these patients who developed recurrence and were eligible for curative reresection was 69 and 10% respectively, with corresponding 5-year survival rates of 50 and 19%. Endorectal ultrasound has been reported to lead to the earlier identification of recurrences and higher rates of curative reresection (111–113). Our group has been using ultrasound performed by a surgeon as part of the routine follow-up, particularly after curative local excision; and our experience suggests that a high proportion of patients with recurrences can be identified while still harboring resectable disease. The ultimate value of careful follow-up in the group of locally treated patients will have to be determined by prospective, randomized trials, but salvage data from the literature does suggest a real benefit.

TABLE 12.15. Treatment Failure and Salvage after Local Surgical Excision as Sole Treatment (No Adjuvant Therapy) with Curative Intent

Series	Patients number	Duration of patient follow-up	Number of treatment failures	Number with distant mets and without local recurrence	Number with distant mets plus local recurrence
Lock, 1978[25] pedunculated	68	minimum 48 months	5	1	2
Lock, 1978[25] sessile	15	minimum 48 months	2	0	0
Morson, 1977[7]	91 T1	>5 years	3	1	0
Morson, 1977[7] Doubtful margins	14	>5 years	2	1 (T1 lesion)	0
Heberer, 1987[16]	42	0-80 months (mean not stated)	7	0	4
Cuthbertson, 1986[65]	28	mean 51 months	6	0	0
Killingback, 1997[14]	60	>5 years	18	1	not stated
Horn, 1989[67]	38	median 42 months 74% >5 years	6	0	0
Nöthinger, 1985[68]	63	>5 years	8	not stated	not stated
Gall, 1988[64]	54	median 5 years, ≥2 y	9	not stated	not stated
Grigg, 1984[6]	16	mean 112 months	1	0	0
Muto, 1991[66]	35	up to 11 years	5	1	1
Hager, 1983[33]	59	T1 median 33 months; T2 median 40 months	8	2 (1 resectable)	0
DeCosse, 1989[69]	48	mean 7.8 years	5	1	1
Gerard, 1989[78]	14	>5 years	2	0	0
Willett, 1989[95]	40	mean 26 months	8	2	4
Jessup, 1992[85]	6	median 25 months	0		
Shafik, 1992[72]	29	>5 years	5	0	0
Stahl, 1993[74]	7	>5 years	2	0	0
Snyder, 1985[75]	24	0.5–8.5 years	8	0	0
Heimann, 1992[76]	36	Mean 48 months	9	0	0
Coco, 1992[77]	36	Median 68 months	3	1	1
Totals	*823*		*122/823 (15%)*	*11/706 (2%)*	*18/646 (3%)*

Number of potentially salvageable failures (isolated local recurrence)	Proportion of potentially salvageable failures salvaged with curative intent	Proportion of failures salvaged with curative intent with all gross disease removed by salvage surgery (grossly disease-free/attempted procedures)	Cancer specific survival of salvaged patients (cured by salvage/ attempted salvages)
2	2/2	1/2 (1 postop death)	1/2 (>5 years)
2	2/2	1/2	1/2 (4 years)
2	2/2	1/2 (1 postop death)	1/2 (>5 years)
1	0/1 (medically inoperable)	0	0
3	3/3	3/3	3/3 (>5 years)
6	6/6	6/6	6/6 (>4 years)
7	7/7	7/7	3/7 (>5 years)
6	4/6	4/4	4/4 (>5 years)
7	5/7	5/5	5/5 (>5 years)
5	5/5	5/5	5/5 (>4 years)
1	1/1	1/1	1/1 (>5 years)
3	1/3	0/1	0/1 (3 years)
7	not stated	not stated	6/7 (unclear)
3	3/3	2/3	2/3 (>5 years)
2	2/2	2/2	2/2 (2 and 5 years)
2	2/2	0/2	0/2 (2 years)
5	5/5	5/5	3/5 (1.5-4 years)
2	2/2	2/2	1/2
8	8/8	8/8	8/8
5	5/5	5/5	4/5
2	2/2	2/2	2/2
81/122 (66%)	*67/74 (91%)*	*60/67 (90%)*	*58/74 (78%)*

TABLE 12.16. Treatment Failure and Salvage after Local Excision with Adjuvant Radiation Therapy (with or without Adjuvant Chemotherapy)

Series	Patients Number	Duration of patient follow-up	Percentage receiving chemotherapy	Number of treatment failures
Jessup, 1992[85] (Deaconess 1988–90)	14	median 25 months	85%	0
Gerard, 1989[78]	4	>5 years	0%	0
Ramming, 1986[88]	8	median 24 months	25%	0
Rich, 1985[84] (Deaconess 1976–83)	14*	median 27 months	21%	1
Ota, 1992[80]	46	median 36 months	17%	8
Bailey, 1992[83]	53	median 44 months	0%	4
Despretz, 1990[86]	25	mean 40 months	40%	6
Read, 1995[87]	22	mean 63 months	13%	2
Deddish, 1974[32]	86	>5 years	0%	7
Wood, 1992[96] (later Mass General series)	20	mean and median 47 months	75%	2
Willett, 1989[95] (earlier Mass General series)	19	Mean 26 months	37%	6
Summers, 1992[95a]	17	mean 64 months	0%	2
Valentini, 1996[81]	21	median 54 months	0%	3
Fortunato, 1995[82]	21	median 50 months	0%	8
Minsky, 1995[5]	22	median 37 months	9%	7
Bleday, 1997[40]	26	Mean 40 months	100%	2
Coco, 1992[77]	16	Median 68 months	0%	2
Rouanet, 1993[89]	37	Median 155 months	0%	2
Frazee, 1995[90]	36	Mean 30 months	0%	3
Mohuiddin, 1994[91]	47	Median 40 months	0%	5
Total	*554*			*70/554 (13%)*

Number with distant mets & without local recurrence	Number with distant mets plus local recurrence	Number of potentially salvageable failures (isolated local recurrence)	Proportion of salvageable failures who had curative operations	Proportion of failures salvaged with curative intent with all gross disease removed by salvage surgery (grossly disease-free/attempted procedures)	Cancer specific survival of salvaged patients (cured by salvage/attempted salvages)
1	0	0			
4	2	2	(not stated)		
1	1	2	2/2	2/2	2/2
1	2	3	3/3	3/3	2/3
0	1	1	1/1	1/1 (only 2 months FU)	1/1
		2	2/2	2/2	2/2
2 (1 resected)	0	1	1/1	1/1 (free of disease at 20 months after resection of liver metastasis)	1/1
2 (1 resected)	0	5	3/5	2/3	2/3
0	0	2	1/2	1/1	1/1
0	1	2	2/2	1/2	1/2
4	0	4	4/4	4/4	3/4
2	2	3	3/3	3/3	3/3 (3 years)
0	0	2	2/2	2/2	0/2
0	0	2	2/2	2/2	1/2
0	0	2	2/2	2/2	2/2
1	0	2	2/2	2/2	2/2
0	0	5	3/5	3/3	3/3
18/554 (3%)	*9/554 (2%)*	*40/70 (57%)*	*33/38 (87%)*	*31/33 (94%)*	*26/33 (79%)*

*excludes 3 patients with carcinoma-in-situ or tumors of unknown depth.
Overall cancer specific survival of patients who fail local excision plus adjuvant radiation (with or without chemotherapy): 26 salvaged and cured/70 local failures = 37%.
Overall cancer specific survival of patients with salvageable recurrences: 26 salvaged and cured/40 potentially salvageable local treatment failures = 65%.

TABLE 12.17. TREATMENT FAILURE AND SALVAGE AFTER ENDOCAVITARY IRRADIATION ALONE

Series	Patients number	Duration of patient follow-up	Number of treatment failures	Number with distant mets without local recurrence	Number with distant mets plus local recurrence
Gerard, 1996[97]	101	Median 61 months	19	4	2
Papillon, 1992[62]	312	>5 years	33	7	7
Sischy, 1991[100]	244	>5 years	22	2	0
Kodner, 1991[106] (ideal patients)	13	>2 years	8	3	0
Kodner, 1991[106] (ideal patients ECR + external beam)	28	>2 years	7	5	0
Reed, 1995[103]	32	Mean 43 months	12	4	2
Frost, 1993[105]	38	Median 38 months	8	0	0
Roth, 1988[99]	72	(not stated)	22	(not stated)	(not stated)
Hull, 1994[104]	126	Mean 52 months	37	10	0
Schild, 1996[101]	20	Mean 55 months	3	1	0
U of MN, 1998[34]	64	Mean 3.4 years	16	1	9
Total	*1050*		*187/1050 (18%)*	*37/978 (4%)*	*20/978 (2%)*

SALVAGE AFTER LOCAL TREATMENT FAILURE

Local therapies for rectal cancer generally do not disrupt conventional surgical resection planes, hence the possibility of performing the standard radical resection for failure of local treatment is appealing. The salvage data from the literature after treatment by local excision alone, local excision with radiation, and ECR are presented in Tables 12.15 to 12.17. The rates of local treatment failure

Number of potentially salvageable failures (isolated local recurrence)	Proportion of salvageable failures who had curative operations	Proportion of failures salvaged with curative intent with all gross disease removed by salvage surgery (grossly disease-free/attempted procedures)	Cancer specific survival of salvaged patients (cured by salvage/ attempted salvages)
15	15/15	15/15	13/15
19	19/19	?15/19	7/19
20	?	?	?15/20
5	?5/5		?3/5
2	2/2	2/2	2/2
6	(not stated)		
8	6/8	?6/6	6/6
?20	(notstated)	(not stated)	12/20
27	23/27	14/23	14/23
2	2/2	2/2	1/2
10	8/10	8/8	5/8
134/187	*80/88*	*62/75*	*78/120*
(72%)	*(91%)*	*(83%)*	*(65%)*

Overall cancer specific survival of patients who fail endocavitary irradiation alone: 78 salvaged and cured/187 local failures = 42%.
Overall cancer specific survival of patients with salvageable recurrences: 78 salvaged and cured/134 potentially salvageable local treatment failures = 58%.

are remarkably similar in the groups in which salvage data are available: 15% after local excision alone; 13% after local excision plus postoperative radiation; and 18% treated solely with endocavitary radiation. The percentage of local treatment failures still considered salvageable is slightly lower in the group that received radiation after local excision: 57% salvageable after failed excision plus radiation as opposed to 66% after failed local excision alone. After failure with endocavitary radiation, 72% of cancers are still considered salvageable. Of patients who are salvaged and those who are not, the overall cancer-specific survival of patients who fail local excision alone is 48%, of those who fail local excision plus radiation, 37%; and of those who fail endocavitary radiation, 42%. These figures are comparable to older data for conventional radical surgery alone in Dukes stage C patients, probably because the incidence of failed local treatment results from selecting out those patients with stage C (node-positive) disease.

THE UNIVERSITY OF MINNESOTA SERIES

The University of Minnesota has been a strong advocate of local therapy for selected rectal cancers based on the literature and on our own results that have shown an 8% local recurrence rate, a 92% cancer-specific survival rate, and a 55% salvage rate selectively using local excision alone (114).

However, a recent review of our current results contradicts our initial encouraging experience (115). Between 1987 and 1996, a total of 180 patients with rectal cancer underwent local treatment at the University of Minnesota. Of those, 85 patients meeting the criteria for local excision (moderately and well-differentiated tumors, no vascular invasion, localized to the rectal wall, etc.), were excised transanally with curative intent. All the tumors were contained within the muscularis propria (uT1, uT2), and were node negative (uN0) by endorectal ultrasound staging. The tumor, along with a margin of normal tissue, was excised in a full-thickness fashion, exposing the perirectal fat. All the tumors were truly T1 or T2 and had negative margins on pathologic examination. None of the patients received any form of adjuvant therapy. The patients have been followed for an average of 52 months according to a protocol of periodic proctoscopic examination and endorectal ultrasonography every 4 months for the first 3 years, then every 6 months for an additional 2 years. The overall recurrence rate is 23% and is lower for the T1 (15%) than for the T2 (39%) tumors. Most recurrences occurred within 2 years after surgery (average of 20 months). The overall and cancer-specific survival rates were 82 and 97% for T1 tumors, and 61 and 84% for T2 tumors, at 55 and 48 months, respectively. The majority of the patients who recurred were salvaged by surgery.

We are puzzled and disturbed by the disparity between our earlier and our most recent experiences and are currently unable to explain these differences. Our results certainly support the addition of chemoradiation for any T2 lesion that is treated for cure by local means.

CONCLUSION

The literature and our experience confirm that local means of therapy for selected rectal cancers are attended by low morbidity and mortality, particularly when compared to low anterior resection and multistaged extended low anterior and coloanal procedures. This lack of morbidity and the favorable results for T1 lesions (9% local recurrence, 4% cancer deaths) suggest that in the face of favorable histologic criteria, local therapy may actually be the treatment of choice for such rectal cancers, even in good-risk patients, particularly because one randomized trial shows no survival difference between total mesorectal excision and conventional radical resection. These data are corroborated by the incidence of nodal metastases found in series of radical resections, i.e., the recurrence rate equals the expected incidence of positive nodes, and the incidence of distant metastases is unaffected. Many patients maintain local control of their primary disease after the development of distant metastases and avoid the morbidity of major surgery. The treatment of T2 lesions is more controversial, but the addition of radiation or chemotherapy appears to lower recurrence rates from 19% (local excision only) to 9% (the same aggregate rate as T1 lesions), with 8% cancer deaths. The three series that used chemotherapy concomitant with radiation after local excision report no recurrences after the treatment of 42 patients. These results compare favorably with conventional resection, especially in high-risk patients. T3 lesions are not appropriate for local therapy alone, except under the most dire circumstances; but it is surprising that the local recurrence rate is virtually the same whether radiation or chemotherapy is added or not (33 vs. 29%), and the cancer-specific survival is also equivalent (28 vs. 39%), in this small number of patients.

The positive or doubtful margin after local excision requires active treatment, because such a pathologic finding is associated with a recurrence rate from 3- to 10-fold higher than with a pathologically negative margin. Limited data suggest that adjuvant radiation is not adequate to deal with the positive margin.

The aggregate experience with local therapy for rectal cancer is a favorable one, but these modalities cry out for randomized trials, and local therapy cannot yet be the standard therapy until at least one or more trials confirm that this is an appropriate course for clearly selected patients. The standardization of pathologic variables (serial sectioning of excised specimens; grading; presence of vascular, lymphatic, and neural invasion) and reporting of these variables are imperative to estimate risk and categorize patients within such studies.

REFERENCES

1. Winde G, Nottberg H, Keller R, et al. Surgical cure for early rectal carcinomas (T1). Transanal endoscopic microsurgery vs. anterior resection [See comments]. Dis Colon Rectum 1996;39:969–976.

2. Finlay IG, Meek D, Brunton F, McArdle CS. Growth rate of hepatic metastases in colorectal carcinoma. Br J Surg 1988;75:641–644.

3. Sitzler PJ, Seow-Choen F, Ho YH, Leong AP. Lymph node involvement and tumor depth in rectal cancers: an analysis of 805 patients. Dis Colon Rectum 1997;40:1472–1476.

4. Brodsky JT, Richard GK, Cohen AM, Minsky BD. Variables correlated with the risk of lymph node metastasis in early rectal cancer. Cancer 1992;69:322–326.

5. Minsky BD, Rich T, Recht A, et al. Selection criteria for local excision with or without adjuvant radiation therapy for rectal cancer. Cancer 1989;63:1421–1429.

6. Grigg M, McDermott FT, Pihl EA, Hughes ESR. Curative local excision in the treatment of carcinoma of the rectum. Dis Colon Rectum 1984;27:81–83.

7. Morson BC. Factors influencing the prognosis of early cancer of the rectum. Proc R Soc Med 1966;59:35–36.

8. Tanaka S, Yokota T, Saito D, et al. Clinicopathologic features of early rectal carcinoma and indications for endoscopic treatment. Dis Colon Rectum 1995;38:959–963.

9. Hermanek P, Gall FP. Early (microinvasive) colorectal carcinoma. Pathology, diagnosis, surgical treatment. Int J Colorect Dis 1986;1:79–84.

10. Huddy SP, Husband EM, Cook MG, et al. Lymph node metastases in early rectal cancer. Br J Surg 1993;80:1457–1458.

11. Dworak O. Number and size of lymph node metastases in rectal carcinomas. Surg Endosc 1989;3:96–99.

12. Cuthbertson AM, Hughes ESR, Pihl E. Metastatic 'early' colorectal cancer. Aust N Z J Surg 1984;54:549–551.

13. Hojo K, Koyama Y, Moriya Y. Lymphatic spread and its prognostic value in patients with rectal cancer. Am J Surg 1982;144:350–354.

14. Killingback M. Local excision of carcinoma of the rectum: indications. World J Surg 1992;16:437–446.

15. Nelson JC, Nimr AN, Thomford NR. Criteria for the selection of 'early' carcinomas of the rectum. Are they valid? Arch Surg 1987;122:533–536.

16. Heberer G, Denecke H, Demmel N, Wirsching R. Local procedures in the management of rectal cancer. World J Surg 1987;11:499–503.

17. Wiggers T, Arends JW, Volovics A. Regression analysis of prognostic factors in colorectal cancer after curative resections. Dis Colon Rectum 1988;31:33–41.

18. Ogiwara H, Nakamura T, Baba S. Variables related to risk of recurrence in rectal cancer without lymph node metastasis [See comments]. Ann Surg Oncol 1994;1:99–104.

19. Blumberg D, Paty PB, Picon AI, et al. Stage I rectal cancer: identification of high-risk patients [See discussion]. J Am Coll Surg 1998;186:574–579.

20. Michelassi F, Ayala JJ, Balestracci T, et al. Verification of a new clinicopathologic staging system for colorectal adenocarcinoma. Ann Surg 1991;214:11–18.

21. Jass JR, Atkin WS, Cuzick J, et al. The grading of rectal cancer: historical perspectives and a multivariate analysis of 447 cases. Histopathology 1986;10:437–459.

22. Saclarides TJ, Bhattacharyya AK, Britton-Kuzel C, et al. Predicting lymph node metastases in rectal cancer. Dis Colon Rectum 1994;37:52–57.

23. Abrams JS. Clinical staging of rectal cancer. Am J Surg 1980;139:539–543.

24. Cohen AM, Wood WC, Gunderson LL, Shinnar M. Pathological studies in rectal cancer. Cancer 1980;45:2965–2968.

25. Lock MR, Cairns DW, Ritchie JK, Lockhart-Mummery HE. The treatment of early rectal cancer by local excision. Br J Surg 1978;65:346–349.

26. Horn A, Dahl O, Morild I. Venous and neural invasion as predictors of recurrence in rectal adenocarcinoma. Dis Colon Rectum 1991;34:798–804.

27. Sticca RP, Rodriguez-Bigas M, Penetrante RB, Petrelli NJ. Curative resection for stage I rectal cancer: natural history, prognostic factors, and recurrence patterns. Cancer Invest 1996;14:491–497.

28. Inoue T, Mori M, Shimono R, et al. Vascular invasion of colorectal carcinoma readily visible with certain stains. Dis Colon Rectum 1992;35:34–349.

29. Sasaki O, Atkin WS, Jass JR. Mucinous carcinoma of the rectum. Histopathology 1987;11:259–272.

30. Umpleby HC, Ranson DL, Williamson RC. Peculiarities of mucinous colorectal carcinoma. Br J Surg 1985;72:715–718.

31. Hoekstra HJ, Verschueren RC, Oldhoff J, van der Ploeg E. Palliative and curative electrocoagulation for rectal cancer. Experience and results. Cancer 1985;55:210–213.

32. Deddish MR. Local excision. Surg Clin North Am 1974;54:877–880.

33. Hager T, Gall FP, Hermanek P. Local excision of cancer of the rectum. Dis Colon Rectum 1983;26:149–151.

34. Finne CO. Endocavitary irradiation: a successful alternative to surgery for selected rectal cancers. In: Schrock TR, ed. Perspectives in colon and rectal surgery. Vol. 10. New York: Thieme, 1988:61–108.

35. Montessori GA, Donald JC. Invasion profile of colorectal carcinoma. Dis Colon Rectum 1978;21:26–28.

36. Greaney MG, Irvin TT. Criteria for the selection of rectal cancers for local treatment: a clinicopathologic study of low rectal tumors. Dis Colon Rectum 1977;20:463–466.

37. Hughes EP Jr, Veidenheimer MC, Corman ML, Coller JA. Electrocoagulation of rectal cancer. Dis Colon Rectum 1982;25:215–218.

38. Haggitt RC, Glotzbach RE, Soffer EE, Wruble LD. Prognostic factors in colorectal carcinomas arising in adenomas: implications for lesions removed by endoscopic polypectomy. Gastroenterology 1985;89:328–336.

39. Nivatvongs S, Rojanasakul A, Reiman HM, et al. The risk of lymph node metastasis in colorectal polyps with invasive adenocarcinoma. Dis Colon Rectum 1991;34:323–328.

40. Bleday R, Breen E, Jessup JM, et al. Prospective evaluation of local excision for small rectal cancers. Dis Colon Rectum 1997;40:388–392.

41. Christiansen J. Excision of mid-rectal lesions by the Kraske sacral approach. Br J Surg 1980;67:651–652.

42. Corman ML. Colon and rectal surgery. Philadelphia: Lippincott, 1989

43. Fielding LP, Goldberg SM. Surgery of the colon, rectum and anus. In: Carter DC, Russell RCG, eds. Rob and Smith's operative surgery. Oxford, UK: Butterworth-Heinemann, 1993: 546–556.

44. Bevan AD. Carcinoma of the rectum: treatment by local excision. Dis Colon Rectum 1986;29:906–910.

45. Mason AY. The place of local resection in the treatment of rectal carcinoma. Proc R Soc Med 1970;63:1259–1262.

46. Allgower M, Durig M, van Hochstetter A, Huber A. The parasacral sphincter-splitting approach to the rectum. World J Surg 1982;6:539–548.

47. Buess G, Hutterer F, Theiss J, et al. [A system for a transanal endoscopic rectum operation.] Chirurg 1984;55:677–680.

48. Mentges B, Buess G, Effinger G, et al. Indications and results of local treatment of rectal cancer. Br J Surg 1997;84:348–351.

49. Heintz A, Morschel M, Junginger T. Comparison of results after transanal endoscopic microsurgery and radical resection for T1 carcinoma of the rectum. Surg Endosc 1998;12:1145–1148.

50. Steele RJ, Hershman MJ, Mortensen NJ, et al. Transanal endoscopic microsurgery—initial experience from three centres in the United Kingdom. Br J Surg 1996;83:207–210.

51. Lezoche E, Guerrieri M, Paganini A, et al. Is transanal endoscopic microsurgery (TEM) a valid treatment for rectal tumors? Surg Endosc 1996;10:736–741.

52. Smith LE, Ko ST, Saclarides T, et al. Transanal endoscopic microsurgery. Initial registry results. Dis Colon Rectum 1996;39:S79–S84.

53. Stipa S, Lucandri G, Stipa F, et al. Local excision of rectal tumours with transanal endoscopic microsurgery. Tumori 1995;81:50–56.

54. Said S, Huber P, Pichlmaier H. Technique and clinical results of endorectal surgery. Surgery 1993;113:65–75.

54a. Turler A, Schafer H, Pichlmaier H. Role of transanal endoscopic microsurgery in the palliative treatment of rectal cancer. Scand J Gastroenterol 1997;32:58–61.

55. Strauss A, SF S, Crawford R, Strauss H. Surgical diathermy of carcinoma of the rectum: its clinical end results. JAMA 1935;104:1480–1484.

56. Jackman RJ. Conservative management of selected patients with carcinoma of the rectum. Dis Colon Rectum 1961;4:429–434.

57. Madden JL, Kandalaft S. Clinical evaluation of electrocoagulation in the treatment of cancer of the rectum. Amer J Surg 1971;122:347–352.

58. Madden JL, Kandalaft SI. Electrocoagulation as a primary curative method in the treatment of carcinoma of the rectum. Surg Gynecol Obstet 1983;157:164–179.

59. Crile G, Turnbull RB. The role of electrocoagulation in the treatment of carcinoma of the rectum. Surg Gynecol Obstet 1972;135:391–396.

60. Salvati EP, Rubin RJ, Eisenstat TE, et al. Electrocoagulation of selected carcinoma of the rectum. Surg Gynecol Obstet 1988;166:393–396.

61. Eisenstat TE, Oliver GC. Electrocoagulation for adenocarcinoma of the low rectum. World J Surg 1992;16:458–462.

62. Papillon J, Berard P. Endocavitary irradiation in the conservative treatment of adenocarcinoma of the low rectum. World J Surg 1992;16:451–457.

63. Sischy B. The use of endocavitary irradiation for selected carcinomas of the rectum: ten years experience. Radiother Oncol 1985;4:97–101.
64. Gall FP, Hermanek P. Cancer of the rectum—local excision. Surg Clin North Am 1988;68:1353–1365.
65. Cuthbertson AM, Simpson RL. Curative local excision of rectal adenocarcinoma. Aust N Z J Surg 1986;56:229–231.
66. Muto T, Sugihara K, Ooya M, Morioka Y. Local excision of rectal tumors—indications and outcome. Coloproctology 1991;8:132–136.
67. Horn A, Halvorsen JF, Morild I. Transanal extirpation for early rectal cancer. Dis Colon Rectum 1989;32:769–772.
68. Nöthinger F. Technique and results of peranal excision of rectal malignoma. Helv Chir Acta 1985;52:325–327.
69. DeCosse JJ, Wong RJ, Quan SHQ, et al. Conservative treatment of distal rectal cancer by local excision. Cancer 1989;63:219–223.
70. Biggers OR, Beart RW Jr, Ilstrup DM. Local excision of rectal cancer. Dis Colon Rectum 1986;29:374–377.
71. Whiteway J, Nicholls RJ, Morson BC. The role of surgical local excision in the treatment of rectal cancer. Br J Surg 1985;72:694–697.
72. Shafik A. Local excision of rectal cancer: report of a technique and results. Eur J Surg Oncol 1992;18:362–367.
73. Stearns MW, Sternberg SS, DeCosse JJ. Treatment alternatives. Localized rectal cancer. Cancer 1984;54:2691–2694.
74. Stahl TJ, Murray JJ, Coller JA, et al. Sphincter-saving alternatives in the management of adenocarcinoma involving the distal rectum. 5-year follow-up results in 40 patients [See discussion]. Arch Surg 1993;128:545–549.
75. Snyder SK. Surgical treatment of low-lying carcinoma of the rectum. Geriatric Clin North Am 1985;1:485–492.
76. Heimann TM, Oh C, Steinhagen RM, et al. Surgical treatment of tumors of the distal rectum with sphincter preservation [See discussion]. Ann Surg 1992;216:432–436.
77. Coco C, Magistrelli P, Netri G, et al. Combined modality therapy in low risk (T2N0) rectal cancer. Rays 1995;20:156–164.
78. Gerard A, Pector J-C, Ferreira J. Local excision as conservative treatment for small rectal cancer. Eur J Surg Oncol 1989;15:544–546.
79. Willett CG, Compton CC, Shellito PC, Efird JT. Selection factors for local excision or abdominoperineal resection of early stage rectal cancer. Cancer 1994;73:2716–2720.

80. Ota DM, Skibber J, Rich TA. M. D. Anderson Cancer Center experience with local excision and multimodality therapy for rectal cancer. Surg Oncol Clin North Am 1992;1:147–152.

81. Valentini V, Morganti AG, De Santis M, et al. Local excision and external beam radiotherapy in early rectal cancer. Int J Radiat Oncol Biol Phys 1996;35:759–764.

82. Fortunato L, Ahmad NR, Yeung RS, et al. Long-term follow-up of local excision and radiation therapy for invasive rectal cancer. Dis Colon Rectum 1995;38:1193–1199.

83. Bailey HR, Huval WV, Max E, et al. Local excision of carcinoma of the rectum for cure. Surgery 1992;111:555–561.

84. Rich TA, Weiss DR, Mies C, et al. Sphincter preservation in patients with low rectal cancer treated with radiation therapy with or without local excision or fulguration. Radiology 1985;156:527–531.

85. Jessup JM, Bothe A, Stone MD, et al. Preservation of sphincter function in rectal carcinoma by a multimodality treatment approach. Surg Oncol Clin North Am 1992;1:137–145.

86. Despretz J, Otmezguine Y, Grimard L, et al. Conservative management of tumors of the rectum by radiotherapy and local excision. Dis Colon Rectum 1990;33:113–116.

87. Read DR, Sokil S, Ruiz-Salas G. Transanal local excision of rectal cancer. Int J Colorectal Dis 1995;10:73–76.

88. Ramming KP, Juillard G, Parker R, Eilber F. Management of carcinoma of the rectum and anus without abdominoperineal resection. Am J Surg 1986;152:16–20.

89. Rouanet P, Fabre JM, Dubois JB, et al. Conservative surgery for low rectal carcinoma after high-dose radiation. Functional and oncologic results. Ann Surg 1995;221:67–73.

90. Frazee RC, Patel R, Belew M, et al. Transanal excision of rectal carcinoma. Am Surg 1995;61:714–717.

91. Mohiuddin M, Marks G, Bannon J. High-dose preoperative radiation and full thickness local excision: a new option for selected T3 distal rectal cancers. Int J Radiat Oncol Biol Phys 1994;30:845–849.

92. Rosenthal SA, Yeung RS, Weese JL, et al. Conservative management of extensive low-lying rectal carcinomas with transanal local excision and combined preoperative and postoperative radiation therapy. A report of a phase I-II trial. Cancer 1992;69:335–341.

93. Wong CS, Stern H, Cummings BJ. Local excision and post-operative radiation therapy for rectal carcinoma. Int J Radiat Oncol Biol Phys 1993;25:669–675.

94. Mendenhall WM, Rout WR, Vauthey JN, et al. Conservative treatment of rectal adenocarcinoma with endocavitary irradiation or wide local excision and postoperative irradiation. J Clin Oncol 1997;15:3241–3248.

95. Willett CG, Tepper JE, Donnelly S, et al. Patterns of failure following local excision and local excision and postoperative radiation therapy for invasive rectal adenocarcinoma [See erratum]. J Clin Oncol 1989;7:1003–1008.

95a. Summers GE, Mendenhall WM, Copeland EM. Update on the University of Florida experience with local excision and postoperative radiation therapy for the treatment of early rectal carcinoma. Surg Oncol Clin N Amer 1992;1:125–130.

96. Wood WC, Willett CG. Update of the Massachusetts General Hospital experience of combined local excision and radiotherapy for rectal cancer. Surg Oncol Clin North Am 1992;1:131–136.

97a. Hermanek P. A pathologist's point of view on endoscopically removed polyps of colon and rectum [Editorial]. Acta Hepatogastroenterol (Stuttg) 1978;25:169–170.

97b. Gérard JP, Ayzac L, Coquard R, et al. Endocavitary irradiation for early rectal carcinomas T1 (T2). A series of 101 patients treated with the Papillon's technique. Int J Radiat Oncol Biol Phys 1996;34:775–783.

98a. Quirke P, Durdey P, Dixon MF, Williams NS. Local recurrence of rectal adenocarcinoma due to inadequate surgical resection. Histopathological study of lateral tumour spread and surgical excision. Lancet 1986;2:996–999.

98b. Parturier-Albot M, Albot G. [2,045 cases of rectal cancer treated by sole, preoperative or palliative endocavitary contact radiotherapy. Statistical results with the help of a modern classification of carcinoma of the rectum]. Ann Gastroenterol Hepatol 1981;17:313–320.

99. Roth SL, Horiot JC, Calais G, et al. Results of endocavitary irradiation of early rectal tumors. Acta Oncol 1988;27:825–827.

100. Sischy B. The role of endocavitary irradiation for limited lesions of the rectum. Int J Colorect Dis 1991;6:91–94

101. Schild SE, Martenson JA, Gunderson LL. Endocavitary radiotherapy of rectal cancer. Int J Radiat Oncol Biol Phys 1996;34:677–682.

102. Lavery IC, Jones IT, Weakley FL, et al. Definitive management of rectal cancer by contact (endocavitary) irradiation. Dis Colon Rectum 1987;30:835–838.

103. Reed WP, Cataldo PA, Garb JL, et al. The influence of local tumor ulceration on the effectiveness of endocavitary radiation for patients with early rectal carcinoma. Cancer 1995;76:967–971.

104. Hull TL, Lavery IC, Saxton JP. Endocavitary irradiation. An option in select patients with rectal cancer. Dis Colon Rectum 1994;37:1266–1270.

105. Frost DB, Wong R, Rao A. A retrospective comparison of transanal surgery and endocavitary radiation for the treatment of 'early' rectal adenocarcinoma. Arch Surg 1993;128:1028–1032.

106. Kodner IJ, Gilley MT, Shemesh EI, et al. Radiation therapy as definitive treatment for selected invasive rectal cancer. Surgery 1993;114:850–857.

107. Kjeldsen B, Kronborg O, Fenger C, Jorgensen O. A prospective randomized study of follow-up after radical surgery for colorectal cancer. Br J Surg 1997;84:666–669.

108. Ovaska J, Järvinen H, Kujari H, et al. Follow-up of patients operated for colorectal cancer. Am J Surg 1990;159:593–596.

109. Vons C, S Houry FL, Huguier M. Treatment of local recurrence after primary restorative resection or Hartmann's operation for carcinoma of the colon and rectum. Int J Colorect Dis 1986;1:227–230.

110. Bozetti F, Bertario L, Rosetti C, et al. Surgical treatment of locally recurrent rectal carcinoma. Dis Colon Rectum 1997;40:1421–1424.

111. Ramirez JM, Mortensen NJ, Takeuchi N, Humphreys MM. Endoluminal ultrasonography in the follow-up of patients with rectal cancer. Br J Surg 1994;81:692–694.

112. Dressing K, Stock W. Ultrasonic endoluminal examination in the follow-up of rectal cancer. Int J Colorectal Dis 1990;5:188–194.

113. Nyst J-F, Janne P, Verjans M, et al. Accuracy of endoscopic ultrasonography (EUS) in the staging of rectal carcinoma and in early diagnosis of local recurrence. Gastroenterology 1991;100(Suppl):A391.

114. Buie WD, Rothenberger DA, Goldberg SM. Local excision of rectal cancer: the importance of complete excision. Paper presented at the Association of Surgeons of Great Britain and Ireland, April 1993.

115. Garcia-Aguilar J, Mellgren A, Sirivongs P, et al. Local excision of early rectal cancer: the Minnesota experience. Unpublished manuscript.

CHAPTER

13

NEOADJUVANT AND ADJUVANT THERAPY FOR ADENOCARCINOMA OF THE RECTUM

DAVID BLUMBERG, M.D.,
AND FRANK G. OPELKA, M.D.

HISTORICAL PERSPECTIVE

Adjuvant therapy is designed to improve both local recurrence and survival rates in patients with clinically resectable rectal cancer. Approximately 75% of all patients with colorectal carcinoma present with clinically resectable disease. Local recurrences or distant metastases develop in 20 to 87% of patients. Recurrences are related to the pathologic stage of the carcinoma. Local recurrence rates for stage I rectal cancer range from 5 to 10%. Stage II recurrence rates rise to 2 to 30%. Stage III rectal cancer has recurrence rates of 50% or higher. Thus several clinical trials have developed in an attempt to limit rectal cancer local recurrences in select groups of stage II and III patients.

Colon and Rectal Cancer, Edited by Peter S. Edelstein, M.D.
ISBN 0-471-35145-8

The major strides in the treatment of cancer of the rectum are largely attributed to the application of multimodality therapy. The two major components of multimodality therapy center around pelvic radiation and fluoropyrimidine based chemotherapy (5-fluorouracil; 5-FU). In the 1980s, the standard of care for patients with a distal rectal cancer was an abdominal perineal resection (APR), which left the patient with a permanent colostomy. Improved surgical techniques and adjuvant therapies have led to sphincter-preserving surgery. Adjuvant radiation therapy can be used in patients, either preoperatively or postoperatively, to decrease local recurrence and increase the possibility of sphincter preservation. Chemotherapy serves to enhance radiation (radiosensitization) and to limit distant metastases.

The efficacy of adjuvant chemotherapy and irradiation for rectal cancer was proven in several national prospective randomized trials from the 1970s and early 1980s. These studies examined the effects of adjuvant 5-FU based chemotherapy and high-dose (4000 to 5400 cGy) pelvic irradiation in patients who had undergone curative surgical resection for Dukes stage B2 and C rectal cancers. In 1975, the Gastrointestinal Tumor Study Group (GITSG) began a four-arm prospective randomized control trial of postoperative adjuvant therapy (1). The GITSG study demonstrated that the use of adjuvant fluoropyrimidine-based chemotherapy in combination with irradiation decreased recurrence rates. At a median follow-up of 80 months, the recurrence rate was 33% for patients treated with chemoradiation compared to 55% in patients treated with surgery alone. In 1988, the National Surgical Adjuvant Breast and Bowel Project (NSABP) published data showing an improved disease-free survival and a trend ($P = .05$) toward improved overall survival in patients treated with adjuvant chemotherapy (2). A trial begun in 1980 by the North Central Cancer Treatment Group and Mayo Clinic was published in 1991 (3). This study compared adjuvant combination chemotherapy and irradiation to adjuvant radiation alone. Patients receiving combination chemotherapy and irradiation had an improvement in both disease-free and overall survival compared to those receiving irradiation alone. Chemoradiation was associated with a reduction in local recurrence by 46%, distant metastasis by 37%, and cancer-related deaths by 36%.

In 1990, adjuvant combined postoperative chemotherapy and radiation became the standard care for the treatment of patients with advanced rectal cancer. The NIH Consensus Conference issued their recommendations that "patients with stage II/III rectal cancer are at high risk for recurrence and warrant adjuvant therapy" (4). This clearly marked a significant change in the care of patients with rectal cancer. Rectal cancer was no longer solely a surgical disease. Multi-modality therapy was established with surgeons, radiation therapists, and medical oncologists all playing an integral part in improving the management, surviva, and quality of life for these patients. Although recurrence rates were reduced and survival was improved with adjuvant chemotherapy and irradiation, this combined therapy was administered in the postoperative setting, which meant that patients with advanced distal rectal cancers were often initially treated with abdominal perineal resection (permanent colostomy). With proven efficacy for chemotherapy and radiation for rectal cancer, the 1990s heralded a decade of studies aimed at using adjuvant therapy preoperatively (*neoadjuvant* therapy) to decrease local recurrence and improve survival. Preoperative treatment may also downstage the primary tumor, facilitating the resection and improving surgical margins. Tumor shrinkage may allow for resection with preservation of the anal sphincter complex, maintenance of continence, and obviate the need for a permanent colostomy.

POTENTIAL BENEFITS OF NEOADJUVANT THERAPY

For a variety of reasons, chemotherapy and irradiation administered in the neoadjuvant setting may offer numerous advantages to chemoradiation therapy delivered postoperatively. First, if therapy is administered preoperatively, the radiated tissues are well vascularized, which theoretically improves the toxic effect of radiation. Second, preoperative therapy allows for greater perfusion of chemotherapy into the tumor and provides a greater oxygen-rich environment for generation of toxic oxygen-free radicals induced by radiation. Because manipulation of tumors during surgical procedures has been associated with tumor seeding and dissemination, neoadjuvant therapy may also reduce the likelihood of surgically manipulated dissemination by reducing the tumor bulk and tumor viability at the time of surgery. Furthermore, examination of surgical specimens in patients who first received neoadjuvant treatment suggests that few if any small lymphatic and venous channels remain patent as routes for intraoperative malignant cell dissemination. Thus neoadjuvant treatment may enable the surgeon to remove the tumor with a wider tumor-free margin with less manipulation of the tumor and with less chance of tumor exfoliation or successful tumor implantation.

Local pelvic recurrence in patients with advanced, bulky rectal cancers may be as high as 35 to 50%. Achieving a microscopic tumor-free circumferential margin is one of the most important factors affecting local pelvic recurrence (5). However, the surgeon's ability to obtain tumor clearance is often challenged by the physical constraints of a narrow pelvis, especially in male patients. Tumor may be adherent to the presacral fascia or the lateral pelvic sidewall, often making dissection with a tumor-free margin difficult. Neoadjuvant therapy offers the advantage of decreasing the size of the tumor before surgical resection, enabling the surgeon a greater chance of obtaining a tumor-free margin. In one study, patients with clinical T3 (transmural) tumors were treated with neoadjuvant chemotherapy and high-dose irradiation (6). The pathologic complete response was 29%, and the local pelvic recurrence was only 4%. Of 23 patients with advanced rectal cancer treated in a phase I trial of neoadjuvant therapy, Minsky et al. (7) demonstrated a clinical response rate in 30% of cases, and 100% of tumors were resectable with negative microscopic margins.

Neoadjuvant therapy may have its greatest immediate effect in patients with advanced rectal cancers By decreasing the size of the tumor, neoadjuvant therapy has enabled many patients previously deemed unresectable to undergo potentially curative surgical resections. One of the earliest studies from the Massachusetts General Hospital showed that radiation treatment is efficacious in downstaging locally unresectable rectal cancers. Of 25 patients with tumors deemed unresectable, 64% of patients were able to undergo surgical resection with negative margins after irradiation (8). More recently, the use of combined chemotherapy and irradiation was studied in 28 unresectable patients at Thomas Jefferson University Hospital (9). These patients had advanced tumors with fixation to the sacrum or the lateral pelvic sidewalls. Chemoradiation allowed for successful grossly negative surgical resection margins in all cases, with 94% demonstrating histopathologic tumor-free margins.

By reducing the tumor size, neoadjuvant therapy has also enabled patients with tumors previously only resectable by APR to undergo curative surgical resection with sphincter preservation. Minsky et al. (10) studied preoperative radiation therapy in 22 patients with distal rectal cancers deemed to require an APR prior to any treatment. Preoperative radiation resulted in significant tumor downstaging, enabling approximately 90% of patients to undergo sphincter preservation surgery. Similarly, Rouanet and Farber (11) used preoperative irradiation to treat 37 patients with rectal cancer thought to require an APR. With this neoadjuvant regimen, sphincter salvage was possible in 78% of patients.

In addition to its tumoricidal effects, adjuvant therapy administered preoperatively may be less toxic to normal host tissues than postoperative therapy. A randomized study comparing preoperative irradiation to postoperative irradiation showed a decreased frequency of grade 3+ toxicity in patients receiving preoperative therapy (12). In patients given radiation therapy preoperatively, a smaller proportion of patients developed small bowel obstructions. A reduction in small bowel toxicity associated with preoperative therapy may be the result of less radiation dosage to the small bowel because it is easier to exclude the small bowel from the radiation field in a pelvis with anatomic boundaries intact and free of surgical adhesions. Preoperative radiation therapy techniques can preclude small bowel from repeated irradiation by properly positioning patients. Postoperative radiation therapy inadvertently targets loops of small intestines that are often low within the pelvis and/or adhesed to the pelvic organs and sidewalls. Small intestine radiation toxicity falls well within the range of radiation dosages for adjuvant therapy (13).

Nonrandomized data suggest that in cases in which intestinal continuity is re-established (such as low anterior resection or coloanal anastomosis), adjuvant therapy given in the preoperative setting also appears to have less adverse effects on long-term bowel function than when administered postoperatively. This may in part be associated with the fact that the radiated rectosigmoid is removed after neoadjuvant therapy, whereas the radiated large bowel remains in vivo after postoperative therapy. In a report by Paty et al. (14), postoperative radiation was associated with increased stool frequency and difficulty with evacuation in patients undergoing sphincter preservation surgery with a coloanal anastomosis. A study from the Mayo Clinic further detailed the adverse effects of postoperative chemoradiation (15). Patients receiving postoperative chemoradiation had a significantly increased (3.5-fold) frequency of daily bowel movements, increased (8-fold) incontinence, and an increased (11.6-fold) use of lomotil or imodium. In contrast to the significant side effects seen with postoperative adjuvant therapy, preoperative radiation therapy appears to have minimal side effects on sphincter function. In 20 patients treated at Barnes Hospital with 4500 cGy of preoperative external beam irradiation, there were no significant differences in anal resting or squeeze pressures after treatment (16). In a second report from this group, 10 patients who were followed for an average of 3 years showed no effect on resting or squeeze pressures from baseline (17). In addition, no patients who were continent (9 of 10) before treatment developed incontinence. Clearly these results compare quite favorably to the high incontinence rates (56% of cases) associated with postoperative adjuvant therapy seen at the Mayo Clinic.

Besides its adverse effects on bowel function, postoperative radiation may result in a greater likelihood of wound complications. In patients undergoing APR, the perineal area must be included in the radiation field to decrease the risk of local recurrence. Because radiated tissues often heal poorly, patients undergoing postoperative treatment after APR may be more prone to perineal wound breakdown. However, this theoretical disadvantage of postoperative radiation compared to preoperative therapy has not been proven.

Although adjuvant therapy administered in the preoperative setting has been shown to downstage rectal cancer, increase resectability, and increase sphincter preservation, we are only just beginning to prospectively evaluate its effects on long-term local recurrence and survival end points. The Swedish Rectal Cancer Trial (18) is the first prospective randomized control study to document that preoperative therapy reduces local recurrence and improves survival.This study randomized 1168 patients with resectable rectal cancer to preoperative radiation or surgery alone. Patients treated with irradiation had an 11% local recurrence compared to 27% for those treated by surgery alone. The overall 5-year survival was 58% for irradiated patients compared to 48% for patients treated by resection alone. Although this study documented efficacy for preoperative therapy, it is believed that considerably larger survival benefits will be seen in current trials being conducted by the NSABP using new and standardized radiation techniques combined with chemotherapy.

Although adjuvant therapy administered in the preoperative setting has been shown to be efficacious and is associated with many more salutary effects than postoperative therapy, proponents of postoperative therapy argue that preoperative therapy may result in overtreatment of a considerable proportion of patients with early stage disease whose surgical pathology would indicate that no radiation therapy was required. Recent refinements in transrectal ultrasound (TRUS) have led to the extremely accurate preoperative staging of rectal cancers, thereby dramatically decreasing the possibility of overtreatment of patients. Several studies have documented that TRUS has an accuracy of 90 to 95% in staging the transmural extent of rectal cancer and up to an 80% accuracy in detection of regional lymph node metastases (19–21). The major limitation of TRUS is that it is not accurate in detecting small lymph nodes that may harbor metastases (21). Newer modalities, such as PET scan imaging, have the potential to be very sensitive techniques for staging patients with rectal cancer. Because PET discriminates between tumor and normal tissue on the basis of metabolic activity, it may be able to detect small pathologic lymph nodes not visible by TRUS.

Clearly, the beneficial effects of adjuvant therapy on tumor downstaging, resectability, sphincter salvage, radiation toxicity, and postoperative bowel function are much more likely to be obtained when chemoradiation is administered in a preoperative fashion. Although neoadjuvant therapy clearly has many advantages compared to postoperative therapy, it must be viewed with some caution. First, neoadjuvant therapy has not prospectively been proven beyond doubt to be of more benefit than postoperative therapy in terms of local recurrence or patient survival rates. However, the long-term clinical efficacy of neoadjuvant chemoradiation awaits prospective evaluation. It is hoped that the current

NSABP trial will confirm that preoperative adjuvant therapy is at least as effective as postoperative therapy in reducing pelvic recurrence and improving patient survival From nonrandomized data, however, it appears that neoadjuvant therapy is efficacious in the treatment of rectal cancer, and neoadjuvant treatment is considered a reasonable alternative to postoperative chemoradiation therapy rectal cancer.

SELECTION OF PATIENTS FOR NEOADJUVANT THERAPY

Selection of patients for neoadjuvant therapy is based on the clinical stage of cancer at the initial preoperative presentation. Preoperative staging should include a complete physical examination, radiographs of the chest, CT scan of the abdomen and pelvis, proctoscopy, and TRUS. Physical examination is focused on auscultation of the heart and lungs, digital examination of the tumor, and palpation of the liver for evidence of metastatic spread. Digital examination of the tumor should attempt to assess the transmural extent of the tumor and determine if the lesion is mobile, tethered, or fixed (clinically T2, T3, or T4, respectively). TRUS is used to complement this examination and much more accurately stage the primary tumor. TRUS may furthermore detect the presence of pathologically appearing lymph nodes. Digital rectal examination is also used along with proctoscopy to determine the intraluminal extent of tumor spread and the distance of the tumor from the anus. Determining the distal extent of the tumor from the anorectal ring is critical in decision making to preserve the anal sphincter. A minimum distal surgical margin of 2 cm is recommended. Radiographs of the chest and CT scan of the liver and pelvis are important for detecting lung, liver, and pelvic metastasis and in delineating presacral tumor extension.

Currently all patients with locally advanced tumors with no evidence of systemic metastases (stage II and III) are candidates for neoadjuvant chemoradiation. This includes patients with transmural tumor invasion as detected by digital examination (tethered or fixed), tumors of advanced stage on ultrasonography (uT3 and uT4 lesions by ultrasound staging nomenclature), and/or patients with sonographically suspicious lymph nodes (hypoechoic and >5 mm in size). Patients with uT1 or uT2 tumors and no suspicious lymph nodes are not usually offered neoadjuvant therapy, because they represent stage I disease and have an approximately 90% or greater rate of survival with primary treatment alone.

Patients with enlarged pelvic lymph nodes or presacral disease noted on CT scan are also candidates for neoadjuvant therapy. Some surgeons prefer neoadjuvant therapy for large tumors to facilitate achieving an adequate tumor-free microscopic surgical margin. Patients with large recurrent rectal cancers should also be considered for preoperative therapy to improve the margins of resection, provided that maximum pelvic irradiation was not administered when treating the initial primary tumor.

In general, patients with uT1 or uT2 rectal cancers with no evidence of suspicious lymph nodes may be considered for initial surgical resection. Postoperative therapy is administered to these patients if the final pathology specimen reveals evidence of improper preoperative clinical staging evidenced by transmural invasion or nodal metastasis, or in the presence of poorer histopathological prognostic factors.

THE STANDARD NEOADJUVANT REGIMEN

In the past, several studies have examined the use of preoperative irradiation alone as a neoadjuvant regimen for the treatment of rectal cancer. One of the earliest studies to prove that preoperative adjuvant therapy is efficacious was a randomized prospective trial conducted by the European Organization for Research and Treatment of Cancer (EORTC). This study randomized patients with T2 to T4 tumors to preoperative radiation with 3450 cGy or to surgery alone (22). Although the radiation dosage was lower than the standard dosage given today, there was a 50% reduction in the local recurrence rate in patients treated preoperatively with radiation. More recently, preoperative radiation combined with chemotherapy has been shown to be more effective than radiation alone. 5-FU has been identified as a radiosensitisizer and acts in part by increasing the susceptibility of tumor cells to the damaging effects of radiation (23). Combined radiation with 5-FU based chemotherapy has been demonstrated in a prospective randomized study to be more efficacious than radiation alone in patients with squamous cell carcinoma of the anus.

Similarly, combined chemoradiation has been shown by Minsky et al. (24) to be more effective than radiation therapy alone as a neoadjuvant regimen in patients with rectal cancer. The authors compared two groups of unresectable patients who were nonrandomly treated with combined chemoradiation or radiation alone. In patients receiving chemoradiation ($n = 20$), there was a higher complete pathologic response than in the 11 patients receiving radiation alone (20 vs. 0%). Chemoradiation was associated with a lower incidence of lymph node metastasis in pathologic specimens, suggesting that it also led to a greater tumor kill of metastasis compared to radiation alone. In addition, the use of combined chemoradiation led to a greater resectability rate, with 90% of patients becoming resectable after therapy, compared to only a 64% resectability rate in patients receiving radiation alone. Studies by Minsky and colleagues (25,26) have formed the basis of the regimen currently being used in a randomized, prospective, national trial comparing preoperative to postoperative multimodality therapy for resectable rectal cancer (27). In general, standard neoadjuvant regimens should include combined chemotherapy (5-FU plus leucovorin) with high-dose pelvic irradiation. 5-FU is administered as a bolus infusion concurrently with pelvic irradiation over a 5- to 8-week period.

For radiation therapy, the patient is placed in the prone position. This prevents the small bowel from entering the pelvis and thus minimizes toxicity. Standard techniques that minimize patient toxicity while providing a high tumor concentration include the use of high-energy linear accelerators, computerized dosimetry, multiple field technique, and fractionation of dosages (180 to 200 cGy). In a study by Fortier et al. (28), a dose response to radiation was observed. Of 60 patients with advanced rectal cancer, local control was 67% with administration of 4000 cGy preoperatively and 91% with a dosage of 5000 cGy. Based on this study as well as others, standard radiation dosage is considered 5040 cGy, with 4500 cGY administered in multiple fractions and 540 cGy given as an additional boost to the tumor. After completion of neoadjuvant therapy, surgery is deferred for 6 to 8 weeks to allow for maximal downstaging of the tumor. Postoperatively, the patient is given several additional cycles of chemotherapy.

Grann et al. (26) prospectively evaluated this regimen in 32 patients. Despite treating advanced stage rectal cancers, initial results were quite favorable. There was a high sphincter preservation rate, and a complete response (pathologic and clinical) was achieved in 22% of patients. There were no local recurrences and a 100% overall 2-year survival rate, with a median follow-up of 24 months. Overall toxicity occurred in 25% of patients, with severe diarrhea in 16% and leukopenia in 12%.

INTRAOPERATIVE ADJUVANT THERAPY

In an effort to improve the results of preoperative radiation, several studies have evaluated the addition of intraoperative radiation therapy (IORT) to neoadjuvant therapy. IORT is administered either by electron beam or brachytherapy. After neoadjuvant therapy and after the resection has been completed, 1000 to 2000 cGy of IORT is given to the tumor bed, which includes the presacral fascia, the lateral pelvic sidewalls, and in the case of an APR, the perineum. Nonrandomized studies suggest that the addition of IORT may be beneficial in reducing local recurrences in select patients. Those most likely to benefit from IORT are patients receiving IORT who have a complete resection with any microscopically positive tumor margin. In the Massachusetts General Hospital series, there was a 31% local recurrence rate in 16 patients treated with IORT who had advanced-stage primary rectal cancers resected with a microscopically positive margin (29). This compares favorably to a 29% local failure rate of patients not receiving IORT with primary rectal cancers resected with microscopically negative margins. Patients with recurrent tumors and those with grossly positive margins have local recurrence rates that are high (50 to 65%) despite administration of IORT. Because none of the studies to date has included a large number of patients or has been randomized, definitive conclusions and recommendations cannot be made. However, it is clear that maximal tumor clearance of at least all gross disease must be obtained to derive significant benefit from IORT.

POSTOPERATIVE ADJUVANT THERAPY

Patients who have early-stage rectal cancers on examination and TRUS do not receive neoadjuvant therapy. However if the surgical pathology specimen subsequently reveals evidence of transmural invasion (pT3 or pT4) and/or nodal metastasis and/or (in some institutions) poor prognostic histopathologic findings, these patients are then eligible for postoperative adjuvant therapy. Like preoperative therapy, postoperative regimens consist of 5-FU-based chemotherapy and high-dose pelvic irradiation. Although radiation dosage of 5040 cGY has become standard, current prospective national trials are evaluating various 5-FU regimens to determine the optimum chemotherapy regimen. The Intergroup 0114 trial (30) compared the efficacy of four drug regimens (5-FU alone, 5-FU plus leucovorin, 5-FU plus levamisole, and 5-FU plus leucovorin plus levamisole). A total of 1696 patients with stage II or III rectal cancers were randomized. With a median follow-up of 4 years, there was no difference in either disease-free or overall survival between any of the four groups. 5-FU alone produced a greater neutropenia compared to each of the other regimens but in general was associated with less diarrhea than the other regimens. The Intergroup trial concluded that no beneficial effect for levamisole was evident and that levamisole should not be included as part of the adjuvant regimen for patients with rectal cancer. The potential benefit of the addition of leucovorin to 5-FU is still being evaluated. In general, the standard postoperative regimen should include one cycle of 5-FU based chemotherapy, an additional one to two cycles of chemotherapy plus irradiation, followed by one or more cycles of chemotherapy alone (30).

SUMMARY

Since the 1980s, major strides have been made in the treatment of rectal cancer. Patients diagnosed with this disease today have a greater chance of survival, a decreased likelihood of local pelvic recurrence with its attendant morbidities, and an opportunity for a better quality of life with sphincter preservation. Although multimodality therapy has improved many facets in the lives of our patients, the future challenges us to develop still more effective regimens for this disease.

REFERENCES

1. Gastrointestinal Tumor Study Group. Prolongation of the disease-free interval in surgically treated rectal cancer. N Engl J Med 1985;312:1465–1472.

2. Fisher B, Wolmark N, Rockette H, et al. Postoperative adjuvant chemotherapy or radiation therapy for rectal cancer: results from the NSABP protocol R-01. J Natl Cancer 1988;80:21–29.
3. Krook JE, Moertel CG, Gunderson LL, et al. Effective surgical adjuvant therapy for high-risk rectal carcinoma. N Engl J Med 1991;324:709–715.
4. NIH Consensus Conference. Adjuvant therapy for patients with colon and rectal cancer. JAMA 1990;264:1444–1450.
5. Quirke P, Durdey P, Dixon MF, Williams NS. Local recurrence of rectal adenocarcinoma due to inadequate surgical margins: histopathological study of lateral tumor spread and surgical excision. Lancet 1986;1:996–999.
6. Rich TA, Skibber JM, Ajani JA, et al. Preoperative infusional chemoradiation therapy for stage T3 rectal cancer. Int J Radiat Oncol Biol Phys 1995;32:1025–1029.
7. Minsky B, Cohen A, Enker W, et al. Preoperative 5-fluorouracil, low-dose leucovorin, and concurrent radiation therapy for rectal cancer. Cancer 1994;73:273–280.
8. Dosertz DE, Gunderson LL, Hedberg S, et al. Preoperative irradiation for unresectable rectal and rectosigmoid carcinomas. Cancer 1983;52;814–818.
9. Chen E, Mohiuddun M, Brodovsky H, et al. Downstaging of advanced rectal cancer following combined preoperative chemotherapy and high dose radiation. Int J Radiat Oncol Biol Phys 1994;30:169–175.
10. Minsky BD, Cohen AM, Enker WE, Sigurdson E. Phase I/II trial of preoperative radiation therapy and coloanal anastomosis in distal invasive resectable rectal cancer. Int J Radiat Oncol Biol Phys 1992;23:387–392.
11. Rouanet P, Farber JM. Conservative surgery for low rectal carcinoma after high dose radiation. Functional and oncologic results. Ann Surg 1995;221:67–73.
12. Pahlman L, Glimelius B. Pre- or postoperative radiotherapy in rectal and rectosigmoid carcinoma: a report from a randomized multicenter trial. Ann Surg 1990;211:187–195.
13. Mohiuddin M. Surgical approaches to minimize risk of radiation-induced small bowel damage. In: Cohen AM, ed. Cancer of the colon, rectum, and anus. 0000 McGraw-Hill, 1995:648–000.
14. Paty PB, Enker WE, Cohen AM, et al. Long-term functional results of coloanal anastomosis for rectal cancer. Am J Surg 1994;167:90–95.
15. Kollmorgen CF, Meagher AP, Wolff BG, et al. The long term effect of

adjuvant postoperative chemoradiotherapy for rectal carcinoma on bowel function. Ann Surg 1994;220:576–582.

16. Birnbaum EH, Dreznik Z, Myerson RJ, et al. Early effect of external beam radiation therapy on the anal sphincter: a study using anal manometry and transrectal ultrasound. Dis Colon Rectum 1992;35:757–761.
17. Birnbaum EH, Myerson RJ, Fry RD, et al. Chronic effects of pelvic radiation therapy on anorectal function. Dis Colon Rectum 1994;37:909–915.
18. Swedish Rectal Cancer Trial. Improved survival with preoperative radiotherapy in resectable rectal cancer. N Engl J Med 1997;336:980–987.
19. Glaser F, Schleg P, Herfarth CH. Endorectal ultrasonography for the assessment of invasion of rectal tumours and lympn node involvement. Br J Surg 1990;77:883–887.
20. Dershaw DD, Enker WE, Cohen AM, Sigurdson ER. Transrectal ultrasonography of rectal carcinoma. Cancer 1990;66:2336–2340.
21. Orrom RJ, Wong WD, Rothenberger DA, et al. Endorectal ultrasound in the preoperative staging of rectal tumors. Dis Colon Rectum 1990;33:654–659.
22. Gerard A, Buyse M, Nordlinger B, et al. Preoperative radiotherapy as adjuvant treatment in rectal cancer: final results of a randomized study of the European Organization for Research and Treatment of Cancer (EORTC). Ann Surg 1988;208:606–614.
23. Rotman M, Aziz H. Concomitant continuous infusion chemotherapy and radiation. Cancer 1990;65:823–835.
24. Minsky BD, Cohen AM, Kemeny N, et al. Enhancement of radiation-induced downstaging of rectal cancer by fluorouracil and high-dose leucovorin chemotherapy. J Clin Oncol 1992;10:79–84.
25. Minsky BD, Cohen AM, Kemeny N, et al. The efficacy of preoperative 5-fluorouracil, high dose leucovorin, and sequential radiation therapy for unresectable cancer. Cancer 1993;71:3486–3492.
26. Grann A, Minsky BD, Cohen AM, et al. Preliminary results of preoperative 5-FU, low dose leucovorin, and concurrent radiation therapy for resectable T3 rectal cancer. Dis Colon Rectum 1997;40:515–522.
27. Hyams DM, Mamounas EP, Petrelli N, et al. A clinical trial to evaluate the worth of preoperative multimodality therapy in patients with operable carcinoma of the rectum. A progress report of National Surgical Adjuvant Breast and Bowel Project Protocol R-03. Dis Colon Rectum 1997;40:131–139.
28. Fortier GA, Krochak RJ, Kim JA. Dose response to preoperative irradia-

tion in rectal cancer: implications for local control and complications associated with sphincter sparing surgery and abdominal perineal resection. Int J Radiat Oncol Biol Phys 1986;12:1559–1563.

29. Wilett CG, Shellito PC, Tepper JE, et al. Intraoperative electron beam radiation therapy for primary locally advanced rectal and rectosigmoid carcinoma. J Clin Oncol 1991;9:843–849.

30. Tepper JE, O'Connell MJ, Petroni GR, et al. Adjuvant postoperative fluorouracil-modulated chemotherapy combined with pelvic radiation therapy for rectal cancer: initial results of Intergroup 0114. J Clin Oncol 1997;15:2030–2039.

TABLE 13.1. POTENTIAL BENEFITS OF PREOPERATIVE NEOADJUVANT THERAPY VERSUS POSTOPERATIVE ADJUVANT THERAPY

Tumor downstaging
Increased tumor resectability
Increased chance of obtaining tumor-free microscopic margins
Increased likelihood of sphincter-preservation
Decreased bowel dysfunction and fecal incontinence
Decreased side effects (hematologic and gastrointestinal)
Decreased chance of tumor seeding during surgery
Greater tumor toxicity in a well-perfused and oxygenated environment

TABLE 13.2. SELECTION OF PATIENTS FOR NEOADJUVANT THERAPY

Advanced stage (uT3 or uT4) on TRUS imaging
Suspicion of metastatic lymph nodes on TRUS imaging
Clinically advanced tumors (tethered or fixed) on digital examination
Large tumors not amenable to surgical resection alone on CT or MRI imaging
Locally recurrent tumors

TABLE 13.3. STANDARD NEOADJUVANT REGIMEN

Combined radiation plus chemotherapy
5-FU plus leucovorin given as bolus
Concurrent irradiation to 5040 cGy
Radiotherapy with high-energy linear accelerator, computerized dosimetry, multiple field technique, and fractionation (180–200 cGy)
Surgery 6–8 weeks after completion of treatment (allows for maximal tumor downstaging before resection)
Additional cycles of 5-FU based chemotherapy postoperatively

CHAPTER

14

Surgical Treatment of Rectal Cancer

Paul E. Bernick, M.D., and
W. Douglas Wong, M.D.

This chapter focuses on the surgical management of rectal cancer including standard surgical procedures, sphincter-sparing operations, laparoscopic surgery, and other important topics. The clinical presentation, patient evaluation, staging, and other relevant clinical matters were discussed in other chapters.

Anatomy

A thorough understanding of basic surgical anatomy of the rectum is paramount to the decision-making process (Fig. 14.1). Management options require a thorough knowledge of surgical anatomy and accurate tumor localization.

For practical purposes, the rectum is divided into three distinct segments in relation to the anal verge. The anal verge is the junction between the perianal skin and the anal mucosa. It is generally the reference point for the measurement of other landmarks and lesions

Colon and Rectal Cancer, Edited by Peter S. Edelstein, M.D.
ISBN 0-471-35145-8

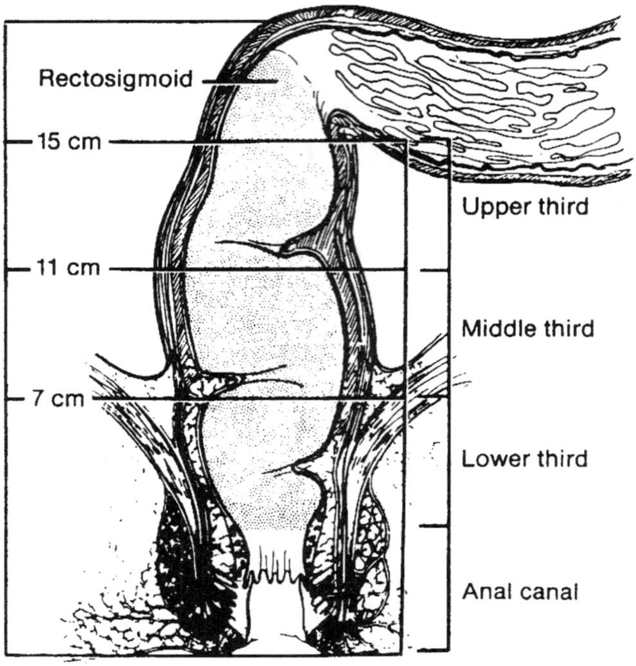

FIGURE 14.1. Anatomy of the rectum. (Reprinted with permission from Ref. 1.)

in the anorectum. The dentate line is located approximately 2 cm proximal to the anal verge and marks the anal transition zone, where the anal crypts originate, and where anal squamous mucosa becomes rectal columnar epithelium.

Though opinions vary, the length of the rectum in adults is approximately 15 cm. The lower third of the rectum extends from the anorectal ring (3 to 4 cm from the anal verge) to 7 cm from the anal verge; the middle third is 7 to 11 cm from the anal verge; and the upper third of the rectum is 11 to 15 cm from the anal verge. For consistency in reporting, it is important to describe the precise location of the rectal tumor in reference to a fixed anatomic position (i.e., the anal verge, dentate line, anorectal ring). Other practical characteristics used to describe rectal tumors include anteroposterior and lateral locations, degree of fixation, mobility, circumferential involvement, degree of ulceration, and exophytic or endophytic features.

An accurate evaluation of the anatomic location of the primary tumor is critical to determining surgical options. For instance, most tumors of the upper third of the rectum are amenable to anterior resection. Tumors of the lower rectum may require abdominoperineal resection with permanent colostomy. A select group of low rectal tumors may be amenable to a variety of local therapies. Sphincter-sparing operations have become significantly more prevalent as surgical expertise has improved for treating lower rectal cancers. This chapter focuses on the surgical options and appropriate indications for the treatment of rectal adenocarcinoma.

Options for Curative Surgery

There are a variety of important goals in the surgical treatment of rectal cancer. Cancer cure and local control are the primary goals of any surgical therapy for rectal cancer. The issue of local control is particularly important because local recurrence is a major cause of morbidity and mortality. It is estimated that up to 50% of patients with local recurrence will die as a result without developing distant metastatic disease. Other important goals of treatment include preservation of sexual, urinary, and sphincter function. It is important that these goals be achieved with acceptable levels of morbidity and mortality.

There is considerable variation in the surgical management of rectal cancer even among colorectal surgeons. Various surgical options exist for curative surgery, each option depending on important clinical information. The most important factors determining the choice of operation are the level of the tumor and the preoperative tumor stage. Preoperative evaluation was discussed in detail in chapter 11, but it must be stressed that accurate preoperative staging is critical to the surgical management of rectal cancer. In this regard, endorectal ultrasound is currently the best modality to assess local tumor stage.

Surgery remains the primary treatment for rectal cancer, and prognosis depends primarily on the stage of the tumor at the time of diagnosis. Surgical technique plays an immensely important role in the management of rectal cancer, particularly in terms of local recurrence. Multimodality therapy has significantly improved outcomes in terms of survival and local recurrence. This chapter highlights the issues in selecting the appropriate surgical options for specific clinical situations.

LOCAL THERAPY

The conventional surgical treatment for patients with potentially curable transmural and/or node-positive rectal cancer is a low anterior resection or abdominoperineal resection. For selected tumors in the distal rectum that are confined to the rectal wall, there has been increasing interest in local therapy as an alternative to more radical resections for elective treatment of early rectal cancers. Local therapy for highly selected tumors, with or without adjuvant radiotherapy and chemotherapy, can achieve favorable cure rates and low recurrence rates. In some situations, local therapy is an effective alternative to more radical resection. It should be stressed that local therapy is suitable only for a minority of patients who present with rectal cancer; in fact, <5% of rectal cancer patients are candidates for local therapy after preoperative evaluation.

Strict selection criteria are critical for choosing the appropriate patient for local therapies (Table 14.1). The criteria for local excision are as follows: tumor size <3 to 4 cm, involvement of less than one third the rectal circumference, location 6 to 8 cm or less from the anal verge, well-differentiated or moderately well differentiated histology, absence of lymphatic or vascular invasion, mobile, and no suspicion of metastatic perirectal or presacral nodes. Endorectal ultrasound has been very useful in selecting tumors appropriate

TABLE 14.1. CRITERIA FOR LOCAL EXCISION

Tumor size < 3–4 cm
<one third of rectal wall involvement
Location 6–8 cm or less from anal verge
Well or moderately differentiated histology
Absence of vascular invasion
Absence of lymphatic invasion
Absence of perineural invasion
Mobile, not fixed
No perirectal or presacral nodes
Endorectal ultrasonography stage uT1N0

for local therapy. Depth of wall invasion can be determined with 80 to 90% accuracy. However, determination of nodal status with endorectal ultrasound is less optimal, with accuracy rates of 60 to 80%. The objective is to select patients for local therapy in whom the tumor is confined to the rectal wall and for whom there is a very low probability of lymph node metastases. Because local excision does not remove the surrounding lymph nodes, it is contraindicated as the sole modality of treatment for patients at high risk of lymph node metastases.

For patients with favorable histology T1 rectal cancers, local therapy alone is sufficient, because the rate of lymph node involvement is 3 to 10%. The 5-year survival exceeds 90% without further adjuvant therapy. Local recurrence rates range from 0 to 11% for T1 lesions. Close clinical follow-up is recommended. Postoperative radiation and chemotherapy may be considered after local excision for patients with T1 tumors and unfavorable histology and for selected T2 tumors with negative margins. The estimated rate of lymph node positivity for T2 lesions is 15 to 20%; and therefore, it is generally not recommended to use local therapy alone for these lesions. T3 tumors clearly have unacceptable local failure rates and should be treated with radical resection and not local therapy. Only under special circumstances should local therapy be considered in patients with T2 and T3 lesions, such as those unfit for or who refuse major surgery.

Procedures used in the local treatment of rectal cancers include transanal excision, trans-sacral/transcoccygeal excision (Kraske), trans-sphincteric excision (York-Mason), transanal endoscopic microsurgery (TEM), and endocavitary radiation (ECR) treatment.

Most small distal rectal cancers that fulfill the criteria for local therapy are amenable to a (Parks) transanal excision, currently the preferred technique (Fig. 14.2). This procedure is generally performed under general anesthesia with patients placed in the lithotomy position for posterior lesions or in the prone-jackknife position for anterior located lesions. Excellent exposure and adequate lighting are essential for successful transanal excision. Using a suitable anal retractor and headlight, the tumor is visualized and excised transanally using electrocautery with approximately a 1 cm gross margin. The excision must be full thickness, exposing the perirectal fat beneath the lesion. The lesion is then pinned out and sent for pathology. The excised defect may be closed transversely with interrupted sutures or even left open to heal secondarily. Morbidity and mortality from this procedure is exceedingly rare. Positive margins require re-resection or a more definitive surgical procedure.

Other approaches used to treat rectal cancers are the posterior transsacral approach (Kraske) and the trans-sphincteric approach

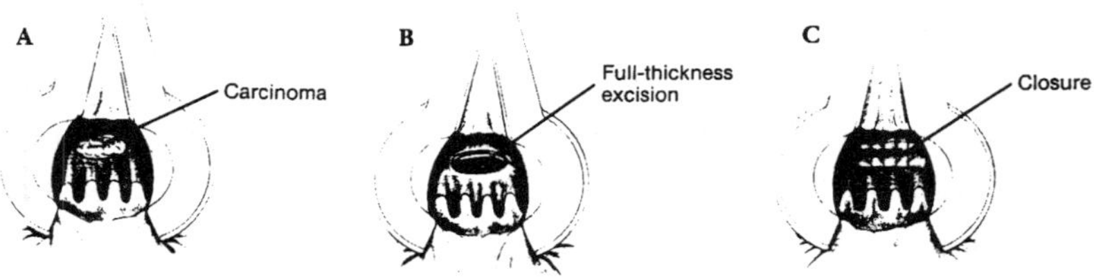

FIGURE 14.2. Transanal excision of carcinoma of rectum. **A**, Exposure of carcinoma. **B**, Full-thickness excision with exposure of perirectal fat. **C**, Completed closure. (Reprinted with permission from Ref. 1.)

(York-Mason). Though not commonly performed, these approaches have been advocated for local excision of some benign sessile and selected malignant tumors. For the Kraske approach the patient is positioned in the prone-jackknife position, and a longitudinal incision is made over the distal sacrum and coccyx. The coccyx is excised and the posterior rectal wall is exposed. The tumor is identified and excised with adequate margins of normal rectal wall, which is then re-approximated with interrupted sutures. The York-Mason approach involves division of the anal sphincters to achieve exposure. After tumor resection, the sphincter complex is then re-approximated with a layered closure. Though sphincter function is usually preserved, concern for possible tumor implantation and local recurrence has deterred the use of the York-Mason procedure by many surgeons. Furthermore, these techniques are often avoided because of the possible complication of a rectocutaneous fistula.

A more recent advance in the local treatment of rectal cancer has been the introduction of TEM. Developed in 1980, TEM uses a sophisticated rigid endoscopic system with binocular optics, suction, and carbon dioxide insufflation of the rectum. Sophisticated instruments are placed through a 40-mm-diameter operating sigmoidoscope that is fixed to the operating room table. The equipment is not readily available in most institutions. The technique of TEM is identical in principle to conventional endoanal excision; however, the procedure is much more technically demanding owing to the nature of the equipment. Currently, formal training is required, and experience with this novel procedure is increasing.

Another technique available for the local treatment of rectal cancer is ECR treatment. ECR may be used with both curative and palliative intent. The main advantage of ECR is that it can be delivered as an outpatient procedure and does not require a general anesthetic. The main disadvantage of this therapy is that the whole specimen is not available for pathologic examination and staging. ECR is particularly useful for patients with tumors amenable to local therapy who cannot tolerate general anesthesia. Currently, endocavitary radiation therapy is available only in selected, specialized centers.

ECR uses a low-voltage, 50-kV machine that delivers radiation locally to the tumor through a specialized proctoscope. Generally, 9,000 to 15,000 cGy of radiation is delivered to the tumor in three to five divided doses at 1- to 2-week intervals. The treatments last 2 to 3 min and require conscious sedation or an anal canal anesthetic block. Attempts are made to deliver radiation to the tumor only, and with particular attention to depth of penetration and voltage, injury to surrounding normal structures is minimized. The limited penetration of this form of radiation permits the use of much larger doses of radiation to the tumor than achieved by external beam irradiation. Results of endocavitary radiation therapy for properly selected patients are similar to transanal excision in terms of local recurrence and survival.

SPHINCTER-PRESERVING THERAPY

Historically, the gold standard surgical treatment for patients with clinically resectable, distal, invasive rectal cancer has been an abdominoperineal resection (APR). Although an APR offers good cure rates, it necessitates a permanent colostomy. In recent years, there has been a trend toward sphincter-preserving operations to avoid the morbidity of abdominoperineal resection. There is ample evidence that this can be accomplished without oncologic compromise.

The introduction of mechanical circular stapling devices has been one of the most important reasons for the increase in sphincter-saving resections. Furthermore, the use of preoperative chemoradiation therapy in selected patients with clinically resectable transmural rectal cancers has increased sphincter preservation while obtaining a high likelihood of local control.

The level of the tumor above the anal verge is the most important factor in determining if a patient is a candidate for a sphincter-preserving resection. Sphincter-preserving procedures are possible for patients with midrectal cancers (7–11 cm from the anal verge) and for highly selected patients with distal rectal cancers (<7 cm from the anal verge). It is generally accepted that for the vast majority of tumors, a 2.0-cm distal margin of resection beyond the distal edge of the tumor is adequate for a curative resection to be performed. The options for sphincter-preservation therapy, including anterior resection, low anterior resection, colonic J-pouch anastomoses, and coloanal anastomoses, will be discussed in the following sections.

ANTERIOR RESECTION An anterior resection is performed for tumors in the upper third of the rectum. Treatment of cancer in the rectosigmoid or intra-abdominal rectum results in cure rates and patterns of recurrence similar to more proximal colon cancers. During an anterior resection, the sigmoid and rectum are first mobilized by division of the lateral peritoneum. The gonadal vessels and left ureter are identified and preserved. The mesentery is divided at the origin of the inferior mesenteric artery (high ligation) or just distal to the origin of the left colic artery (low ligation). If a high ligation of the inferior mesenteric artery is performed, then the left colon and anastomosis will be perfused by the middle colic artery via collateralization through the marginal artery. Retrospective studies have not shown that high ligation of the inferior mesenteric artery confers any significant survival benefit.

During anterior resection, the splenic flexure may require mobilization to achieve a well-vascularized and tension-free anastomosis. Mobilization of the splenic flexure may be difficult if the flexure is closely applied to the spleen or if there are adhesions between the greater omentum and the splenic capsule. Care must be taken in mobilizing the splenic flexure to avoid traction on the attachments to the spleen and subsequent iatrogenic splenic injury. The rectum is transected distally to achieve at least a 2-cm distal margin of resection. The anastomosis for an anterior resection is above the peritoneal reflection, within the peritoneal cavity.

LOW ANTERIOR RESECTION By definition, a low anterior resection represents a rectal resection in which the anastomosis is below the peritoneal reflection and within the sacral hollow. This anastomosis is truly intrapelvic, in contradistinction to an anterior resection in which the anastomosis is above the peritoneal reflection and within the peritoneal cavity. The majority of low anterior anastomoses are performed using circular stapling devices, but anastomoses may also be hand sewn. The choice to use stapled or hand-sewn anastomoses depends on surgeon preference. Clinical trials and a recent meta-analysis have shown no major clinical differences between hand-sewn and stapled anastomoses.

Local recurrence rates after rectal cancer surgery may vary considerably between different centers and different surgeons. The best reported surgical results in terms of local recurrence have been achieved using a technique called total mesorectal excision (TME). This technique, popularized by Heald and Ryall (2) involves the complete removal of the envelope of fibrofatty and lymphatic tissues (the so-called mesorectum) that encompass the rectum from the sacral promontory to the pelvic floor (Fig. 14.3) (3). Pathologic studies have shown that local recurrences often result from incomplete excision of tumor at the circumferential resection margins. These studies have also demonstrated that distal mesorectal spread often extends farther than intramural spread. Total mesorectal excision attempts to decrease local recurrence rates by obtaining maximal circumferential resection margins. Heald and Ryall (2) have reported remarkably low local recurrence rates (<4%) using TME without the use of adjuvant radiotherapy. This low rate of local recurrence from a single surgeon's personal experience has gained worldwide attention and enthusiasm for this technique. However,

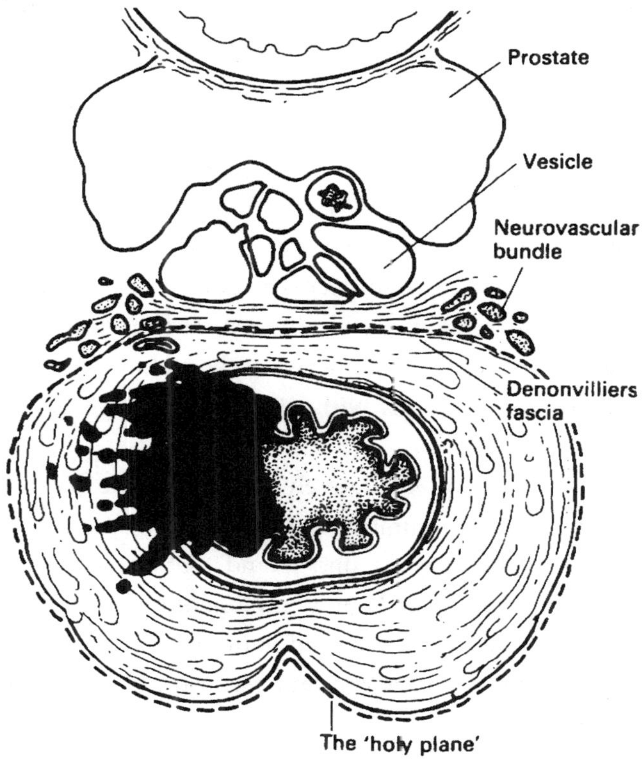

FIGURE 14.3. The relationships of the mesorectum to the anatomical structures in the male. The neurovascular bundle contains the nerves responsible for erection and ejaculation and aspects of bladder function (Reprinted with permission from Ref. 3.)

TME has been associated with somewhat higher leak rates (>17%), and proximal diversion is often performed.

Another important consideration in rectal cancer surgery is autonomic nerve preservation of urinary and sexual function. Identification, dissection, and preservation of the pelvic autonomic nerves are critical and allow for optimal preservation of urinary and sexual function in combination with TME and sphincter preservation. Autonomic nerve injury may lead to erectile dysfunction and retrograde ejaculation in males. Results of autonomic nerve preservation in conjunction with TME and sphincter preservation have been reported. From these reports, approximately 85% of male and female patients can expect to have preserved sexual and urinary function after surgery.

COLOANAL ANASTOMOSIS AND COLONIC J-POUCH Most patients with cancers in the midrectum may be treated with a low anterior resection with sphincter preservation. For more distal tumors in the lower rectum, surgery is technically more challenging and sphincter preservation can be difficult. However, low anterior resection with a coloanal anastomosis can be technically performed for certain low rectal lesions without compromising cancer treatment.

Often one cannot preoperatively determine the feasibility of performing an adequate, curative resection with a sphincter-preserving operation. Patients must understand that decisions to resect and reconstruct are often made only intraoperatively. Patients must, therefore, be prepared for an abdominoperineal resection and permanent colostomy if resection and reconstruction are not technically possible.

Indeed there are situations in which the use of the coloanal anastomosis is not a suitable option and is contraindicated. Proper patient selection for coloanal anastomosis and reconstruction is essential. Clearly, compromised preoperative sphincter function will lead to impaired postoperative continence and a failed procedure. Sphincter invasion by tumor is an obvious contraindication to coloanal anastomosis and demands abdominoperineal resection. Essentially, for sphincter-preserving therapies to be recommended, they must be performed with cancer cure and local recurrence rates equivalent to that of abdominoperineal resection.

Although distance from the anal verge, body habitus, patient gender, and prostate size are all factors affecting reconstructive options, the distance from the lower edge of the tumor to the anorectal ring is the major determinant of sphincter preservation. For consideration of a coloanal anastomosis, the lower edge of the tumor should be a minimum of 2 cm above the anorectal ring. This level allows for an adequate 2-cm distal margin of resection without anal sphincter injury.

Historically, a 5-cm distal margin was cited in surgical textbooks as being the minimal adequate distal surgical margin; however, more recent data do not support the need for such a generous margin. The optimal length of the distal margin for cancer cure and prevention of local recurrence has been evaluated, and distal margins in excess of 2 cm do not appear to reduce the risk of suture line or local recurrence. In fact, <2% of patients will have intramural spread of >2 cm, and generally these patients have very advanced, poorly differentiated cancers that are incurable by surgery alone. Thus surgeons attempt to obtain at least a 2-cm distal margin for resection. Furthermore, the extent of circumferential clearance and lateral margins is particularly important in terms of limiting local recurrence. Quirke et al. (4) showed convincing evidence that local recurrence is mainly the result of lateral spread of tumor within the mesorectum when inadequate surgical resection is performed.

Even selected patients harboring tumors as low as 2 cm above the anorectal ring who, when preoperatively treated with radiation, demonstrate excellent clinical regression are candidates for low anterior resection with coloanal anastomosis. In fact, studies have shown that in selected patients with low rectal tumors, high-dose preoperative chemoradiation may downstage the tumor enough to permit resection of the primary tumor with a high rate of sphincter preservation. Such treatment results in survival rates similar to those observed with more radical surgery without increasing the risk of pelvic or perineal recurrence. Low-lying anaplastic and poorly differentiated rectal adenocarcinomas should be treated with abdominoperineal resection and not a sphincter-preserving operation.

The introduction of circular stapling devices has considerably increased the rate of very low anastomoses after low anterior resection for rectal cancer. As anastomoses are being created more distally, the functional results of the conventional straight coloanal anastomosis have been compromised. Although fecal continence is preserved with sphincter preservation, frequency of bowel movements and episodic urgency have significantly affected the ultimate long-term results for patients with very low colorectal or coloanal anastomoses. It is thought that the loss of capacitance and reservoir function of the resected rectum is responsible for the altered functional status in patients with straight coloanal anastomoses.

As a result of the success achieved with the ileoanal pouch anastomosis in the treatment of inflammatory bowel disease, the colonic J-pouch anastomosis was first described in 1986 in France by Lazorthes et al. (5,6) and Parc et al. (7) (Fig. 14.4). Reports have since been described in the literature that have demonstrated improved functional outcomes with use of the colonic J-pouch in selected situations. Creation of a J-pouch increases the capacity of the constructed neorectum by creating a reservoir; superior functional

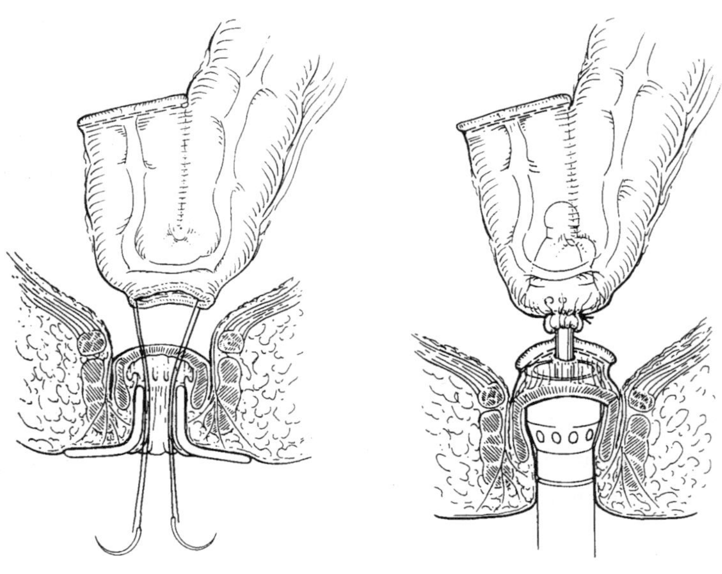

FIGURE 14.4. Colonic J-Pouch with coloanal anastomosis. **A**, Handsewn anastomosis. **B**, Stapled anastomosis. (Reprinted with permission from Ref. 8.)

results have been shown compared to the straight anastomoses, particularly in the 1st postoperative year.

Initial reports with the colonic J-pouch described early evacuation problems, necessitating the use of enemas in up to 25% of patients. The early colonic J-pouches were made with colonic limbs measuring 10 to 12 cm. The size of optimum reservoir size has been studied prospectively, and a 6- to 8-cm pouch has been advocated as the optimal size to provide improved functional outcome.

The clinical leak rate from the colonic J-pouch anastomosis is considerable (>15%); hence the majority of patients generally require a temporary diverting stoma. Coloanal anastomosis with colonic J-pouch provides similar rates of long-term survival and local recurrence as does low anterior resection without coloanal anastomosis. Although there is some evidence to suggest that the addition of a colonic pouch improves functional outcome after proctectomy with coloanal anastomosis, the straight coloanal anastomosis is still the more common operation used currently for sphincter-preservation therapy for low rectal tumors.

INDICATIONS FOR TEMPORARY FECAL DIVERSION

There are certain situations in which a temporary defunctioning stoma is recommended after low anterior resection, coloanal anastomosis, or colonic J-pouch. Diverting stomas are performed for concern of anastomotic disruption, pelvic sepsis, and subsequent poor function secondary to pelvic fibrosis, rigidity, and noncompliance. Factors contributing to increased risk of anastomotic leakage include preoperative radiation, a low level of anastomosis, chemotherapy, steroids, diverticular disease, and technical problems. Generally, a temporary defunctioning stoma is elected if the anastomosis is <5 cm from the anal verge or if any adverse factors exist.

Effective fecal diversion reduces the risk of significant sequelae related to anastomotic leak. One cannot overemphasize the importance of preoperative consultation with an enterostomal therapist for patient education and appropriate stoma site marking. Colostomy or ileostomy sites should be marked preoperatively, with attention to the belt line and skinfolds. Temporary stomas are generally closed electively any time >2 to 3 months after surgery, provided radiographic contrast studies confirm a well-healed anastomosis.

HARTMANN PROCEDURE

The Hartmann procedure is currently most commonly used in the setting of complicated diverticular disease; however, it is an important option in the treatment of advanced, obstructed, or perforated rectal cancer. Because of the increased risk of anastomotic leakage, resections with anastomoses have traditionally not been performed in the presence of obstruction or perforation. In addition, for noncomplicated, resectable rectal cancer, the Hartmann procedure has an occasional role in both curative and palliative surgery as an alternative to abdominoperineal resection.

A Hartmann procedure involves resection and colostomy with the potential for delayed anastomosis. At operation, the tumor is resected with adequate proximal and distal margins, and the proximal colon is brought to the skin as an end colostomy. The distal rectum is sutured or stapled closed and referred to as the Hartmann's pouch. This Hartmann's pouch is completely defunctioned from the fecal stream but may continue to produce small amounts of mucus, which may occasionally be passed. Intestinal continuity may be re-established during a second operation whereby the Hartmann procedure is reversed and the colostomy is closed. Generally, at least 3 to 6 months pass before reversing the Hartmann procedure. Patients may not wish to have a second operation and may elect not to have their colostomy reversed; in fact, owing to advanced patient age and associated co-morbidities, 40 to 50% of patients do not undergo Hartmann reversal and have a permanent colostomy.

Occasionally, the Hartmann procedure has a role as an alternative to an abdominoperineal resection for some advanced low rectal cancers. There are situations in which rectal resection may be performed with an adequate margin, yet re-anastomosis is inappropriate. The Hartmann procedure has less overall morbidity compared to an abdominoperineal resection, primarily because of the absence of perineal wound complications and pain.

ABDOMINOPERINEAL RESECTION

Despite increased trends in the use of local therapies and sphincter-preserving resections for the treatment of rectal cancer, abdominoperineal resection (APR) may be necessary for many distal rectal cancers. An APR removes the rectum and neighboring lymph node–bearing tissues and the anal sphincters. Although APR was at one time the most common operation for all rectal cancers, APR is now performed less frequently. With the increased use of sphincter-sparing operations for rectal cancer, APR is required in approximately 10% of patients with midrectal cancers and 50 to 60% of patients with distal rectal cancers.

There are two phases to the operation: an abdominal phase and a perineal phase. The rectum and its mesorectum are mobilized to the pelvic floor initially by the abdominal approach; the anus and rectum are then removed via the perineal route. Posterior vaginectomy with or without vaginal reconstruction should be considered in women with anterior tumors that may involve the rectovaginal septum. A two-team or synchronous excision is performed by many surgeons and permits shorter operating room times. There are a variety of factors that influence the decision to perform an abdominoperineal resection or attempt a sphincter-preserving resection. Management decisions regarding operability and resectability should be made clinically, considering a variety of important factors.

Clearly, there may be tumor factors present that necessitate APR for potential cure. Tumor location and depth of invasion are the two most important variables influencing the decision to perform an APR. As discussed earlier, there are established criteria that have been developed for the use of local therapies for treatment of distal rectal cancers; patients who do not meet such criteria and are not candidates for sphincter preserving therapies will generally require an APR. Distal rectal cancers that invade the anal sphincter and/or vagina are best treated with an APR.

There are also a variety of patient variables that influence the choice of operation. In certain situations, even though a sphincter-sparing operation may be technically possible in a particular patient, the use of APR may be more appropriate. For example, patients with poor preoperative sphincter function and continence may not tolerate a low rectal anastomosis and may be better served by a colostomy. Furthermore, certain disabilities, such as blindness, severe arthritis, mental or psychologic incapacity and paraplegia or quadriplegia, may influence the use of APR.

There are certain technical factors that are important for the decision to perform an APR. Some tumors that may be very accessible in the gynecoid pelvis may be very difficult to resect and anastomose in the male android pelvis. The surgeon must take into consideration all of these factors, often intraoperatively, in deciding whether to perform an abdominoperineal resection.

The results in terms of morbidity and mortality for abdominoperineal resection have improved significantly since the operation was first described by Miles (9) in 1908. However, morbidity and mortality continues to be significant because the APR is a very major operation. Currently, operative mortality varies from 0 to 6% and has remained quite stable over the past few decades.

Morbidity is significant for this operation. Cardiorespiratory complications are common and account for the majority of operative mortality. Bladder dysfunction; sexual dysfunction (including impotence and retrograde ejaculation in males); and urethral, ureteral, and bladder injury can be major sources of patient morbidity. Perineal complications do occur and are second in frequency only to the more common urologic complications. Perineal complications include wound abscess, hemorrhage, delayed healing, and chronic perineal sinus. Perineal hernias may occur but are fortunately uncommon. Colostomy problems such as prolapse, retraction, stenosis, and pericolostomy hernia can occur and may necessitate reoperative repair. Many of these colostomy complications may be avoided with careful attention to operative technique and appropriate preoperative stoma marking.

PELVIC EXENTERATION

There is a small but significant number of patients with locally advanced rectal cancers that are potentially curable only with radical surgery and combined multimodality therapy. For curative surgery, a pelvic exenteration may be necessary for males with rectal tumors invading the prostate or base of bladder and for women with invasion of the bladder after prior hysterectomy. Although this procedure is not commonly performed, retrospective studies suggest that a radical approach in selected patients can be done with acceptable morbidity and mortality.

Total pelvic exenteration involves the en bloc removal of the rectum, bladder, prostate, lower ureters, uterus, ovaries, the perineum, draining lymph nodes, and pelvic peritoneum. A sacrectomy may be indicated for rectal cancers that locally invade the sacrum posteriorly. Both a permanent colostomy and a urostomy are necessitated.

For those who are candidates for curative pelvic exenteration, this aggressive operation has resulted in reported 5-year survival rates of 30 to 50% for primary colorectal cancers confined to the pelvis. Indications for exenteration for recurrent colorectal carcinoma are less well defined. Central recurrences may be amenable to pelvic exenteration with curative intent. In addition, there may be a palliative role in selected patients. Median survival ranges from 17 months to 3 years, with 5-year survival rates of 10 to 20% for patients treated with recurrent rectal cancer. Median hospital stay after surgery is 26 to 60 days. Overall operative morbidity ranges from 25 to 85%, with operative mortality rates in the 2 to 8% range. Although pelvic exenteration carries with it substantial morbidity and mortality, in expert centers increased experience has significantly decreased morbidity and mortality rates.

INTRAOPERATIVE RADIATION THERAPY

Issues regarding the use of preoperative and postoperative external beam radiation therapy have been addressed in other chapters. This section briefly addresses the current use of intraoperative radiation therapy (IORT) in the treatment of rectal cancer.

IORT refers to either intraoperative electron radiation therapy (IOERT) or to brachytherapy. The advantage of IORT is that it can deliver precise, localized, high-dose radiation treatment to areas at high risk of local recurrence while minimizing the dose of radiation to adjacent normal tissues. Doses of between 1000 and 2000 cGy to one or more fields are delivered, depending on the area of margin involved. Single-dose radiation treatments may be biologically equivalent to two to three times the same quantity delivered as external-beam radiation therapy. Structures that are sensitive to radiation injury such as the small bowel and ureters, are protected by displacement from the IORT field. Brachytherapy is an alternative to external beam radiation therapy and consists of locally placing catheters embedded in a flexible plastic pad onto areas of presumed residual disease. In small series, local control and disease-free survival have been improved with the use of brachytherapy. Both IOERT and brachytherapy are equivalent modalities of administration of intraoperative radiation therapy.

Although currently only used in a limited number of centers, combined modality therapy with high-dose preoperative radiotherapy and IORT appears to improve local control of locally advanced or initially unresectable rectal cancers. Morbidity owing to early and late pelvic complications has been somewhat higher in IORT-treated patients. Pelvic soft-tissue complications such as abscess, wound infection, and delayed healing have been higher in IORT-treated patients. Myocutaneous flaps are now often used during reconstruction to decrease morbidity related to the problems associated with delayed pelvic wound healing.

SMALL BOWEL EXCLUSION

Classically, radiation therapy has been given postoperatively after final pathology and accurate staging are determined. Different centers use different strategies for radiation therapy. Postoperative adjuvant combined modality therapy has been shown to decrease local recurrence rates for stage II and III rectal cancer and improve survival. After abdominoperineal resection or low anterior resection, the small bowel descends into the pelvis, where it is at risk from the effects of postoperative radiation therapy used to treat the pelvis. Radiation-induced enteropathy has been the major limiting factor in the use of adjuvant postoperative radiation therapy for patients with advanced rectal cancer.

In an attempt to limit small bowel toxicity from radiation therapy, small bowel exclusion techniques are often used when postoperative radiation therapy is anticipated. There are several methods that have been described that exclude the small bowel from the pelvis and thus minimize small bowel injury from pelvic radiation. Cystopexy may be performed by approximating the bladder to the peritoneum at the sacral promontory, preventing the small bowel from prolapsing into the pelvis during the early postoperative period. Retroversion of the uterus has also been used to exclude the small bowel from the pelvis. Furthermore, the small bowel may be excluded from the pelvis by creating a hammock using a pedicle of greater omentum, without the need for foreign synthetic material. Others have used mesh slings using synthetic, absorbable polyglycolic mesh that is attached to the pelvic brim to exclude the small bowel from the pelvis. In addition, another technique uses saline-filled tissue expanders that are temporarily placed in the pelvis to protect the small bowel from radiation. Although these techniques are not routinely performed at all centers using postoperative radiation therapy, they have produced a significant reduction small bowel toxicity when used.

EXPERIMENTAL NEOSPHINCTER RECONSTRUCTION

Despite considerable advances in the use of sphincter preservation for low rectal cancers, there are situations in which preservation of continence and sphincter function is not possible. APR remains the gold standard operation for low rectal cancers and is absolutely indicated in certain situations. Usually these situations include rectal cancers that are locally advanced and involve the sphincter mechanism or cancers that are so low that adequate tumor clearance cannot be ensured to preserve sphincter function. Under such circumstances, the only way to avoid a permanent colostomy is to perform a total anorectal reconstruction (Fig. 14.5).

Currently, 50 to 60% of patients with distal rectal cancers need to undergo an APR for adequate cancer treatment. All of these patients require a permanent colostomy and must adjust to the change in body image that an ostomy produces. There is a significant acute psychological effect for cancer patients undergoing abdominoperineal resection. Quality of life of patients has been assessed comparing APR to sphincter-sparing operations. Despite problems with increased frequency of bowel movements, decreased continence to flatus, and the increased need for bowel motility–altering medications, patients with sphincter-saving procedures were found to have a better quality of life compared to those treated with an abdominoperineal resection and permanent colostomy.

In an attempt to create a normal continence mechanism in patients undergoing APR, surgeons in Europe have reconstructed the rectum and pelvic floor using a perineal colostomy supported by either a single or bilateral transposed gracilis muscles (graciloplasty).

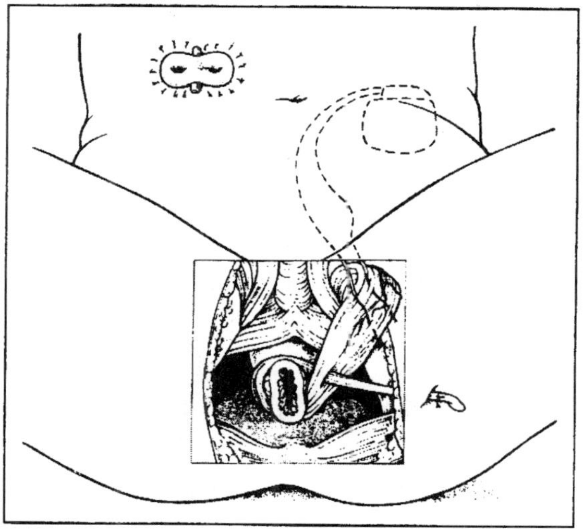

FIGURE 14.5. Total anorectal reconstruction after APR with stimulated graciloplasty. (Reprinted with permission from Ref. 10.)

Using transposed gracilis muscle wrapped around a perineal colostomy, a neosphincter is created that attempts to re-create normal continence. Because the gracilis muscles used to create a "neosphincter" are fast-twitch, fatigue-prone skeletal muscles, investigators have used external intermittent electrical stimulation with pacemakers to convert them to slow-twitch, fatigue-resistant muscles that allow continuous contraction and tone.

Currently, European groups have used the dynamic graciloplasty with reconstruction after APR for cancer in >100 patients with good to excellent continence in >90% of subjects. Overall morbidity in the early experience has been 41%. There have been no perioperative deaths. Complications have declined as experience has increased with the procedure. This innovative technique has the advantages of a standard abdominoperineal resection while avoiding a permanent colostomy and establishing a neosphincter.

Laparoscopic Surgery

Laparoscopic techniques are increasingly being used in many areas of abdominal surgery, including in the treatment of various benign colorectal problems, such as diverticular disease, inflammatory bowel disease, benign polyps, and rectal prolapse. The role of laparoscopic surgery in the treatment of colon and rectal cancer remains highly controversial. The feasibility of laparoscopic colon surgery has been well documented. Experience with laparoscopic-assisted anterior resection and abdominoperineal resection has been described. Advantages of laparoscopic surgery may include decreased length of hospital stay, decreased postoperative pain, and improved cosmesis. Note that early reports of port-site tumor recurrences after laparoscopic colorectal surgery have significantly challenged the role of laparoscopy in the treatment of cancer.

An international registry has been established to follow patients undergoing laparoscopic colorectal surgery for cancer. Currently, laparoscopic surgery for colorectal cancer is being performed in a national, multicenter, prospective clinical trial. Important issues regarding cancer cure, recurrence rates, outcomes, and efficacy need to be addressed before widespread use of laparoscopy for colorectal cancer can be recommended.

Complicated Rectal Cancer

Rectal cancers may be complicated by obstruction, hemorrhage, and perforation. Tumors may be locally advanced and cause neurologic or pressure symptoms. Malignant fistulization may occur. Metastatic disease, most commonly to liver and lung, may alter surgical options.

Malignant obstruction owing to colorectal cancer is the most common cause of large bowel obstruction. Therapeutic options are challenging, because obstructing tumors are frequently advanced at the time of diagnosis. Surgeons are often reluctant to perform a resection and primary anastomosis because the proximal colon is often dilated, unprepared, and may be edematous. Attempts may be made to convert an obstructed lesion to a near-obstructed lesion through bowel rest, nasogastric suction, and intravenous fluid hydration. This may allow for a semielective operation. Selected patients may be candidates for placement of self-expanding stents, which may relieve the obstruction and permit bowel cleaning before definitive surgery.

Complete large bowel obstruction secondary to obstructing rectal cancer generally requires prompt surgical therapy. There are several options for surgical management, and selection of the appropriate operation requires surgical judgment. Traditionally, obstructed tumors have been treated with a staged procedure involving an initial proximal defunctioning stoma, followed by resection with anastomosis, and finally by stoma closure. Although this three-stage approach is not commonly performed for obstructing colon cancer, it continues to be used for obstructing rectal cancer because these lesions are often locally advanced and generally benefit from preoperative chemoradiation treatment to increase resectability. Hence the first stage of treatment is proximal diversion with either a loop ileostomy or transverse colostomy. After diversion, a course of preoperative chemoradiation therapy is administered. The second operative stage involves definitive resection of the primary tumor and low anastomosis. Stoma closure occurs during the third stage. Alternatively, the Hartmann procedure with resection and end sigmoid colostomy is an option if the primary tumor is resectable at initial presentation but circumstances for anastomosis are unfavorable. Another option is primary resection with anastomosis. Primary resection may be combined with an on-table bowel lavage with or without proximal-diverting stoma.

Although an uncommon presentation, rectal cancer may be complicated by perforation. The area of perforation may be within the tumor itself or more proximally located in an area of dilatation secondary to the distal obstruction. Perforation of a tumor is associated with a particularly poor prognosis. Patients may present with peritonitis, and surgical treatment is emergent. The objectives of treatment are control of sepsis and removal of the tumor. The Hartmann procedure with end sigmoid colostomy is appropriate in this setting, because anastomoses are not favored in the presence of sepsis and peritonitis.

Hemorrhage from rectal cancer is seldom significant enough to require emergent treatment. Intermittent rectal bleeding is the more common presentation. Massive lower gastrointestinal bleeding is more often the result of diverticulosis or angiodysplasia. Occasionally, rectal tumors bleed significantly and require prompt treatment. Generally, patients are managed medically, with attention to fluid resuscitation and blood transfusions as necessary. Angiographic embolization is an option to control significant hemorrhage, usually in a palliative setting. Only in rare situations is emergent surgery necessary for the treatment of hemorrhage owing to rectal cancer.

PALLIATIVE PROCEDURES

The management of locally advanced and metastatic rectal cancer may be very challenging. There are rare situations in which palliative procedures are appropriate for the treatment of incurable rectal cancer. The presence of distant metastatic disease affects the choice of operation. Patients with unresectable lung or liver metastases but small primary tumors may best be treated with local therapies. Large primary tumors have the potential to obstruct, bleed, or cause significant local symptoms owing to invasion of contiguous structures. Large, unresectable tumors with significant local invasion that cause obstruction may best be treated by proximal colostomy and palliative radiation therapy. Electrocoagulation, laser and photodynamic therapy, and internal stents have been used in some centers for the palliation of bleeding and obstruction. Experience with these techniques is rather limited. In selected patients, palliative low anterior resection, APR, or the Hartmann procedure is justified to minimize potential for future morbidity.

COMPLICATIONS OF SURGERY

The specific risks and complications of rectal cancer surgery depend on the extent of procedure performed. The more common complications include infection, hemorrhage, and anastomotic problems. Perineal wound infection, dehiscence, and delayed perineal healing are potential complications of abdominoperineal resection. Conventional resections for rectal cancer in men are associated with postoperative erectile dysfunction and retrograde ejaculation in up to 25 to 75% of cases. Attention to autonomic nerve preservation with total mesorectal excision can significantly reduce the morbidity associated with sexual dysfunction.

Anastomotic leakage is one of the most serious complications after rectal resection with anastomosis. Anastomotic leak rates for colorectal anastomosis are higher than for ileocolic or colocolic anastomosis. Leak rates for anterior resection vary considerably in the literature, from 1 to 30%. The clinical leak rate is 5 to 10%, with the subclinical leak rate demonstrated radiographically in 30 to 50%. There are a variety of factors that influence leak rates, including technical and surgeon-related factors. Studies in the literature have investigated leak rates with stapled and hand-sewn anastomoses; the conclusion from a variety of analyses is that there is no difference in regard to leakage. The level of the anastomosis is the most important factor influencing anastomotic leak rates.

The management of anastomotic leaks is variable and depends on the clinical situation. Diagnosis may be confirmed with a gentle enema using water-soluble contrast. Patients may present with minor symptoms or with signs of peritonitis and overt septic shock. The stable patient without peritonitis may be managed conservatively. Pelvic abscesses may be drained percutaneously. The patient with peritonitis and signs of sepsis requires prompt reoperation, usually with proximal diversion and pelvic drainage.

Mortality rates from radical surgery for rectal cancer range from 2 to 6%, with the highest mortality occurring in the elderly. Mortality rates are similar for sphincter-preserving procedures and abdominoperineal resection. Mortality rates with the use of local therapies for rectal cancer are minimal.

RESULTS OF TREATMENT

Data from retrospective series, using conventional low anterior resection or APR before the widespread use of adjuvant therapy, report approximately a 50% 5-year survival for rectal cancer. This survival rate for rectal cancer is somewhat lower than the overall survival rate for colon cancer (55 to 75%). Clearly, the probability of survival depends on the stage of disease, with 5-year survival rates of 80, 60, and 35% for rectal cancer stages I, II, and III, respectively.

In terms of overall local recurrence, rates have been reported between 4 and 30% for curative rectal cancer operations. Most recurrences become apparent during the first 2 years after surgery, supporting more intensive follow-up during this period. Despite curative intent surgery, up to 50% of patients develop a recurrence, either local, distant, or a combination of both. Clearly the role of technical factors, type of operation, and use of adjuvant multimodality therapy requires continued study to evaluate the best strategies to minimize local recurrence and maximize cure.

THERAPY RECOMMENDATIONS BY STAGE

Because preoperative staging determines therapy, it is instructive to summarize and discuss the surgical management of rectal cancer based on the preoperative staging of specific rectal cancers (Table 14.2).

TABLE 14.2. PREFERRED AND ACCEPTABLE THERAPY FOR CURE FOR RECTAL CANCER BASED ON PREOPERATIVE ULTRASOUND STAGING[a]

Stage	Preferred Treatment	Acceptable Treatment
uT1N0M0	Transanal excision[b]	ECR for medically unfit Radical resection for high lesions or poor histologic features TEM for high lesions in medically unfit
uT2N0M0	Radical resection	ECR for medically unfit Transanal excision + XRT if medically unfit or colostomy unacceptable TEM + XRT for high lesions in medically unfit
uT3N0M0		
Superficial	Radical resection	Transanal excision + XRT for medically unfit TEM + XRT for high lesions in medically unfit
Deep	Preoperative chemotherapy/XRT + radical resection	Radical resection + postoperative chemotherapy/XRT, depending on surgeon preference Transanal excision + XRT for medically unfit

(continued)

TABLE 14.2. (CONTINUED)

Stage	Preferred Treatment	Acceptable Treatment
uT4N(any)M0	Preoperative chemotherapy/XRT + radical en bloc resection	Radical en bloc resection + postoperative chemotherapy/XRT, depending on surgeon preference
uT(any)N1M0	Preoperative chemotherapy/XRT + radical resection + postoperative chemotherapy	Radical resection + postoperative chemotherapy/XRT, depending on surgeon preference

[a] Modified from Ref. 11.
[b] Tumor must meet appropriate criteria for local therapy (Table 14.1).
XRT, radiation therapy.

T1N0M0 (Stage I)

T1 tumors are the most favorably staged rectal cancers. T1 lesions involve the mucosa and submucosa but do not invade the muscularis propria. Predicted lymph node involvement with T1 tumors is reported to range between 3 and 10%. Local therapy, if technically possible, is the preferred treatment for T1 lesions that have favorable histologic features. Well or moderately differentiated tumors without lymphovascular invasion and that are located within 8 cm of the anal verge are ideally treated for cure by transanal excision. Local recurrence rates are 0 to 11%, with cancer-specific survival rates >90%. Postoperative radiation therapy is considered for patients with poorly differentiated tumors or lymphovascular invasion who decline radical surgery; local excision alone is acceptable treatment for patients with T1 tumors and favorable histology.

Endocavitary radiation (ECR) is an alternative therapy for T1N0M0 cancers. ECR therapy does not require general anesthesia and thus is a good option for patients who cannot have surgery under a general anesthetic. The results of ECR are similar to transanal excision in terms of local recurrence and survival.

For T1N0M0 lesions proximal to 10 cm above the anal verge, anterior resection may be required. TEM is another option, although available in only a few experienced centers.

T2N0M0 (Stage I)

T2 lesions partially invade the muscularis propria without involvement of the serosa or perirectal fat. Lymph node metastases occur in 15 to 20% of patients with T2 tumors. Most patients with T2 tumors should not be treated with local therapies alone; T2 tumors are best treated with a sphincter-sparing resection or abdominoperineal resection, depending on the distance of the tumor from the anal verge. However, there are some situations in which local therapy with transanal excision is appropriate treatment for T2 lesions. Some patients with superficial T2 lesions demonstrated by endorectal ultrasound are candidates for transanal excision. Local therapy is particularly appropriate for patients with significant medical comorbidities who would not tolerate a larger operation; furthermore, local therapy is appropriate for patients who require an APR but refuse a permanent colostomy. When local therapy is used for the treatment of T2 lesions, postoperative radiation treatment is recommended to lower the risk of local recurrence.

T3N0M0 (Stage II)

T3 tumors penetrate the muscularis propria and invade the perirectal fat. Incidence of lymph node metastases in T3 tumors is 30 to 50%. Patients with superficial T3 lesions by endorectal ultrasound undergo radical anterior resection or APR. Adjuvant therapy is based on final pathologic staging and the status of surgical margins. Patients with deeply invasive T3 lesions determined by endorectal ultrasound should receive preoperative (neoadjuvant) combined chemotherapy and radiation therapy. Surgery is scheduled 4 to 8 weeks after radiation treatment, allowing time for the maximal effects of radiation to occur. Local therapies are not appropriate for T3 lesions.

T(1,2)N1M0 (Stage III)

Patients with unequivocal node-positive rectal cancer on preoperative endorectal ultrasound are treated with preoperative (neoadjuvant) combined chemotherapy and radiation therapy. In the situation in which endorectal ultrasound does not identify positive lymph nodes with a high degree of certainty, patients are best treated initially by surgical resection, and if node-positive disease is verified on the final pathology, then postoperative adjuvant chemoradiation therapy is administered.

T3N1M0 (Stage III)

Patients with T3N1M0 rectal tumors are treated with preoperative neoadjuvant chemotherapy and radiation therapy. Surgery with low anterior resection or APR is scheduled 4 to 8 weeks after this preoperative treatment, allowing time for the radiation's maximal effects to be attained. Additional postoperative chemotherapy is given for 4 to 5 months after surgery. Preoperative neoadjuvant therapy can shrink the primary tumor, downstage the patient, sterilize lymph nodes, and decrease the rate of local recurrence, while also decreasing the toxicity rates of pelvic irradiation. Resection followed by definitive pathology and postoperative radiation therapy is an alternative for patients and surgeons who do not wish to delay surgery with preoperative chemoradiation, but this may limit resectability of larger lesions, diminish the ability to preserve the anal sphincters, and increase the risk of radiation toxicity.

T4N(0,1)M0 (STAGE II, III)

T4 cancers are locally invasive into contiguous structures. They are often fixed or tethered. Organs commonly invaded include the uterus and adnexa, posterior vaginal wall, bladder, and prostate. T4 rectal cancers can be resected for cure in less than half of cases. Contiguous organ involvement occurs in up to 16% of patients with rectal cancer. Organs involved with tumor invasion should be removed en bloc with the primary rectal cancer. The use of preoperative (neoadjuvant) radiation therapy often can shrink the primary tumor and allow for increased resectability with decreased local recurrence rates. IORT is used in some highly specialized centers and, when used in combination with high-dose preoperative radiotherapy, appears to improve local control of locally advanced or initially unresectable rectal cancers. Rectal cancers with contiguous organ involvement have a poorer prognosis compared to tumors without contiguous organ invasion.

T(ANY)N(ANY)M1 (STAGE IV)

The presence of metastatic disease significantly influences treatment options. Preoperative evaluation and imaging are important to detect potentially resectable metastatic disease. Patients with potentially resectable liver or lung metastases should have the primary rectal cancer treated by standard resection, using preoperative neoadjuvant therapy if appropriate. Repeat evaluation and imaging should be performed postoperatively to determine if the metastases remain stable and resectable. If stable and resectable, metastatic resection is recommended at a second operation. Surgery for resectable liver metastases has been associated with a reported 5-year survival of 25 to 42% in current series. Similarly, resection of isolated pulmonary metastases from colorectal cancer results in reported 5-year survival of 21 to 43%. Mortality rates in current series are <5%. Occasionally, in very specialized centers, concomitant resection of a rectal cancer and solitary liver metastasis may be appropriate at a single operation.

Unfortunately, patients with metastatic rectal cancer more commonly have multiple and incurable metastases. Treatment options are limited for patients with diffuse metastatic disease. Clearly, good clinical judgment is necessary in managing patients with metastatic rectal cancer. Palliation of the symptoms of obstruction, bleeding, and pain is the goal of treatment. Narcotic analgesics are often necessary and may aggravate constipation and obstructive symptoms. Blood transfusions may be required to palliate symptoms owing to profound anemia. Surgery with a proximal loop sigmoid colostomy may be advised for patients with circumferential rectal cancers that are likely to obstruct. Often, elective colostomy may allow the patient to die without the pain and morbidity of a large bowel obstruction. Despite incurable, slowly progressive metastatic disease, the primary tumor may cause significant patient morbidity such that palliative surgical procedures, including low anterior resection and APR, are occasionally justified.

SUMMARY

The surgical treatment of rectal cancer is a challenging area for the surgeon. Pelvic surgery can be technically demanding. Local therapies play an important role in select cases that meet specific criteria. Sphincter-sparing procedures are being performed more commonly as expertise in pelvic surgery improves. Preoperative evaluation and good surgical judgment are required to select the appropriate surgical approach for the appropriate clinical situation. Because there are a variety of options for the surgical treatment of rectal cancer, physicians should be familiar with these options and the various multimodality therapies used to improve patient outcome.

REFERENCES

1. Gordon PH. Malignant neoplasms of the rectum. In: Gordon PH, Nivatvongs S., eds. Principles and practice of surgery for the colon, rectum and anus. St. Louis: Quality Medical, 1992:591–653.
2. Heald RJ, Ryall RDH. Recurrence and survival after total mesorectal excision for rectal cancer. Lancet 1986;1:1479–1482.
3. Heald RJ, Moran BJ. Embryology and anatomy of the rectum. Semin Surg Oncol 1998;15:66–71.
4. Quirke P, Dixon MF, Durdey P, Williams NS. Local recurrence of rectal adenocarcinoma due to inadequate surgical resection—histopathological study of lateral tumour spread and surgical excision. Lancet 1986;2:996–999.
5. Lazorthes F, Fages P, Chiotasso P, et al. Resection of the rectum with construction of a colonic reservoir and colo-anal anastomosis for carcinoma of the rectum. Br J Surg 1986;73:136–138.
6. Lazorthes F, Gamagami R, Chiotasso P, Istvan G, Muhammad S. Prospective, randomized study comparing clinical results between small and large colonic J-pouch following coloanal anastomosis. Dis Colon Rectum 1997;40(12):1409–1413.
7. Parc R, Tiret E, Frileux P, et al. Resection and colo-anal anastomosis with colonic reservoir for rectal carcinoma. Br J Surg 1986;73:139–141.
8. Nicholls RJ. Surgery for rectal carcinoma. In: Nicholls RJ, Dozois RR, eds. Surgery of the colon and rectum. New York: Churchill Livingstone, 1997:427–474.
9. Miles WE. A method of performing abdominoperineal excision for carcinoma of the rectum and of the terminal portion of the pelvic colon. Lancet 1908;2:1812–1813.
10. Rosen HR, Novi G, Zoech G, et al. Restoration of anal sphincter function by single-stage dynamic graciloplasty with a modified (split sling) technique. Am J Surg 1998;175:187–193.
11. Shelton AA, Wong WD. Colorectal cancer In: Cameron JL, ed. Current surgical therapy. 6th ed. St. Louis: Mosby, 1998:217–227.

CHAPTER
15

Post-Treatment Follow-Up and Treatment of Recurrent Disease in Adenocarcinoma of the Rectum

Kathleen M. Manning, M.D., and
Peter S. Edelstein, M.D.

Unlike the situation after the initial treatment of the patient with colon cancer, the follow-up of the patient who has undergone initial treatment of a rectal cancer is not limited to metastatic disease surveillance. This is because a locoregional (pelvic) recurrence rate of approximately one in three still exists for patients who have completed apparently curative treatment for their rectal cancers. When found early, a second curative attempt is sometimes possible for rectal cancer patients whose recurrence is limited both to and within the pelvis. When evaluating for evidence of potentially curable rectal cancer recurrence, it is important to remember that curability always requires complete surgical resectability. Thus if a recurrence, whether local or distant, is not amenable to complete operative extirpation, curability is an impossibility. This chapter is

Colon and Rectal Cancer, Edited by Peter S. Edelstein, M.D.
ISBN 0-471-35145-8

designed to assist in the selection of rectal cancer patients who are appropriate for aggressive follow-up and to provide for the creation of a logical, comprehensive approach aimed at identifying local, metastatic, and metachronous lesions when still potentially resectable. This strategy must be tailored to the individual's grade and stage of cancer and to the timing and type of adjuvant treatment, as well as to the specific operation initially performed. The follow-up approach may also be modified for patients who are poor candidates for reoperation but who may still benefit from aggressive palliative medical therapy of their recurrent disease. Techniques useful (or not) for patient follow-up are discussed. Although tactics for identifying distant metastases is addressed, the reader is referred to Chapter 3, which is entirely devoted to the evaluation and treatment, both curative and palliative, for both metastatic colon and metastatic rectal cancer. This chapter focuses primarily on surveillance for and curative and palliative treatment of rectal cancer that recurs locally.

There is no specific algorithm on which there is uniform agreement that is used to follow treated rectal cancer patients. Every approach, from the nihilistic no follow-up to the performance of a physical examination, chest x-ray, and abdominal/pelvic CT scan every 3 months, can be found in clinical practice. The reason for this tremendous variability is multifactorial. A major factor concerns the continuing evolution in the initial treatment options for rectal cancer. Adjuvant therapy has been introduced and proven effective for stage II and stage III disease. More recently, the role of neoadjuvant therapy has grown exponentially. Both the use of preoperative radiation and the development of circular stapling devices has meant that abdominoperineal resection, once the mainstay of rectal cancer surgery, has been supplanted by low anterior resection and, even more recently, by sphincter-sparing complete proctectomy with coloanal anastomosis. Currently, less than one third of operations performed for rectal cancer are abdominoperineal resections. A second evolution in the surgical treatment of rectal cancer is the total mesorectal excision (TME), based on evidence that the vast majority of local recurrences are secondary to the persistence of tumor within unresected mesorectal tissue after primary operation. Thus most local recurrences present within 2 years of initial treatment and arise from remaining mesorectal and lateral margins and do not involve the mucosa except secondarily. After TME, local recurrence rates as low as 3% have been reported. The constantly changing (and hopefully improving) initial approaches to rectal cancer does not allow for one uniform, obvious follow-up strategy for all patients.

A second reason for the inconsistent approach to patient follow-up is the overall dismal and depressing reported outcomes after the attempted curative treatment of recurrent disease. Although many physicians lecture on the encouraging success rates of resection for recurrent rectal adenocarcinoma, when the overall recurrence and true resectability rates are honestly analyzed, it is clear at present that actual success in curing recurrent disease is extremely uncommon. Thus, given the shrinking number of available health care dollars, some argue that once a rectal cancer patient completes his or her initial treatment, there is no indication for any regular patient follow-up, or at least not before the development of symptoms that suggest recurrence. Such nihilistic attitudes are based on published data that, unfortunately, suggest no significant survival benefit in patients with colorectal cancer when closely followed after initial treatment compared to those not regularly followed.

Still, given our constantly growing armamentarium in the war against recurrent disease, surgical, radiotherapeutic, and chemotherapeutic, and given our rapidly improving radiologic techniques for detecting early recurrences, it seems reasonable to allow for follow-up of at least those rectal cancer patients who are participating in recurrent disease evaluation and/or treatment protocols. Furthermore, human beings, and perhaps physicians in particular, have great difficulty in surrendering to disease, especially when on rare occasion a patient with recurrent rectal cancer can in fact truly be cured. Thus, although difficult, identifying patients with disease recurrence who are good candidates for attempted curative treatment and then defining an aggressive follow-up strategy for those patients will allow for the greatest opportunities to further improve our success in curing rectal cancer.

THE CAUSE AND TIMING OF RECTAL CANCER RECURRENCE

Rectal cancer recurrence occurs relatively early after initial treatment. Approximately 75% of recurrences are diagnosed within the first 2 years after treatment of the primary disease, and a full 95% are detected within 5 years. The pattern of recurrence can be local/regional (pelvic), metastatic, or a combination of the two. Historically, local recurrence was believed to be secondary to insufficient initial bowel resection, with viable cells remaining and then growing at the anastomosis. Although such anastomotic recurrences secondary to inadequate bowel resection do indeed occur, this is an extremely rare event. A large volume of published data now suggest that the overwhelming majority of pelvic recurrences arise from viable cells within mesorectum (including lateral tissue) which are left behind at initial resection. These persistent malignant cells develop into a radiographically and/or grossly detectable recurrent cancer, usually within 18 months of initial resection. Thus, in actuality, cancer recurs outside of the anastomosed bowel, within the surrounding perirectal tissue. In many instances, the recurrence grows along the previously dissected surgical planes and penetrates through the new anastomosis, giving rise to the long-held belief that all recurrences originated in the anastomotic line. Unfortunately, by the time a recurrent cancer has penetrated into the mucosa, it has often obtained an unresectable size and/or has penetrated beyond curability into other pelvic organs or into the sacrum.

The evolving understanding of the cause of pelvic recurrence is the basis of the inclusion of total mesorectal excision and wide circumferential margins into the primary operative approach to rectal adenocarcinoma, as described in Chapter 14. When properly performed, TME has led to a reported drop in local recurrence rates from >30% for some disease stages to as low as 3%.

Metastatic rectal cancer most frequently targets the liver, with the lungs as the second most frequent site of malignant spread. Carcinomatosis is less common, and metastasis to the bones or brain, although an occasional occurrence, is uncommon. Of note (and of significant frustration), approximately one-half of all patients who succumb to rectal cancer have recurrent disease confined to the pelvis.

HISTORY AND PHYSICAL EXAMINATION

Unfortunately at present, by the time a rectal cancer recurrence is detectable by history or physical examination, the overwhelming majority cannot be resected for cure. This incurability is based on the central role played by complete surgical resection in any cure. By the time most recurrences are detectable either to the patient (as symptoms) or to the physician (as signs on examination), the tumors are quite large. Even small local recurrences are frequently only incompletely resectable, because they are growing along the upper sacrum, invading into unresectable pelvic bony structures, or involving the major vessels of the pelvis or extremities.

LOCAL RECURRENCE

Local recurrence most often presents with vague abdominal or deep pelvic pain. Some patients become partially obstructed, complaining of constipation and/or diarrhea, narrowing stool caliber, and occasionally of bloating. Patients may also experience rectal bleeding. Often patients do not themselves realize that a subtle but significant change in bowel habits has occurred. Therefore, it is vital that the physician ask detailed questions concerning the frequency and characteristics of bowel movements in an attempt to specifically elicit any seemingly minor yet important hint to the presence of local recurrence. Even when patients admit to an alteration in their diet as the probable cause of changed bowel habits, the evaluating physician must always suspect and rule out a local recurrence.

The most frequent sign of local recurrence on physical examination is the presence of a palpable lesion, most often fixed, but rarely mobile, detectable on digital rectal or vaginal examination. It is important for the examiner to aggressively sweep the palpating digit posteriorly over the puborectalis muscle. This will allow for evaluation of the distal presacral space, a common origin for rectal cancer recurrence, especially in patients whose mesorectum was incompletely excised. Large posterior recurrences, however, require no such diligent search, because they are clearly palpable as solid, extrinsic masses compressing the rectum and not infrequently actually invading into or through the bowel wall. Some recurrences spread within the presacral space without exerting a significant mass effect on the bowel. These are more difficult to identify on digital examination, presenting more as a feeling of fullness in the pelvis than as a discrete mass. Lateral and anterior recurrences in women may be detectable on posterior vaginal examination, but in the male patient, these tumors may be difficult to palpate until quite large. Frequently, stools are guaiac positive, and such a finding should generate a search for recurrence despite the fact that many low colorectal and coloanal anastomoses also produce small quantities of bright red blood with defecation. It is rare for recurrent tumor to actually produce significant anemia through luminal blood loss.

METASTATIC DISEASE

Metastatic disease is often significantly more difficult to detect by history or physical examination than is local recurrence. Again, patients may be entirely unaware that any subtle changes have occurred, let alone that these changes are of significance. Thus the task of weeding out important clinical information falls to the physician, whose inquiries must include a complete review of systems. Metastatic disease to the liver, the most common site of distant spread, may produce a sense of abdominal fullness, bloating, or dull ache. Occasionally, but certainly not always in this situation, the disease is bulky enough to produce palpable hepatomegly. Jaundice is most often a late finding, carrying with it a grave prognosis. Like most hepatic metastases, spread of tumor to the lungs is usually asymptomatic, at least until there is extensive pulmonary involvement, when the patient may present with hemoptysis and for dyspnea. Auscultation of the chest is unlikely to ever detect an early recurrence. Bone metastases may produce focal pain in the area of the tumor spread. On the other hand, the patient may complain only of a nonspecific severe joint or muscle ache. Physical examination may be able to identify a specific skeletal area suspicious for metastatic disease if focal, reproducible bony tenderness is demonstrable. Headaches, vertigo, nausea and vomiting, blurred vision, and syncope are common symptoms of metastatic spread to the brain. Balance and visual changes are not difficult to identify on adequate physical examination.

If a physician chooses to discard the nihilistic approach to rectal cancer, especially if patients are to be entered into recurrent disease evaluation and/or treatment protocols, then regularly obtaining a patient history and performing a physical examination is a relatively simple and inexpensive approach to routine follow-up. Given the timing of recurrences, it is reasonable to suggest frequent earlier evaluations, especially during the first 2 years (as often as every 2 or 3 months), for a total of 5 years (every 6 to 12 months over the final 3 years) after initial treatment. Any concerning finding on physical examination, and selected suspicious patient complaints even when not associated with physical findings, should then lead to further, more objective evaluation in the form of imaging and laboratory studies.

LABORATORY STUDIES

Laboratory studies (blood tests), although safely, rapidly, and easily obtained, play only a limited role in the early diagnosis of recurrent rectal cancer. The CBC is virtually never of any diagnostic benefit, because anemia is uncommon and changes in white blood cell count are only rarely associated with recurrence presenting as an abscess or fistula. Liver function test (LFT) abnormalities are usually nonspecific, with changes occurring only when hepatic involvement is extensive. Still, despite no data to support their use (other than some reports concerning alkaline phosphatase), routine CBC and LFT analysis is often performed but cannot be specifically recommended. Carcinoembryonic antigen (CEA) is the only blood test that has been demonstrated to be useful in the early detection of recurrent disease in a specific subset of patients. Although quite sensitive in that subset, determining which patients fit into this category can be difficult.

CARCINOEMBRYONIC ANTIGEN

When first identified, CEA was touted hopefully as the blood test that would detect cancer. Unfortunately, CEA is now known to be very nonspecific; but the blood test is still of great use for certain patients. Recent data suggest that in selected patients, CEA is able to detect a recurrence 3 months earlier than CT scan and 6 months earlier than physical examination. Although previous reports revealed that patients followed with CEA had no better outcome than those not followed with CEA, these studies were too general, including all colorectal cancer patients, rather than analyzing only the subset of patients in whom CEA was elevated preoperatively, dropped to normal levels immediately postoperatively, and then subsequently rose again. Such a second rise in a patient with a known CEA-producing primary tumor appears to be quite sensitive for the detection of recurrence. Recommendations for obtaining CEA levels in such patients vary, with most suggesting CEA testing every

4 to 8 weeks during the first 2 post-treatment years, and continued, albeit less frequent, testing during the following 3 years. Patients whose CEA was high before treatment, then fell to normal after treatment, but then rise again should undergo further evaluation (radiographic) in an attempt to identify any site of recurrence. Unfortunately, although a CEA elevation may be a sensitive indicator of recurrence in this group of patients, a normal CEA in these same patients is a very insensitive indicator of no recurrent disease. That is, in a patient whose elevated CEA normalizes after initial treatment, continuing normal CEA levels does not ensure the absence of recurrent cancer, because many recurrent tumors do not produce detectable elevations of CEA even when the primary lesion did. In patients whose primary tumor did not produce elevated CEA, monitoring blood CEA levels seems unnecessary and wasteful, because the occurrence of CEA-producing metastases in such patients is a rarity. Likewise, following CEA levels in patients whose elevated CEA did not normalize after initial therapy is of no apparent benefit. Obviously the key to using CEA levels in such a fashion depends on obtaining a CEA level before and then following treatment of the primary rectal tumor.

RADIOLOGIC EVALUATION

LOCALLY RECURRENT DISEASE

A variety of radiologic imaging studies can be used in the follow-up of rectal cancer patients. However, for a number of reasons there is currently no uniformly accepted protocol for the use of imaging studies. Even which technique is the most appropriate has not been established, as the use of different modalities varies along with the changing treatment approaches for the primary disease. For example, as the frequency of abdominoperineal resection, an operation leaving no intraluminal access to the pelvis, diminishes in favor of low anterior and coloanal anastomoses, both of which leave the anus intact and in continuity with the large bowel, the role of endorectal ultrasonography (ERUS) in the follow-up of rectal cancer has grown significantly. In addition, as some data emerge to demonstrate curability if local or metastatic recurrence is identified while at a limited stage, new radiologic approaches, such as PET, are concurrently evolving in an attempt to achieve earlier detection. Finally, even relatively older imaging techniques, such as CT scanning, continue to dramatically improve, requiring reassessment.

CT Scan Imaging

Historically, the CT scan has played the major role in post-treatment evaluation of rectal cancer patients. CT can be used in routine surveillance, when there is no clinical suspicion of local or distant recurrence. When used in this fashion, a baseline CT of the pelvis (and of the abdomen, if not obtained before treatment) should be performed no earlier than 3, and usually at 6, months after operation. This time period allows for resolution of the pelvic inflammation associated with treatment, particularly surgical resection. Once the inflammation has resolved, the CT will establish the appearance of the pelvis with what will likely remain as the individual patient's pattern of pelvic scarring. Further imaging, as frequently as every 3 to 6 months, can be compared to this "baseline" scan for evidence of changes in the pelvic tissues, suggesting local recurrence, given that benign scar tissue does not continue to grow. A suspicious increase in pelvic tissue can be further evaluated by other imaging techniques or via percutaneous biopsy. However, it is important not to rely exclusively on CT surveillance, because when used in this fashion, CT is only 60 to 85% sensitive, having significant difficulty differentiating between true recurrence and scar. Thus even in the presence of an equivocal or unchanged CT, new patient symptoms require further investigation. It is also important to remember that at present, there are no collective studies to demonstrate an association with CT detection of recurrence and improved patient outcome. It is hoped that as imaging techniques improve further, a significant curability rate will be clearly demonstrated with earlier detection of recurrence.

MRI

When local pelvic recurrence is suspected based on CT, the scan not infrequently overpredicts potential resectability. Thus following a suspicious CT scan, MRI is often beneficial in evaluating true resectability. Sagittal MRI views, in particular, are much more accurate in answering the important surgical questions, especially by demonstrating the proximal level of sacral involvement and the extent of lateral pelvic sidewall involvement (Fig. 15.1). Although virtually all soft tissue of the anterior pelvis (bladder, prostate, vagina) can be resected en bloc with the recurrence (pelvic exenteration), the extent of resection of these structures (sacrum, iliac vessels, pelvic skeleton) is limited. Although significantly better than CT, MRI also overpredicts disease resectability.

PET

Even when, following a CT scan, MRI suggests surgical resectability, the physician should consider one additional imaging study to rule out the presence of unidentified extrapelvic disease (which makes the patient's recurrence incurable). For this task, PET imaging is now proving valuable. PET is a nuclear medicine study based on the increased use of glucose by malignant cells. Fluorine 18-2-fluoro-2-deoxy-D-glucose (FDG) is the form of radioactive glucose most often used for imaging. The patient fasts for 4 hr, 10 μCi FDG is injected, and images are obtained after waiting for approximately 60 min. Uptake is measured in standardized uptake ratio (SUR) after the areas of maximal uptake are correlated to their anatomic location on CT or MRI. The larger the SUR, the more likely the area of uptake represents malignant tissue. As a nuclear medicine modality, PET provides only very crude anatomic imaging and, therefore, in no

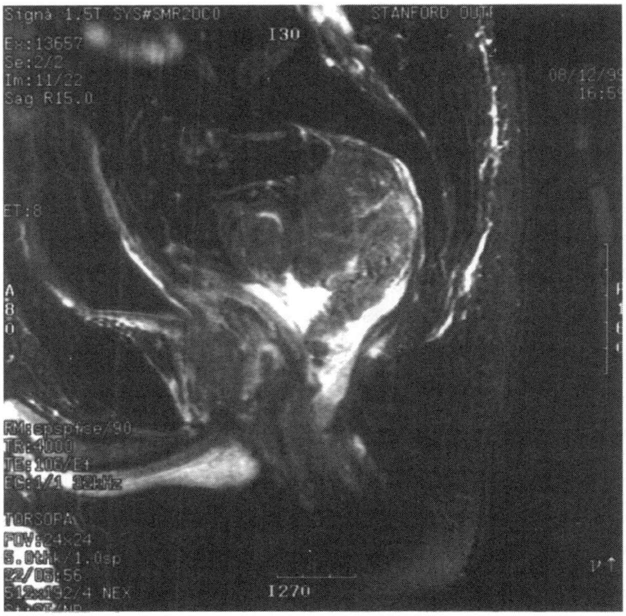

FIGURE 15.1. Sagittal MRI (anterior to left) demonstrating large rectal cancer recurrence (bright, heterogeneous mass) within the presacral space, invading in the region of previous low rectal anastomosis (bowel lumen is black), and lining the anterior sacrum from approximately S2 to S5.

way replaces CT or MRI. However, PET scan can be an adjunct study to further support the diagnosis of recurrence when suspected on CT and/or MRI and when biopsy is not obtainable or has failed to yield malignant tissue. But PET scanning is probably even more useful in situations in which CT and MRI suggest only local recurrence. PET scan may support this conclusion, encouraging attempted resection for cure (Fig. 15.2). PET may, however, detect extrapelvic areas of uptake suggesting previously unidentified metastatic disease outside of the pelvis, for instance in the paraaortic lymph nodes. These sites of metastatic spread are frequently too small to be detected by CT and MRI, leading those studies to the erroneous conclusion that the recurrence is limited to the pelvis. Although unfortunate for the patient, the finding of extrapelvic disease on PET

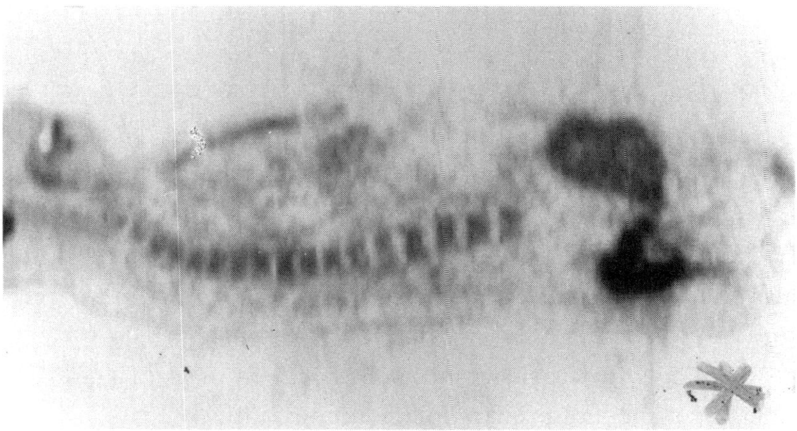

FIGURE 15.2. Sagittal PET scan image (anterior to right) demonstrating large presacral rectal cancer recurrence (darkest collection) with extension anteriorly toward normal bladder (lighter collection). This study did not identify any extra-pelvic disease, and the patient underwent attempted curative re-resection.

imaging avoids a major surgery, with the associated morbidity and mortality, that would ultimately (and often rapidly) prove unsuccessful at curing the recurrent disease.

Unfortunately, PET scan imaging is not available in every medical center, but the information potentially provided by PET for selected patients makes an extra visit to an institution that has the capability worthwhile. As a primary surveillance technique, PET is not currently recommended, because there are as of yet no clinical studies demonstrating its ability to diagnose recurrence significantly earlier than either CT or MRI.

ERUS

ERUS has been available for more than a decade. Currently ERUS has supplanted all other imaging modalities for the initial evaluation of primary rectal tumors and pelvic lymph nodes, based on its superiority relative to CT (as discussed in previous chapters). But because abdominoperineal resection is more and more frequently replaced by low anterior resection and by proctectomy with coloanal anastomosis, ERUS may also prove to be extremely useful in detecting early pelvic recurrence. Even in women who have undergone abdominoperineal resection, use of ERUS transvaginally may still allow for accurate imaging of the pelvic soft tissues. The combination of accuracy in identifying very minor changes in the perirectal tissues (relative to CT and standard MRI), ease of imaging, and low cost and availability, as well as the potential to perform ERUS-guided transluminal biopsy of suspicious areas, makes ERUS quite appealing as a primary follow-up modality.

In limited studies, ERUS has a >90% sensitivity in identifying locally recurrent rectal cancers. ERUS has also been shown to be the most reliable method for diagnosing asymptomatic local recurrences. In these studies, ERUS detected recurrences not identified by physical examination, CT, endoscopy, and laboratory testing. Furthermore, in the cases in which recurrent disease was identified by one or more of these other approaches, ERUS also demonstrated recurrent cancer. For these reasons, ERUS is quickly becoming a primary radiologic technique both for surveillance and evaluation of suspected recurrent rectal cancer. Currently, the timing and frequency of ERUS evaluation after initial treatment of rectal cancer is unclear. In all likelihood, the first post-treatment "baseline" ERUS study should be performed no earlier than 3 months, and perhaps as late as 6 months after initial resection, as is recommended for CT imaging, to allow for resolution of the acute postoperative pelvic inflammation. Given its ease of performance, it is not unreasonable to suggest ERUS examinations as frequently as every 2 to 3 months thereafter, particularly in first 2 years after treatment, although there is no clear evidence to support this schedule.

There is also a known significant learning curve for the use of preoperative ERUS, and thus it seems likely that there is an even greater such learning curve for those who wish to use ERUS to evaluate the pelvis after irradiation and surgical resection. However, no doubt there will soon be a significant volume of literature concerning ERUS in this setting, and it is hoped that these reports will clarify the best use of this technique.

Metastatic Disease

For patients followed by surveillance CT scan in hopes of detecting local recurrence at an early stage, the liver, the major target of metastatic spread, is included in the routine imaging studies. Clinical evidence of hepatic metastasis, whether in the form of symptoms, palpable hepatomegaly, or elevated liver function tests, is virtually always associated with unresectable liver disease. Thus if there were to be any chance of metastatic resection for cure, liver disease must be identified when extremely limited. Unfortunately to date there has been no conclusive body of evidence demonstrating a significant survival benefit for rectal cancer patients followed by CT imaging for hepatic metastases. Still, until more accurate methods of detecting early hepatic spread are developed, the routine surveillance CT may rarely identify a patient with resectable metastatic disease to the liver. If potentially resectable disease is suggested by CT, percutaneous biopsy can frequently confirm the malignant nature of the lesion. If biopsy fails to confirm tumor metastasis, PET scan is often quite helpful in supporting the CT diagnosis while also searching for small areas of extrahepatic spread unidentified by CT that classify the patient as unresectable for cure.

Surveillance imaging to identify metastasis to less common sites is not routinely performed, because such follow-up has never been demonstrated to improve patient survival and is clearly not cost-effective. Imaging of these less common sites is based on patient symptoms or, less frequently, on physical examination findings. Thus patients whose complaints are suspicious for bony disease undergo bone scan imaging. Those whose symptoms or physical findings suggest brain metastasis undergo head CT or MRI. The only common exception to this approach is the use of annual chest x-ray for 5 years after initial rectal cancer treatment. Those whose chest films are suspicious for metastases undergo chest CT. This recommendation, too, is controversial, because the frequency of isolated, resectable pulmonary metastasis is 1 to 2% at best. However, although finding such patients with isolated, resectable lung metastasis is rare, the results after surgery are encouraging enough that most physicians believe the cost of annual chest x-ray is worthwhile. Despite this general feeling, it is important to remember that no cohort of studies has demonstrated cost-effective benefit to such routine use of chest x-rays. If the identified metastatic disease appears resectable for cure, patients should undergo further imaging studies, PET scan in particular, to identify any other sites of unsuspected cancer spread which would prevent an unnecessary and doomed "curative" resection attempt.

TUMOR MARKERS

Currently, a number of investigators are attempting to develop methods to differentiate between more aggressive and more indolent tumors. The purpose of this search is not only to assist in determining individual patient prognosis but also to identify patients for whom more aggressive therapy is warranted (e.g., stage II colon and stage I rectal cancers, which carry a greater risk of recurrence than is usually associated with most similarly staged lesions). Another reason for defining the biologically aggressive level of an individual tumor is to aid in determining the approach to patient follow-up. Thus patients with more aggressive lesions may be appropriate for more frequent imaging studies in hopes of identifying recurrence while still resectable, whereas those with less hostile lesions may require less frequent radiologic studies. The range of biologic markers currently being investigated is impressive, including quantifying the total amount of nuclear antigen within a proliferating cancer cell, measuring the extent of microvasculature within a tumor, identifying the presence of mutations within tumor-suppressor genes, and detection of chromosomal deletions. Many of the markers are still in the research phase but are becoming increasingly available in cases in which aggressive treatment or retreatment is being considered.

GENE DELETIONS

Colorectal cancer genetics is discussed in Chapter 1. However, we will briefly mention the tumor-suppressor gene *p53*, which has been well-studied in a variety of malignancies. *p53* is on chromosome 17p. Loss of heterozygosity at this allele has been associated with disease progression in colorectal cancer patients. Actually, a number of negative clinical tumor characteristics have been shown to increase in the presence of *p53* deletion. These include (but are not limited to) neoplastic transformation, progression through cell cycle, and metastatic spread. It is furthermore becoming apparent that an increase in microvasculature (angiogenesis) is also associated with *p53* deletion.

Another gene deletion, called deleted in colorectal cancer (DCC), has a significant negative prognostic effect when loss of heterozygosity occurs. This gene, on chromosome 18q, appears to code for a cell adhesion molecule. Data demonstrate that patients in whom the DCC gene is functionally deleted through mutation have an increased risk of liver metastasis. Clinically, overall survival in patients with stage II (node-negative) colorectal cancer who display loss of heterozygosity at the DCC gene decreases to 54% compared to 93% for stage II patients without the DCC deletion. However, given the significant number of tumor-suppressor genes on 18q, whether this dramatic worsening in prognosis is truly secondary to the DCC gene or possibly to a neighboring tumor-suppressor gene is currently under investigation. What is clear at present is that the determination of loss of heterozygosity at 18q can significantly affect the decision on how aggressively stage II patients should be followed after initial treatment.

ANGIOGENESIS

Since Folkman and co-workers' (1) 1989 article in *Nature*, the role played by angiogenesis in tumor growth and metastatic spread has come under intensive study. Tumor growth depends on both external blood supply and on the microvascular structure within the tumor itself. How tumors promote and maintain their own microvasculature is an area of ongoing investigation. The level of quantification of microvasculature within a tumor is defined as the intratumoral microvessel density (IMD). A preponderance of literature suggests that in colorectal cancer patients, an elevated IMD may predict increased potential for invasion and hemotogenous metastasis, and an overall poorer prognosis. Although further research and clinical trials are necessary, any patient treated for cure who has a high IMD should be followed particularly closely, because there appears to be an increased likelihood of local and/or metastatic recurrence. Included in some recommendations for such aggressive patient follow-up is the performance of a thoracoabdominal CT scan every 6 months in hopes of identifying pulmonary or hepatic spread while still resectable.

PROLIFERATING CELL NUCLEAR ANTIGEN

One marker that appears to aid in assessing the level of tumor bioaggressiveness is proliferating cell nuclear antigen (PCNA). This antigen is a cyclin required in order for a cell to pass through the S-phase and into the proliferative G2 stage of the cell cycle. PCNA can be quantified in the laboratory using immunofluorescence techniques. Along with another cyclin, Ki-67, elevated PCNA has been associated with an increased rate of cellular proliferation. However, there are conflicting data as to whether this increased proliferative rate correlates with a significant increase in the rate of tumor recurrence. At present, PCNA appears to be a valuable marker of malignant cell aggressiveness and thus may be helpful in determining responsiveness to radiation. Further PCNA investigation is necessary before this marker can be recommended as a routine factor in directing patient follow-up.

METACHRONOUS LESION SURVEILLANCE

One aspect of patient follow-up on which there is uniform agreement concerns the need for colonic surveillance. Metachronous large bowel cancers are not rare, and these new malignancies can occur at any time after treatment of the initial rectal lesion, including after the 5-year point that is used to mark a cure from the rectal primary. Thus colonoscopy plays a major role in the follow-up of rectal cancer patient, but its use is distinct in that it is not primarily used to detect recurrent disease (although rarely endoscopy will first identify locally recurrent disease invading through the anastomosis). Rather, colonoscopy is recommended to identify and treat any metachronous neoplasms, i.e., new adenomatous polyps and/or cancers that develop after the treatment of the original tumor. Relative to the general population, the incidence of developing a metachronous adenoma or cancer is significantly greater in patients who have previously been diagnosed with colorectal cancer, at approximately 50 and 7%, respectively. Interestingly, at least one-half of metachronous cancers are discovered during the first 2 years after initial treatment, raising questions about the true incidence of missed adenomas during the colonoscopic evaluation that originally diagnosed the cancer. Even in rectal cancer patients who have undergone abdominoperineal resection and thus have permanent colostomies, colonoscopy via the stoma is necessary and easily performed. Although some physicians still prefer to screen for metachronous lesions with the combination of flexible sigmoidoscopy and barium enema, given the incidence of new neoplasm formation, colonoscopy will still be required frequently enough for treatment in these patients that it is probably most cost-effective and convenient for colonoscopy to be the initial procedure of choice for follow-up. Barium enema alone is not acceptable, based on the reportedly high false-negative rate for the left colon.

The timing of colonoscopic follow-up is a source of controversy, but surveillance should be lifelong and probably no less frequent than every 5 years. The overwhelming majority of rectal cancer patients can and should undergo colonoscopy before treatment. Most physicians recommend performing the first post-treatment surveillance colonoscopy at 1 year. If no lesions are identified, some recommend a second annual endoscopy, but many feel that a delay of 3 to 5 years is acceptable, given the known rate of polyp formation and malignant transformation. Any bowel symptoms that develop between routine examinations should be immediately evaluated endoscopically. If adenomas are identified and resected via the colonoscope, most physicians would recommend annual colonoscopic examinations until there are two sequential examinations where no adenomas are identified. It then seems reasonable to decrease the frequency of evaluation, usually to 3 years initially, and then to every 5 years, if the 3-year examination is negative. If for any reason (usually large bowel obstruction) a complete colorectal evaluation was not performed before rectal cancer resection, a colonoscopy should be performed immediately after the postoperative recovery (usually at 2 to 3 months). There are little solid data to guide such recommendations, but again, the physician should remember the true rate of adenoma proliferation (estimated at 5 to 10 years) and malignant transformation (estimated to be 5 additional years) before excessively recommending annual colonoscopy in patients harboring no metachronous polyps. Individual physician style and judgment currently play key roles in this aspect of patient follow-up. Patients who are diagnosed with a metachronous adenocarcinoma should undergo aggressive treatment, which usually involves the resection of all remaining large intestine based on the patient's propensity for developing colorectal malignancies.

Many physicians routinely perform annual rigid proctoscopy in rectal cancer patients who have undergone resection and anastomosis. While there are no data demonstrating that such follow-up detects local recurrence at an earlier stage, there is minimal risk and discomfort involved. However, rigid endoscopy should in no way replace imaging (such as ERUS and/or CT) as a tool for local recurrence surveillance.

SUMMARY OF POST-TREATMENT FOLLOW-UP

Unfortunately, as stated in the introduction to this chapter, it is difficult at present to recommend one specific protocol for the routine post-treatment evaluation of rectal cancer patients. Much of this problem is based on the current reality that no collection of data has demonstrated any clearly significant survival (or even quality of life) benefit in post-treatment rectal cancer patients followed closely for recurrent disease. Thus nihilistic physicians can suggest that no laboratory evaluations, imaging studies, or even physical examinations need be performed unless (or until) a patient develops symptoms suggestive of recurrence. Then imaging will identify the rare patient who is a candidate for attempted curative resection. To many, such an attitude and approach are horrific. But we must be realistic, given the current limitations on health care dollars. Thus such a nihilistic approach is no more foolish than the frequent use of multiple blood tests, CT and MRI studies, and endoscopy. Such an excessive approach to patient follow-up is not uncommon and clearly does not take into account our knowledge of recurrence patterns and curability.

So it seems that even in this day of amazing medical technologic advances, much of the decisions regarding rectal cancer patient follow-up fall to the physician's personal style and beliefs. Understanding the natural history of local and distant rectal cancer recurrence aids in the development of a rational follow-up strategy, with the most frequent and intensive evaluations performed during the first 2 years and further investigations continuing over the next 3 years. Modifying follow-up strategies will be greatly assisted by ever-improving tumor marker techniques, which help identify cancers with more aggressive biologic activity. Here, we respectively highlight some suggestions:

1. Patients should be closely followed through the routine performance of history and physical examinations. This clinical evaluation process is a safe, inexpensive, and reasonable tactic. New patient symptoms and/or physical findings are still frequently the first indication that a local recurrence has developed. Such clinical changes require further evaluation, usually in the form of imaging studies.

2. Imaging studies, especially CT and ERUS, will likely be useful in evaluating any new patient complaints or physical examination findings. In order for such imaging studies to be of benefit, however, baseline studies are necessary. Thus rectal cancer patients should have a baseline CT and ERUS (when technically possible) at 3 to 6 months after their initial surgical treatment, and one or both studies should be repeated any time that suspicious signs or symptoms develop.

3. Unfortunately, routine surveillance CT imaging has not as of yet conclusively demonstrated significant beneficial effect for rectal cancer patients. Thus the regular performance of CT scan imaging in a patients without new symptoms or clinical findings suspicious of recurrence does not at present appear warranted unless a patient is enrolled in a research protocol requiring CT. The use of surveillance ERUS, however, has not yet been adequately analyzed as part of routine patient follow-up. Furthermore, ERUS is rapid, safe, and relatively inexpensive. To further evaluate the efficacy of ERUS, it is reasonable to recommend the imaging study every 3 to 6 months after performance of the initial baseline study, prefer-

ably as part of a controlled trial. Only through use, experience, and subsequent analysis can we learn more about the effectiveness of ERUS in the early identification of locally recurrent disease. ERUS changes suspicious for recurrence should lead to the performance of a CT or MRI and to biopsy.

4. Annual chest radiograph is a safe and relatively inexpensive method of screening for pulmonary metastasis, despite the rarity of identifying resectable disease. New findings should lead to the performance of a chest CT scan. However, based on the unfortunate rarity of finding resectable lung metastasis, the exclusion of chest x-ray from routine follow-up is also acceptable.

5. Routine blood tests should be limited to CEA analysis, and even this assay should be performed only for those patients who had elevated pretreatment CEA levels that normalized after initial treatment.

6. Tumor marker analysis, when available, should be used, especially on protocol. Along with pathohistologic findings, tumor markers may identify individual lesions with greater biologic aggressiveness. Patients harboring such cancers may require even more frequent and intensive follow-up.

7. Surveillance colonoscopy, timed as described, is required to identify and treat both benign and malignant metachronous lesions.

Again, the use of clinical research protocols, for everything from surveillance imaging to tumor marker analysis, is the approach most likely to lead to improvement in our ability to identify recurrent rectal cancer at an earlier stage, with the ultimate goal of increasing resectability and survival from recurrent disease. Thus it is vital that physicians involved in the initial evaluation and treatment of patients with rectal cancer keep apprised of local, regional, and national protocols into which their patients may be enrolled.

SURGERY FOR RECURRENT RECTAL CANCER

In as much as the approach to follow-up of rectal cancer patients after initial therapy is far from uniform, there is also lack of consensus concerning reoperation for locally recurrent disease. One fact is clear: complete surgical resection of all gross recurrent disease is required in order for there to exist any chance of cure. Unfortunately, curative operations performed for local recurrence have produced disappointing results, with well less than 40% long-term survival even in highly selected patients. Furthermore, operations for symptom palliation are associated with significant morbidity and mortality rates. Despite these negatives, the grim prognosis and devastating symptomatology of locally recurrent rectal cancer still makes radical re-resection an important option, the results of which may be viewed as beneficial for patients who are chosen with extreme care. Depending on an individual patient's previous treatment regimen, the addition of IORT can further aid in both curative and palliative surgical efforts.

Any patient being considered for re-resection for cure must meet several criteria. First, the patient's overall health and comorbid conditions must be such that the patient can tolerate a major surgical undertaking. Next, the pelvic tumor burden must by physical examination and by all imaging studies appear to be completely resectable. Finally, a thorough investigation for metastatic disease must be undertaken before any attempt at curative resection. Metastatic disease is most commonly found in liver, lungs, or in both sites. Many oncologic physicians feel that any metastatic disease outside of the pelvis is a contraindication to attempted curative resection. Others, however, are willing to attempt combined pelvic and metastatic resection for cure if the metastases are discrete and resectable, although the true potential for cure in this setting is extremely minimal, and the morbidity and mortality of the procedure, along with the patient's likely limited lifespan (which is best spent outside of the hospital), must be carefully weighed against the minuscule possibility of benefit to the patient. If the metastatic disease is unresectable, either based on location or extent, the patient is a candidate only for palliation.

RE-RESECTION FOR CURE

During re-resection, the most important determinant of potential curability is complete removal of the recurrent cancer. Overall survival and disease-free survival rates drop precipitously when any macroscopic tumor remains within the pelvis at completion of the operation. When all gross disease is removed, IORT has been demonstrated to significantly improve survival rates, most likely via ablation of residual microscopic disease. Unfortunately, even when CT, MRI, ultrasound, and PET scan imaging suggest resectable local recurrence, at least 30 to 40% of these patients who return to the operating room for curative surgery are found at surgery to have unresectable disease. Even in the presence of imaging studies suggesting resectability, physical findings that indicate truly unresectable disease include sciatic nerve pain, tumor fixity to the pelvic sidewalls or the proximal sacrum on rectal or pelvic examination, and lower extremity swelling.

Determining the type and extent of resection required for cure is based on the location of all locally recurrent disease. In a patient with a limited, early recurrence who has previously undergone a low anterior resection or proctectomy with coloanal anastomosis, a standard abdominoperineal resection (with consideration of IORT) may suffice. If the recurrence extends anteriorly into vagina, prostate, and/or bladder, a limited or complete pelvic exenteration is performed. Pelvic exenteration includes the en bloc removal of the tumor along with any organs involved by malignancy via local extension, optimally with a 2-cm circumferential margin. Attempts should also be made to resect the lymphatic drainage of all involved organs if the patient is to be given the best chance for cure. When recurrent tumor invades posteriorly into the sacrum, a partial sacrectomy is performed en bloc with the tumor, again with a margin if possible. For vertebral column bony stability, at least the upper half of both S2 vertebrae should be left intact. If at least one S3 sacral nerve root is spared (and some authors believe that only one S2 nerve root is necessary), many patients have adequate bowel and bladder control, although voluntary abdominal muscle contraction may be required to void. Furthermore, given that many of these patients require colostomy, bladder resection, and urinary diversion, there is no need to protect the sacral nerves regulating bowel and bladder function. Erectile dysfunction is common after proximal sacrectomy, but lower extremity weakness is usually avoidable. Abdominosacral resection is a long and arduous surgical undertaking and should be performed only by an experienced surgical oncologist, frequently with the assistance of an orthopedic or neurologic surgeon. Once again, the addition of IORT should be seriously considered. Despite the difficulty of the procedure for both surgeon and, especially, patient, 5-year survival can be increased from <5% in those treated nonoperatively to 20 to 30% in resected patients.

PALLIATIVE RE-RESECTION

A tumor that extends laterally onto the pelvic sidewalls has a poorer surgical prognosis. If the cancer has truly invaded into the bone, it cannot be resected for cure. If the iliac vessels are encased, the tumor is also unresectable. Either malignant invasion causing ureteral obstruction proximal to the ureteral-vesical junction or involvement of the sciatic nerve also precludes curative resection. Of the several indications for palliative operation, such as pain, obstruction, fistulization, and infection, pain is by far the most devastating and most common indication for palliative reoperation. Pain that cannot be controlled medically is usually secondary to local recurrence within the presacral space with compression or invasion of the sacrum. Although additional external beam irradiation is possible for many, the response to this nonoperative approach is short-lived and less effective. The pain from sacral invasion is often so severe that "prepalliative" surgery should be considered in asymptomatic patients with known unresectable presacral recurrence, because the probability that symptomatic sacral invasion will soon occur is high, and given that these patients are better surgical candidates before the development of debilitating symptoms. Resection of all areas of involved sacrum is the most effective means of alleviating the intense pain. However, even incomplete removal of invaded sacral bone (when the proximal sacrum is also involved but cannot be resected) may be effective in significantly reducing or even eliminating the patient's most severe pain, especially when surgery is combined with IORT.

Large bowel obstruction in patients who were reanastomosed at their initial operation is most easily treated via proximal diversion, unless accompanied by pain. In the latter setting, operation in the form of abdominoperineal resection, with sacrectomy if indicated, is required to palliate both symptoms. When the small intestines have not been excluded from the pelvis at initial operation, loops of ileum that fell into and adhered to the pelvic brim and sidewalls may be invaded by recurrent rectal cancer, producing small bowel obstruction and, on occasion, significant intestinal bleeding. Such obstruction requires either diversion or resection, whereas resection may be the only option for hemorrhage. Pelvic recurrence also has a propensity for fistulization, usually presenting as a lower abdominal wall or perineal abscess. Drainage relieves the infectious symptoms, but many of these malignant tracts either remain open permanently or recur, requiring repeated drainage. There is rarely a role for major surgical intervention in such cases. Fistulization into the bladder may lead to urinary tract infection and even urosepsis. In this setting, resection of the involved bladder may be indicated.

RISKS OF OPERATING

Unfortunately, by the time most patients are diagnosed with locally recurrent rectal cancer, their overall health, especially their nutritional status, is often quite poor. Thus many patients, even those whose local recurrence appears on imaging to be resectable for cure, are not candidates for surgical intervention, given their extremely high perioperative morbidity and mortality. Even in those whose operative risk is believed to be acceptable, reported morbidity rates, most often in the form of pelvic infection or sepsis, are significant, ranging from 30 to 70%. Poor wound healing, especially in the area of previous irradiation (lower back and abdomen, perineum), is also a source of significant morbidity. Perioperative mortality, again most often secondary to pelvic sepsis, can surpass 10%. Immunologic compromise secondary to poor nutritional status plays a major role in all of these complications and deaths. Thus improving a patient's nutritional status, preferably enterally (even if a feeding tube is required) or, if necessary, via TPN, is essential to maximize the potential for a successful operation and to minimize the risk of complications. Such nutritional replenishment may be required preoperatively (often for days or even weeks) as well as postoperatively.

Intraoperative radiation therapy is proving to be beneficial both in resection for cure and for palliation. The concept of IORT is to deliver minimal radiation to uninvolved tissue surrounding a recurrence site while administering a larger dose more accurately to the tissue at greatest risk of harboring residual disease. Many centers now have dedicated operating rooms where IORT can be delivered directly into the open surgical wound after resection. Although individualized for each patient, 1000 to 3000 cGy are administered to one or more intracorporeal at-risk sites. Surrounding, uninvolved tissue can be shielded with small, lead strips placed by the surgeon before initiation of IORT. Unfortunately, a few patients have previously received maximal external beam radiation doses as part of their original cancer treatment and, therefore, are not candidates for additional IORT. Fortunately, the majority of rectal cancer patients, even those having previously undergone radiation treatment, are still eligible to receive IORT, given its ability to limit the areas irradiated. In resection for cure, IORT targets areas suspected of still harboring microscopic disease at the completion of operation. Studies of the efficacy of IORT, while retrospective and limited to small numbers of patients, demonstrate a trend toward increased cure rate, longer disease-free survival, and improved overall survival compared to patients treated by surgical resection alone. As a complement to palliative resection (when IORT is delivered to areas of remaining gross disease), studies also suggest a trend toward increasing disease-free and overall survival compared to patients palliated by surgery alone.

IORT is not without its complications. The most serious is the contribution of IORT to poor wound healing, which has a significant effect on patient morbidity and even mortality. Other morbidities attributed to IORT include ureteral obstruction (approximately 30% of cases), peripheral and pelvic neuropathy (approximately 50%), and small bowel enteritis (approximately 40%). Many of these complications may be averted or greatly diminished by surgical mobilization of the ureters and bowel before irradiation, use of lead shielding, and the guidance of experienced IORT personnel at the time of radiation administration. Furthermore, the majority of IORT complications can be palliated without significant difficulty or risk. Thus, although studies monitoring quality of life have yet to be undertaken, the IORT data are encouraging enough that the risk of related complications is usually felt to be acceptable given the apparent improvement in patient survival and palliation.

REFERENCE

1. Folkman J, Watson K, Ingber D, Hanahan D. Induction of angiogenesis during transition from hyperplasia to neoplasia. Nature 1989;339:58–61.

PART

IV

METASTIC DISEASE

CHAPTER

16

Treatment for Metastatic Disease of the Colon and Rectum

ALAN F. HORGAN, M.B.B.C.H., AND
JOHN H. PEMBERTON, M.D.

Metastatic disease from colorectal cancer (CRC) remains a major cause of death in the developed world despite advances in operative technique and adjuvant therapy. Complete eradication of the primary disease at the time of initial surgery remains the best, and in most cases the only, opportunity for cure of patients with colorectal cancer. Nonetheless, 25% of CRC patients will be found to have distant metastases at the time of diagnosis, and a further 25% will subsequently develop metastases. Up to 95% of CRC metastases occur in the absence of locally recurrent disease. Complete resection of metastases is compatible with long-term survival in 30 to 40% of patients, and surgical intervention must, therefore, always be considered when metastases are discovered preoperatively, intraoperatively, or during follow-up of patients with colorectal cancer.

Colon and Rectal Cancer, Edited by Peter S. Edelstein, M.D.
ISBN 0-471-35145-8

Without surgical intervention, the median survival time is 9 months for patients with CRC liver metastases. An equally poor prognosis has been reported for surgically untreated metastases to other sites such as bone (10 months), lung (10.5 months), brain (5.5 months), and multiple sites (10 months).

Attention has been focused on the use of new imaging modalities in an attempt to diagnose metastases at an earlier stage and to more accurately stage patients under consideration for resectional surgery. In addition to the more established imaging modalities, such as CT scanning and transabdominal ultrasound, a number of newer techniques have shown potential; these include intraoperative, laparoscopic, and transanal ultrasound; MRI; PET scan; and targeting imaging strategies using radiolabeled monoclonal antibodies.

Systemic chemotherapy has been reported to be helpful in delaying the onset, or preventing the development, of distant metastases after surgical treatment of the primary tumor. However, once established, only 20% of patients with hepatic metastases will respond to such treatments; and once distant metastases develop, long-term survival is rare. In view of the toxicity and cost associated with administration of all chemotherapy regimes, there has been increasing interest in identifying subgroups of patients at high risk of developing systemic metastases after surgery so that systemic therapy can be targeted to this high-risk population. Techniques such as the immunohistochemical detection of micrometastatic deposits in bone marrow aspirates of patients with CRC may be useful in this situation. The demonstration of such deposits may represent true residual disease or cell shedding with metastatic potential. The persistence of micrometastatic deposits after resection of gastric tumors has been shown to be associated with a significant increase in the development of metastases during follow-up. The prognostic value of micrometastatic deposits in CRC patients, however, remains to be determined.

New methods of delivering adjuvant treatment are also being explored. Studies are under way of new chemotherapeutic agents and new routes to deliver more established agents. Oxaliplatin, a platinum analogue, when combined with 5-FU and FA, has been associated with a significant increase in tumor response rates. Time to treatment failure appears to be further prolonged when the same combination of drugs are administered as a chronomodulated infusion (administered to coincide with relevant circadian rhythms). This method of administration not only increases response rates but also appears to be less toxic than a constant infusion; 3-year survival rates, however, are not affected.

Attempts have been made to influence long-term survival of patients with CRC by early identification of metastases. The value of intensive follow-up of patients after surgery for colorectal cancer, however, remains unclear. A recent randomized study has shown that annual colonoscopy, together with CT and chest radiography, fails to increase 5-year survival of these patients when compared to standard follow-up. Annual liver CT did result in earlier detection of hepatic metastases but did not increase the number of curative hepatic resections. The use of routine carcinoembryonic antigen (CEA) estimation for monitoring patients with resected colon cancer has also been questioned. In one multicenter study, 59% of 417 colon cancer recurrences were preceded by an elevation in CEA levels. CEA appeared to be most sensitive for liver and retroperitoneal recurrences. However, 16% of patients without recurrence showed a false-positive CEA elevation. Of 115 patients who underwent surgical exploration, <50% were resected with curative intent. Survival 1 year after surgery for recurrent colon cancer was similar whether or not metastases had been detected by CEA-elevation.

After detection of colon cancer recurrences by whatever method, long-term disease-free survival remains possible. A multi-institutional study followed up 547 patients with recurrent disease out of 1247 patients with resected stage II and stage III colon cancer. Further surgery was carried out in 41% of these patients, with curative intent in 20%. The 5-year disease-free survival after surgery with curative intent was fully 23%.

HEPATIC METASTASE

INCIDENCE

It has been estimated from studies of tumor-growth kinetics that the time from metastatic implantation to the clinical appearance of liver metastases may be 2.5 to 5 years. Liver metastases are found at the time of initial diagnosis of CRC in up to 35% of patients and will develop during follow-up in a further 8 to 30%. A total of 25% will have a recurrence that is confined to the liver, and in turn <20% of these will be suitable for curative surgical resection (approximately 5000 cases per year in the United States). The median survival of patients with untreated hepatic metastases is <12 months, and survival beyond 5 years occurs in <3%. Fluorouracil-based chemotherapy regimens have prolonged median survival and improved quality of life, but rarely produce 5-year survivors.

TREATMENT

Surgical resection remains the only potentially curative treatment for metastatic colorectal carcinoma. As early as 1963, Woodington and Waugh (1) published the Mayo Clinic experience of CRC hepatic metastases resection and reported a 20% 5-year survival in selected patients. Since then, most of the larger series report a gradual improvement in perioperative mortality (0 to 14%) and morbidity (8 to 46%) with better understanding of hepatic anatomy, advances in anesthesia, and improvements in technology. Now 5-year survival rates of >30% are frequently reported for unilobar tumors with free surgical margins. In addition, survival appears to plateau at about 5 years with the surviving patients having a life expectancy approaching that of controls (Figs. 16.1 and 16.2). Further evidence that the natural history of these cancers is altered by hepatic resection is seen by the fact that recurrences have been increasingly observed in unusual sites such as bone and lung. Adjuvant chemotherapy is routinely offered to patients after resection of hepatic metastases in

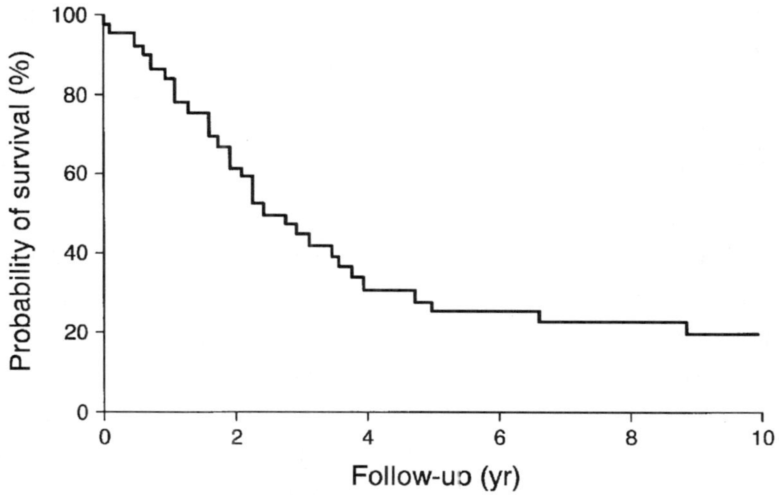

FIGURE 16.1. Overall survival after hepatic resection for metastases from colorectal cancer.

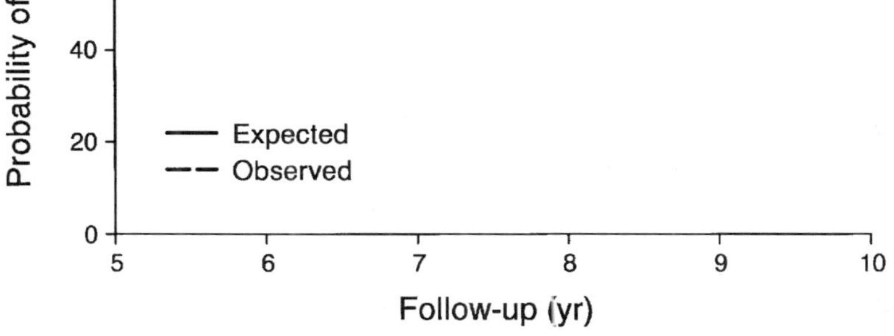

FIGURE 16.2 Comparison of observed survival beyond 5 years after hepatic resection for metastases from colorectal cancer with expected survival of an age- and sex-matched population.

most institutions. There is, however, little evidence to show that it influences survival.

Resectability and Prognostic Factors

Accurate preoperative and intraoperative staging are mandatory to avoid unnecessary surgery. As experience and technology develop, factors that had previously been thought to be a contraindication to surgery are now considered acceptable. The absolute number of metastases has become less important, assuming there is adequate residual functioning liver. There is evidence that estimated residual hepatic tissue of 35% or greater on preoperative assessment is associated with a good outcome. Uncontrolled primary disease, extensive hepatic or extrahepatic disease, and invasion of the inferior vena cava or portal structures remain contraindications for resection.

Poor prognostic factors include extensive hepatic parenchymal disease, bilobar distribution of metastases, extrahepatic malignant disease, or involvement of periportal or celiac lymph nodes. Factors that do not appear to influence prognosis include the number and size of the metastases, the disease-free interval, and the stage of the primary CRC. The type of hepatic resection does not appear to be important as long as clear surgical excision margins are achieved. Data from the Registry of Hepatic Metastases showed that a margin of 1 cm or greater is associated with a 5-year survival of 45%, which fell to 23% if the resection margin was <1 cm.

Despite initial suggestions that synchronous metastases (discovered at the time of the original surgery) have a worse prognosis than metachronous metastases (discovered during follow-up), multivariate analysis suggests that outcome does not depend on the time of diagnosis. It would seem appropriate, therefore, to resect metastases discovered at the time of initial laparotomy for resection of the primary CRC, provided that adequate expertise, equipment, and postoperative care are available. Lesions detected at surgery for the primary disease should be resected if simple wedge resection is all that is required, because this limited procedure is associated with minimal morbidity and may spare the patient further surgery. More complex lesions require a full assessment of the liver, including intraoperative ultrasound, and a great deal of technical expertise to achieve adequate resection margins with low morbidity and mortality. In general, although concomitant resection is certainly possible and effective, in anything other than the simple metastasis situation we advise allowing the patient to recover from the initial surgery, then reassess the liver in conjunction with a suitably trained surgeon. The appropriate liver resection can then be performed after a full discussion with the patient, provided the criteria for resectability are met.

SURGICAL TECHNIQUES

Although details of surgical technique are outside the scope of this chapter, several principles are worth emphasizing.

- The availability of newer imaging modalities, such as CT portography and intraoperative ultrasound, allows detection of small lesions and definition of their relationship to the vascular structures; preoperative angiography is no longer considered routinely necessary.

- Precise knowledge of hepatic anatomy enables a relatively bloodless procedure to be performed and leads to a significant reduction in perioperative morbidity and mortality.

- Use of the ultrasonic dissectors has allowed multiple segmental resections to be performed safely, maximizing residual hepatic tissue.

- Margin of resection appears to be the most important prognostic variable; patients with positive resection margins have a median survival approaching that of patients who do not undergo any surgical intervention.

- The surgical results for liver metastases are only as good as one's ability to exclude extrahepatic disease.

Recurrence after Resection of Hepatic Metastases

Survival after resection of hepatic metastases has been reported as high as 95%, 65%, and 49% at 1, 3 and 5 years respectively. Of those that develop recurrence (lungs, liver, and locally, in that order), 20 to 40% of patients develop recurrence that is confined to the liver. Complete repeat hepatic resection has been possible in about half of those who underwent surgery, with a 5-year survival as high as 44% after the second hepatectomy. The presence of extracapsular disease decreases this survival to <20% and is, therefore, regarded as a relative contraindication to resection. Repeat resections are technically more difficult. Adhesions can distort the anatomy and make exposure more difficult. Vascular control at the portal pedicle can also be difficult, and the hepatic parenchyma can be fibrotic and friable. Despite this, some series report morbidity and mortality rates similar to those for the primary hepatic surgery.

Hepatic Artery Infusion

The route of spread of colorectal cancer cells to the liver is via the portal vein. However, once >1 mm in diameter, liver metastases appear to derive their blood supply exclusively from the hepatic artery while normal hepatocytes continue to derive their nutrition via the portal vein. This provides a unique opportunity to target liver metastases via the hepatic artery with levels of chemotherapy that would be toxic if administered systemically. Fluorodeoxyuridine (FUDR) is considered the drug of choice, because its uptake and extraction by the liver is significantly greater than that of 5-FU (90 vs. 19 to 55%). A high pump complication rate was initially reported with percutaneous devices. This problem was largely eliminated by the use of a totally implantable pump, which can be refilled by percutaneous needle injection.

The use of hepatic artery infusion (HAI) has been shown to markedly reduce systemic side effects such as alopecia, nausea, diarrhea, and vomiting. HAI is not, however, without side effects, the most frequent of which are hepatic toxicity and peptic ulcer disease. Chemical cholecystitis, which occurred in up to 33% of patients, has been eliminated by the inclusion of prophylactic cholecystectomy at the time of pump implantation. Elevated bilirubin levels, which occur in 24% of patients, usually respond to temporary discontinuation of the therapy, followed by reintroduction at a lower dose once bilirubin levels have returned to normal.

Several randomized studies comparing hepatic artery infusion of FUDR with systemic 5-FU for the treatment of CRC hepatic metastases have demonstrated superiority of HAI in terms of tumor response rates. Survival advantage could not, however, be demonstrated in the majority of these studies owing to inadequate sample size. In a small number of cases, HAI has led to "down-staging" of the metastases, making subsequent resection possible.

CRYOTHERAPY

Cryotherapy uses insulated probes containing liquid nitrogen, which destroys metastases by freeze–thaw cycles. Side effects include thrombocytopenia, the risk of which increases with an increasing number of cycles. Application currently requires a laparotomy and intraoperative ultrasound guidance, although laparoscopic cryotherapy has been used in an animal model with some success. Cryotherapy was initially used solely for unresectable metastases but has been used more liberally by some groups with a reported 3-year survival approaching 30%. Survival appears to be increased if cryotherapy is combined with hepatic artery infusion of 5-FU and FA.

Chemoembolization

Use of an occluding substance in conjunction with regional administration of cytotoxic agents causes interruption of the hepatic artery blood flow and increases the exposure time of the metastatic tumor to the infused chemotherapeutic agent. Vaso-occlusive substances that have been used include starch microspheres, gelfoam, angiostat, and polyvinyl alcohol particles. Superselective catheterization of the branches of the hepatic artery that feed the tumor is required to prevent excessive damage to normal liver tissue. Selective internal radiation, embolizing microspheres of yttrium 90 into the hepatic circulation, has also been used with some success.

Isolated Liver Perfusion

Recirculating perfusion of a vascularly isolated liver allows for the delivery of doses of chemotherapeutic agents that would be fatal if administered systemically. Some groups have reported clinical response, but this response has generally been poor and the administration technically difficult.

Immunotherapy

Use of immunostimulants, such as interleukin 2, as neoadjuvant therapy or use of monoclonal antibodies, such as F19, which is highly sensitive for CRC liver metastases, is currently under trial and may prove useful in the future both as therapy for hepatic metastases and for imaging smaller metastatic lesions. Active immunization with vaccines (autologous irradiated metastasis-derived tumor cells) after surgery for CRC liver metastases is also under investigation.

Pulmonary Metastases

Despite advances in systemic chemotherapy, resection of metastases localized to the lungs remains the only mode of curative treatment in these patients. The lung has been reported as a site of recurrence after surgery in 12% of rectal cancers and 4% of colon cancers. Half of the lesions will appear within 32 months of surgery for rectal tumors and within 22 months of surgery for colonic tumors. Approximately 2% of patients who undergo surgery for CRC will develop metastases that are confined to the lung. Prognosis after resection of pulmonary metastases does not appear to be affected by the site of the primary tumor, the size of the primary tumor, the disease-free interval, the type of original surgery for the primary, or prior resection of hepatic metastases. the 5-year survival may, however, be influenced by the number of metastases resected and can be as high as 62% for solitary lesions, 35% for two lesions, but 0% for greater than four metastases. Other studies have found no relationship between number of metastases and survival, but did find that radicality of resection was a significant prognostic factor.

CT scan accurately detects most lung metastases. Patient selection is guided by the control of the primary tumor, ability to resect all gross tumor, and the presence of an adequate cardiorespiratory reserve. The extent of resection is primarily determined by the location of the metastatic tumor. Wedge resections are well tolerated by most patients, necessitating removal of a minimal amount of lung tissue, and do not significantly reduce total lung capacity. The majority of resectable metastases can be removed as peripheral wedges and are well suited to the use of a stapling device. Use of electrocautery may preserve more lung tissue but is more time-consuming and has been associated with increased morbidity, such as air leaks and increased blood loss. If lobar vessels or bronchi are invaded, a lobectomy is necessary to achieve clear surgical margins. If a main vessel or bronchus is invaded, a pneumonectomy is required, provided respiratory reserve is adequate. The addition of mediastinal lymphadenectomy is routinely performed in the case of primary lung tumors. This provides staging information and is thought to be therapeutic. There is, however, no proof that mediastinal node dissection improves prognosis in metastatic CRC, and it is.

therefore, not routinely performed. Repeat pulmonary resection for recurrent metastases has been performed in a number of centers and is associated with long-term survival in up to 50% of the small number of patients who are deemed suitable for such surgery. There is no evidence to suggest that the addition of systemic chemotherapy increases survival or decreases the chance of recurrence after surgery for pulmonary metastases.

Other Sites of Metastatic Spread

CRC accounts for 8% of cerebral metastases. The majority of these patients (82%) have concomitant extracerebral metastases, especially in the lungs. The 1-year survival was reported in one study to occur in only 16%, and of these patients, 92% had solitary metastases. Treatment options are limited. Median survival for those treated with steroids alone was 1 month, for those treated with radiotherapy alone was 3 months, and for those suitable for surgical treatment was 9 months. Survival rates were similar in those receiving surgery with radiotherapy compared to those receiving surgery alone. Early onset of metastases, older age, concomitant bone metastases, and memory loss were all poor prognostic signs. Survival, whatever treatment option is chosen, is dismal, and craniotomy is rarely indicated except in cases with minimal neurologic impairment, a long previous disease-free interval, a solitary metastasis, and no extracranial disease.

Bone metastases have been reported to be present in 10 to 23% of autopsy cases of patients with CRC. Primary tumor sites commonly included the rectum and cecum; and bone metastases were more frequently found in younger patients and in those with signet-ring tumors. They are rarely found as isolated metastases. Treatment options include radiotherapy and internal fixation as required for stabilization.

SUMMARY

Surgery for CRC metastases in the absence of uncontrolled primary disease remains these patients' only hope of cure. The vast majority of such patients will not be candidates for resectional surgery in view of failure to meet the above-mentioned criteria or because of co-existing morbidity. Unresectable patients may achieve some increase in survival time and quality of life with the administration of regional or systemic adjuvant therapy. Survival in patients who do meet the criteria for surgical resection, however, is as high as 40%. Encouragingly, morbidity and mortality associated with resectional surgery continues to decrease with improvements in technique, equipment, and perioperative care.

REFERENCE

1. Woodington GF and Waugh JM. Results of resection of metastatic tumors of the liver. Ame J Surg 1963;105:24–29.

Part

V

Unique Issues

CHAPTER

17

LAPAROSCOPIC SURGERY FOR MALIGNANT DISEASE

JOHN D. F. ALLENDORF, M.D.;
NEIL R. GLEASON, B.A.; AND
RICHARD L. WHELAN, M.D.

The recent introduction of the laparoscope with video camera projection has revolutionized general surgery. In a very brief period of time, laparoscopic cholecystectomy has become widely accepted as the standard of care for benign disease of the gallbladder. Although consistent and reproducible benefits of the laparoscopic approach in terms of length of hospital stay, cosmesis, time to return to work, operative blood loss, and postoperative pain have been demonstrated after colon surgery, the approach has not been widely accepted. The major indication for colon resection in the United States is malignancy, and the concerns about laparoscopic colon resection center around oncologic issues, including adequacy of resection, local and metastatic recurrence rates, and port site tumor recurrences.

This chapter first reviews the physiologic, immunologic, and oncologic consequences of laparoscopic surgery vis-à-vis open surgery. It then examines the adequacy of tumor margins and

Colon and Rectal Cancer, Edited by Peter S. Edelstein, M.D.
ISBN 0-471-35145-8

lymph node harvest after laparoscopic colon resection. The issue of port site tumor recurrences is explored by reviewing the available laboratory and human data. The final section describes several ongoing trials designed to evaluate the possible benefits of laparoscopic colon resection.

BASIC SCIENCE REVIEW

PHYSIOLOGY

Laparoscopic surgery alters cardiovascular and pulmonary function. Carbon dioxide pneumoperitoneum has both mechanical and metabolic effects on the patient. Insufflation raises abdominal pressure, which impedes venous return to the heart from the lower extremities. This reduction may be severe enough to cause intraoperative hypotension, which usually responds to volume administration. Insufflation also limits downward excursion of the diaphragm, decreasing tidal volumes, increasing airway pressures, and decreasing minute ventilation. Decreased ventilation is compounded by the absorption of the insufflated carbon dioxide gas across the peritoneum. These two factors together contribute to intraoperative acidosis, which can be overcome by increasing minute ventilation via increased respiratory rate. Thus the immediate intraoperative mechanical and metabolic effects of carbon dioxide pneumoperitoneum seem to be well tolerated and easily compensated for in most patients. Better pulmonary function postoperatively is thought to be the result of less pain associated with laparoscopic surgery, allowing for better ventilation.

IMMUNOLOGY

Investigators have studied a variety of parameters in an effort to characterize the effects of laparoscopic surgery on immune defenses. Cell-mediated immune function can be grossly assessed by delayed-type hypersensitivity (DTH) testing, which involves the intradermal injection of an antigen to which the host has previously been exposed. The area of induration of the resulting wheal is measured 24 to 48 hr after the challenge and can be used as an index of the host's ability to mount an immune reaction. Using this technique in rats, we demonstrated better preservation of cell-mediated immune function after laparoscopic versus open bowel resection through postoperative day 5 (1). Expanding on evidence from small animal experiments, we (2) measured DTH responses in healthy controls and in patients after laparoscopic-assisted and open colon resection. All subjects were challenged preoperatively, intraoperatively, and on postoperative day 3. There were no differences in the preoperative responses among the three groups. As expected, the open surgery group responses were significantly diminished postoperatively compared to their own preoperative responses. Interestingly, a significant postoperative reduction in the area of induration was not seen in the laparoscopic group, suggesting that cell-mediated immune function was better preserved in the laparoscopic cohort.

Other authors have studied more specific components of immune function. Horgan et al. (3) demonstrated preservation of mouse T-cell mitogen response after laparoscopy and a decreased response after laparotomy. Southall et al. (4), in a similar experiment, determined the time course of the diminished lymphocyte proliferation rate (LPR) after laparotomy and confirmed that CO_2 insufflation did not result in such changes. Significantly decreased LPR results were noted on postoperative days 2, 3, and 4. By the 7th day after surgery, the LPR had returned to normal. Redmond et al. (5) demonstrated significantly increased monocyte release of superoxide ion and tumor necrosis factor, and neutrophil release of superoxide ion and chemotaxis in patients who underwent open versus laparoscopic cholecystectomy. Watson et al. (6) compared the ability of isolated monocytes to phagocytize *Candida albicans* 24 hr after laparotomy and CO_2 insufflation in mice. Postoperative monocyte phagocytosis was impaired in the laparotomy group but preserved in both the insufflation and control groups. In the same study, expression of MAC-1(CD11b), an important receptor in recognition of opsonized particles before phagocytosis, was significantly less in the laparotomy group than in both the insufflation and control groups. These results suggest that lymphocyte, macrophage, and neutrophil function may be better preserved after laparoscopic intervention.

ONCOLOGY

Several researchers have investigated the effect of laparoscopic and open intervention on tumor behavior. We (7) demonstrated that existing dermal tumors in mice grew significantly larger after laparotomy than after peritoneal insufflation with CO_2 gas. In the same study, tumors were more easily established and grew larger after laparotomy versus insufflation. Our subsequent investigations demonstrated that the differences in tumor establishment and growth persisted in the setting of a bowel resection (8).

Lee et al. (9) examined pre-existing dorsal tumors in mice for rates of apoptosis and cell proliferation after sham laparotomy and insufflation. The tumors from the laparotomy group mice had significantly greater proliferative rates than the insufflated group tumors. Conversely, the laparotomy group tumors had significantly lower rates of apoptosis than the tumors from the insufflation group. Additional investigation suggests that a serum transferable factor is responsible for the differences in tumor cell proliferation (10).

Although the factors influencing tumor proliferation after open surgery are not yet well defined, it appears that laparotomy induces factors that stimulate tumor growth and inhibit apoptosis. These derangements are seen to a lesser extent after laparoscopic intervention.

TECHNICAL ISSUES

Concern over the adequacy of tissue margins and lymph node harvest coupled with the specter of port site recurrences have generated considerable hesitancy on the part of many surgeons to apply the technique of laparoscopic colon resection in the setting of malignant disease. In regard to length of resection, tumor margins, and lymph node harvest, several trials have demonstrated the same or better results after laparoscopic than after open resection. One study involving 76 patients who underwent laparoscopic colon resections demonstrated an average distal bowel margin of 4.5 cm and an average lymph node harvest of 8.5, which was not significantly different from their institution's open colectomy average (11). A second study involving 415 patients (224 open resections and 191 laparoscopic resections) stratified patients according to the type of resection performed. Within stratification groups, the total length of resection was somewhat longer in the open group; however, the distal margin was greater in the laparoscopic group, and lymph node harvest was essentially the same for both groups (12). A third study involving 408 patients (203 open and 205 laparoscopic) demonstrated that total length of resection, proximal and distal margins, and number of lymph nodes harvested were the same for both the open surgery and the laparoscopic groups (13). Two small, randomized, and prospective trials comparing open and laparoscopic colectomy for cancer, which together involved >300 patients, demonstrated that there were no differences in regard to size of specimen, proximal or distal margins, length of mesentery resected, and lymph node harvest (14,15). In summary, the evidence suggests that, given the requisite laparoscopic skills, the laparoscopic approach allows for as radical a colonic resection as can be accomplished via an open technique.

Inability to palpate the lesion intraoperatively has also been a concern and has resulted in laparoscopic resection of the wrong portion of bowel. This has been overcome by improved pre-operative localization. The site of the lesion can be pre-operatively tattooed colonoscopically with India ink, or if concern persists, the lesion can be endoscopically identified intraoperatively.

PORT WOUND TUMOR RECURRENCE

Incisional tumor recurrence after open surgery occurs infrequently. Hughes et al. (16) performed a retrospective review of 1603 colon cancer patients and found the incidence of tumor recurrence at the incisional site to be 0.68% and identified an overall abdominal wall tumor incidence of 1%. The local recurrence of cancer at the port wounds is a frightening development that has been well documented. Of concern, authors have reported port site tumor recurrences with all stages of disease, and recurrences occur both at the site used for removal of the specimen and at remote port sites. The reported incidence of port wound tumors varies widely. Berends et al. (17) reported a rate of 21% (3/14), whereas Lacy et al. (14) and Lord et al. (11) each found no port site recurrences in series of >100 patients. The incidence of port wound tumor recurrence reported by large nonrandomized and smaller prospective randomized studies with a mean follow-up of >2 years is between 0 and 1.2% (12–14,18,19). A survey of the surgeons participating in the NCI Clinical Outcomes of Surgical Therapies (COST) study was presented in 1996 (20). The surgeons reported on their pretrial patient follow-up. In 372 combined patients, the incidence of port wound tumors was about 1%. The mean follow up was 22.6 months (range 15 to 45 months). It appears that the rate of port site recurrences, although still slightly higher, may be approaching the incidence of open incisional recurrences reported by Hughes et al.

For port wound tumors to develop there must be free, viable cancer cells within the abdominal cavity and a means of transporting the cells to the port wounds. Port wound tumors are unlikely to result from hematogenous or lymphatic spread based on anatomical grounds. In a study of specimens after open colectomy for cancer, Turnbull et al. (21) demonstrated that liberated tumor cells are often present in the blood contained in the specimen. Other investigators have found tumor cells in the blood from the operative field. Liberated tumor cells have also been found in peritoneal fluid samples after open colectomy using standard cytology (22–25). More sensitive immunohistochemical and microbiologic methods have found cancer cells in blood from the operative field in 43 to 100% of patients (26). No matter the mechanism involved, it seems clear that tumor cells are shed into the operative field during colon resection. Direct implantation of cancer cells shed during bowel mobilization and resection seems the most likely mechanism by which tumor cells migrate to port sites. Liberated tumor cells may be transported to the port wounds via CO_2 desufflation events (which may carry cells to the wound in fluid droplets or as an aerosol), specimen extraction through the enlarged port incision, contaminated instruments and trocars, and finally via peritoneal fluid, which may contain tumor cells during the procedure or after closure. Although the true incidence and effect of port site tumor recurrences continue to be evaluated in several prospective randomized trials, numerous investigators using several different animal models have carried out many studies in an attempt to determine the factors influencing port wound tumor development.

Although a large volume of data has been published on this topic, little can be said conclusively about the clinical situation. Studies by Hewitt et al. (27) using a cell suspension model in pigs demonstrated that contaminated instruments and trocars could be the avenue by which tumor cells enter port site wounds. Further studies by Lee et al. (28) using a mouse model in which isolated splenic tumors were established and then resected demonstrated that rough handling of the primary tumor resulted in tumor spillage and abdominal wall recurrences in both open and laparoscopic groups, re-emphasizing the importance of meticulous surgical technique. The presence or absence of a CO_2 pneumoperitoneum, in this study, had no effect on the incidence of port tumors.

Several in vitro studies have been conducted to examine the effect of pressurized gasses on cancer biology and as a possible means of disseminating cancer cells within the abdomen. Jacobi et al. (29) found that cancer cells incubated with CO_2 gas grew more rapidly than those incubated with helium. The same group (30) investigated the effects of pressure and demonstrated that in vitro tumor cell growth was depressed in pressures of 5, 10, and 15 mm Hg. Further work by us (31) using a rigid chamber with an expandable latex pouch was unable to demonstrate aerosolization of tumor cells from a liquid cell suspension after multiple manipulations. We did demonstrate, however, that droplets of cell suspension carrying viable tumor cells could be transported via sudden desufflation. In an in vivo study, Wittich et al. (32) attempted to transport viable tumor cells via aerosolization from a cell suspension in one animal to a second animal through a 2.5-cm plastic cannula connecting the animals. None of the recipient animals developed tumors.

Recognizing that tumor spillage is an inevitable consequence of colon resection, several investigators have examined ways to reduce the tumor cell load and to protect the port site wounds from tumor cell implantation. In mice, Eshraghi et al. (33) demonstrated that port wound irrigation with 5-flourouracil was associated with significantly less port wound tumor formation than port site treatment with sterile water, saline, heparin, or nothing. Jacobi et al. (34) found that intraperitoneal injection of heparin caused a decrease in peritoneal tumor growth, whereas intraperitoneal injection of taurolidine reduced both peritoneal and port wound tumor establishment. The results of this study have encouraged its authors to perform standard postoperative lavage with 0.2% taurolidine and 5000 i.E/L heparin. Lee et al. (35) demonstrated a reduction in abdominal wall recurrences when the abdomen was irrigated with a 0.25% betadine solution before removal of the laparoscopic instruments in mice. Similarly, Schneider et al. (36), in a large animal survival study, demonstrated a significant reduction in port tumors when betadine irrigation was used at the end of the case.

Because tumor cells can be liberated during surgery, laparoscopic techniques have been modified to reduce port wound tumor recurrence. To date, wound protectors, limitation of instrument exchange, avoidance of inadvertent desufflation events, and port anchoring techniques are being practiced routinely in some centers. Some surgeons are also routinely irrigating the abdomen with tumoricidal agents.

CURRENT TRIALS

Several large studies are under way both in the United States and abroad that are designed to compare laparoscopic to open resection for colonic malignancies (Table 17.1). Franklin et al. (12) enrolled 415 patients in a prospective study comparing laparoscopic and open resection for colon cancer. The laparoscopic arm included 166 patients with stage I to III tumors and the open arm recruited 202. The conversion rate from laparoscopic to open resection was 4.18%. The complication rates were lower in the laparoscopic (17%) than in the open (23%) group. This study also noted a significantly shorter length of stay in the laparoscopic group. No significant differences in

TABLE 17.1. CURRENT TRIALS

	Number of Patients	Lymph Node Retrieval		
Year	Laparoscopic/Open	Laporoscopic	Open	Reference
1998	55/54	19	25	15
1996	32/49	9	7.1	11
1996	189/217	15.3	13	12
1995	25/25	6	10	37
1994	80/53	8	6.1	38
1994	18/24	10.6	7.9	39

the total length of bowel resected, proximal and distal margins, and lymph node harvest were noted between groups when stratified based on the segment of colon resected. At last report, with about a 30-month mean follow-up, no abdominal wound tumor recurrences had been noted in either group. The intra-abdominal recurrence and distant metastatic tumor rates, as well as the survival rates, were similar for both the open and minimally invasive groups.

Lacy et al. (14) carried out a single-center trial in Barcelona, Spain. An interim report regarding the short-term results of 91 trial patients documented a significant length of stay benefit as well as significantly shorter time to return of bowel function. No port site tumors were noted with an average follow-up of about 2 years.

Milsom et al. (15) reported on 99 patients who underwent either laparoscopic (55) or open (54) colon resection. The indication for operation was cancer in 76 and 70%, respectively. The complication rate was 15% for each group, and there was one perioperative mortality in each group. After a mean follow-up of 36 months in each group, no port wound tumors were found in the laparoscopic group, but two abdominal wall recurrences were found in the open group. This study reported a shorter hospital stay for the laparoscopic than for the open group (6 vs. 7 days); however, this was not statistically significant.

The study that promises to best characterize both the risks and benefits of laparoscopic colon resection for cancer is the COST study comparing laparoscopic and open techniques for curative resection. This is a randomized, multicenter trial that plans to enroll 1200 patients with primary colon cancer. The length of follow-up will be up to 8 years. The goals of the study are to determine rates of disease-free survival and relative rates of mortality and morbidity. To date, 590 patients have been enrolled, but no data on mortality or morbidity are yet available. One report revealed that total length of bowel resected, proximal and distal margins, and the average number of lymph nodes harvested is the same in both groups thus far (13).

The members of the COST study group conducted a retrospective analysis of the patients they had operated on before initiating the trial (their early experience). A total of 16 of the 32 study members had operated on 372 patients with stage I to IV cancer. The conversion rate in this analysis was 15%, the perioperative mortality was 2%, and the overall port wound tumor recurrence rate was 1.3% (19).

SUMMARY AND RECOMMENDATIONS

Laparoscopic colon resection, in experienced hands, can be performed safely and reliably with many potential benefits to the patient. Length of stay has consistently been demonstrated to be less for laparoscopic than for open surgery patients. Other potential, but less conclusively demonstrated, benefits include improved cosmesis, better preservation of cell-mediated immune function, reduced tumor cell proliferation, more rapid return of bowel function, decreased need for analgesics, and a decreased rate of adhesion formation. Despite these benefits, laparoscopic colon resection for cancer continues to be viewed skeptically within the colorectal community. Initial concerns about the adequacy of resection have been resolved by several large studies; however, the threat of port site tumor recurrences remains an important concern. Data from randomized, prospective, multicenter trials will, it is hoped, settle this issue.

REFERENCES

1. Allendorf JD, Bessler M, Whelan RL, et al. Better preservation of immune function after laparoscopic-assisted vs open bowel resection in a murine model. Dis Colon Rectum 1996;39(suppl):S67–S72.
2. Whelan RL, Franklin M, Donahue J, et al. Postoperative cell mediated immune response is better preserved after laparoscopic versus open colectomy in humans. Surg Endosc 1998;12:586.

3. Horgan PG, Fitzpatrick M, Couse NF, et al. Laparoscopy is less immunotraumatic than laparotomy. Minim Invasive Ther 1992;1:241–244.
4. Lee SW, Southall J, Gleason NR, Huang EH, Bessler M, Whelan RL. Time course of differences in lymphocyte proliferation after laparotomy vs. insufflation. Surg Endosc 2000;14:145–148.
5. Redmond HP, Watson WG, Houghton T, et al. Immune function in patients undergoing open vs laparoscopic cholecystectomy. Arch Surg 1994;129:1240–1246.
6. Watson RWG, Redmond HP, McCarthy J, et al. Exposure of the peritoneal cavity to air regulates early inflammatory responses to surgery in a murine model. Br J Surg 1995;82:1060–1065.
7. Allendorf JDF, Bessler M, Kayton ML, et al. Increased tumor establishment and growth after laparotomy vs. laparoscopy in a murine model. Arch Surg 1995;130:649–653.
8. Allendorf JD, Bessler M, Horvath KD, et al. Increased tumor establishment and growth after open versus laparoscopic bowel resection in mice. Surg Endosc 1998;12:1035–1038.
9. Lee SW, Gleason NR, Senymanturno K, et al. Colon cancer tumor proliferative index is higher and tumor cell death rate is lower in mice undergoing laparotomy vs. insufflation. Surg Endosc 1998;12:514.
10. Lee SW, Gleason NR, Allendorf JD, et al. A heat labile serum soluble factor(s) stimulates tumor growth following laparotomy in a murine model. Surg Endosc 1999;13(suppl 1):S6.
11. Lord SA, Larach SW, Ferrara A, et al. Laparoscopic resections for colorectal carcinoma: a three year experience. Dis Colon Rectum 1996;39:148–154.
12. Franklin ME, Rosenthal D, Abrego-Medina D, et al. Prospective comparison of open vs. laparoscopic colon surgery for carcinoma: five year results. 1996;39:S35–S46.
13. Stocchi L, Nelson H. Laparoscopic colectomy for colon cancer: trial update. J Surg Oncol 1998;68:255–267.
14. Lacy AM, Delgado S, Garcia-Valdecasas JC, et al. Port site metastases and recurrence after laparoscopic colectomy. A randomized trial. Surg Endosc 1998;12:1039–1042.
15. Milsom JW, BartholomÄus B, Hammerhofer KA, et al. A prospective randomized trial comparing laparoscopic versus conventional techniques in colorectal cancer surgery: a preliminary report. J Am Coll Surg 1998;187:46–57.

16. Hughes ESR, McDermott FT, Polgase AL, et al. Tumor recurrence in the abdominal wall scar after large bowel cancer surgery. Dis Colon Rectum 1983;26:571–572.

17. Berends FJ, Kazemier G, Bonjer HJ, Lange JF. Subcutaneous metastases after laparoscopic colectomy [Letter]. Lancet 1994;344:58.

18. Lacy AM, GarcÍa-Valdecasas JC, PiquÉ JM, et al. Short-term outcome analysis of a randomized study comparing laparoscopic vs open colectomy for colon cancer. Surg Endosc 1995;9:1101–1105.

19. Reilly WT, Nelson H, Schroeder G, et al. Wound recurrence following conventional treatment of colorectal cancer. Dis Colon Rectum 1996;39:200–207.

20. Fleshman JW, Nelson H, Peters WR, et al. Early results laparoscopic surgery for colorectal cancer: retrospective analysis of 372 patients treated by Clinical Outcomes of Surgical Therapy (COST) Study Group. Dis Colon Rectum 1996;39:S53–S58.

21. Turnbull RB, Kyle K, Watson FR, et al. Cancer of the colon: the influence of the no touch isolation technique on survival rates. Ann Surg 1967;166;420–427.

22. Horattas MC, Evasovich MR, Tophan N. Colorectal carcinoma and the relationship of peritoneal cytology. Am J Surg 1997;174:334–337.

23. Martin JK Jr, Goellner JR. Abdominal fluid cytology in patients with gastrointestinal malignant lesions. Mayo Clin Proc 1986;61:467–471.

24. Murphy PD, Wadhera V, Griffin, et al. Free peritoneal tumor cell identification in patients with gastric and colorectal cancer. J R Coll Surg Edinb 1993;38:28–32.

25. Solomon MJ, Egan M, Roberts RA, et al. Incidence of free colorectal cancer cells on the peritoneal surface. Dis Colon Rectum 1997;40:1294–1298.

26. Leather AJ, Kocjan G, Savage F, et al. Detection of free malignant cells in the peritoneal cavity before and after resection of colorectal cancer. Dis Colon Rectum 1994;37:814–819.

27. Hewett PJ, Thomas WM, King G, Eaton M. Intraperitoneal cell movement during abdominal carbon dioxide insufflation and laparoscopy: an in vivo model. Dis Colon Rectum 1996;39:S62–S66.

28. Lee SW, Southall J, Allendorf M, et al. Traumatic handling of the tumor independent of pneumoperitoneum increases port site implantation rate of colon cancer in a murine model. Surg Endosc 1998;12:828–834.

29. Jacobi CA, Ordemann J, Wenger F, et al. The impact of elevated intraabdominal pressure during laparoscopy on tumor growth and trocar metastases in a rat model [Abstract]. Surg Endosc 1998;12:513.

30. Jacobi CA, Ordemann J, Bohm B, et al. Inhibition of peritoneal tumor cell growth and implantation in laparoscopic surgery in a rat model. Paper presented at international meeting of Animal Laparoscopic Researchers, Frankfurt, Germany, 1997.

31. Whelan RL, Seller GJ, Allendorf JDF, et al. Trocar site recurrence is unlikely to result from aerosolization of tumor cells. Dis Colon Rectum 1996;39:S7–S13.

32. Wittich P, Bonthuis F, Marquet RL, et al. Port-site metastases: is Aerosolization a pivotal factor [Abstract]? Surg Endosc 1998;12:519.

33. Eshraghi N, Bax T, Bair A, et al. The effect of laparoscopic port site irrigation on the incidence of wound site metastases [abstract]. Surg Endosc 1998;12:512.

34. Jacobi CA, Wuildbredt P, MÜller JM. Influence of gases and intraperitoneal instillation of different agents in the prevention of metastases during laparoscopy [Abstract]. Surg Endosc 1999;13(suppl):S18.

35. Lee S, Gleason N, Bessler M, Whelan RL. Peritoneal irrigation with betadine solution following laparoscopic splenectomy significantly decreases port tumor recurrence in a murine model. Dis Colon Rectum 1999;42:319–326.

36. Schneider C, Reymond MA, Tannapfel A, et al. Port site metastases can be largely prevented [Abstract]. Surg Endosc 1998;12:517.

37. Saba AK, Kerlakian GM, Kasper GC, Hearn AT. Laparoscopic assisted colectomies vs open colectomy. J Laparoendoscopic Surg 1995;5:1–6.

38. Hoffman GC, Baker JW, Fitchett CW, Vansant JH. Laparoscopic-assisted colectomy. Initial experience. Ann Surg 1994;219:732–740.

39. Musser DJ, Boorse RC, Madera F, Reed JF. Laparoscopic colectomy: at what cost? Surg Laparoscopy, Endoscopy & Percutaneous Tech 1994;4:1–5.

CHAPTER

18

UNCOMMON TUMORS OF THE COLON AND RECTUM

JAIME L. MAYORAL, M.D., AND
CHITTAMURU V. SURENDRANATH, M.D.

Although adenocarcinoma of the colon and rectum is the most common malignancy seen in clinical practice, sometimes the clinician comes across other less common malignancies that provide variety and challenge to his or her clinical and surgical skills. Often such lesions are difficult to clinically differentiate from routine adenocarcinomas, and it is the pathologist who first calls into attention the pathologic variation. Understanding the natural course and biology of these less common lesions assists the clinician in modifying the therapeutic interventions.

These tumors are better understood by defining the tissue from which they originate. They are thus categorized as originating from malignant epithelial, lymphoid, mesenchymal, vascular, or neural tissue or as metastatic from a primary malignancy outside of the large intestine (Table 18.1).

Colon and Rectal Cancer, Edited by Peter S. Edelstein, M.D.
ISBN 0-471-35145-8

TABLE 18.1. UNCOMMON TUMORS OF THE COLON AND RECTUM CATEGORIZED BY TISSUE OF ORIGIN

Malignant epithelial tumors
- Carcinoid
- Malignant melanoma
- Squamous cell carcinoma
- Adenosquamous carcinoma/stem cell carcinoma
- Neuroendocrine carcinoma
- Cloacogenic carcinoma

Lymphoid tumors
- Primary malignant lymphoma
- Extramedullary plasmacytoma

Mesenchymal tumors
- Fibrosarcoma
- Malignant fibrous histiocytoma
- Leiomyosarcoma
- Liposarcoma
- Rhabdomyosarcoma

Vascular tumors
- Kaposi's sarcoma

Neural tissue tumors
- Ganglioneuromas

Metastatic tumors

MALIGNANT EPITHELIAL TUMORS

CARCINOID TUMOR

Next to adenocarcinomas, carcinoids are the most common malignant intestinal lesions, although the incidence of lymphoma is rising. Carcinoids originate from the Kulchitsky or basogranular cells and can be found anywhere along the course of the gastrointestinal tract. The relative frequency of occurrence of carcinoid in the different gastrointestinal organs is appendix, small bowel, rectum, stomach, and colon. Women are diagnosed with intestinal carcinoid tumors twice as frequently as are men. Because of the potential for carcinoid to metastasize, these lesions were believed to behave like most carcinomas until it was realized that the usual course of these tumors is relatively benign. Carcinoid of the large bowel is most commonly found in the right colon and the rectum. The colonic carcinoids are usually larger in size than their small bowel counterparts and are frequently associated with metastases, likely owing to the fact that they are relatively asymptomatic in the colon until they achieve a greater size. Carcinoids of the appendix are usually found incidentally on pathologic examination after routine appendectomy. Carcinoids of the rectum tend to be smaller when they are first discovered as compared to the colonic lesions, possibly owing to the more frequent use of sigmoidoscopy than of colonoscopy or barium enemas in cancer screening.

Pathologic evaluation shows midgut carcinoids (ligament of Trietz to midtransverse colon) to be both argentaffin and argyrophil positive, and $<10\%$ of these patients have carcinoid syndrome symptoms caused by the overproduction of serotonin, 5-hydroxytryptamine (5HT). Hindgut carcinoids (distal transverse colon, left colon, and rectum) are only very rarely argyrophil and argentaffin positive, and hindgut tumors are not associated with the carcinoid syndrome. Therefore, evaluation of serum levels of 5-HIAA (a serotonin metabolite) may be of benefit in defining metastatic disease for patients with midgut carcinoids but is of no assistance for those with rectal carcinoids. Carcinoids are associated with an increased incidence of either synchronous or metachronous malignancies in other areas of the gastrointestinal tract. We have found a carcinoid of the small bowel and a synchronous adenocarcinoma of the rectum in a patient evaluated for bright red blood per rectum.

Unfortunately, large bowel carcinoids are usually asymptomatic until they attain a large size. Pain, bleeding, and change in bowel habits are the most common complaints and may mimic those of colorectal adenocarcinoma. The presence of a palpable mass and symptoms suggestive of the carcinoid syndrome, such as diarrhea, may signify that the lesion has spread. Appendiceal carcinoids are usually asymptomatic and rarely actually cause appendicitis.

All patients suspected of having a carcinoid tumor should have an endoscopic examination of the entire colon and rectum. Colonoscopy will identify the carcinoid and rule out any other synchronous lesions; and determining the size of the carcinoid also assists in determining the initial management of the tumor. Rectal carcinoids are usually palpable on digital examination. On proctoscopy, the tumor appears as a small, circumscribed, yellowish, submucosal nodule. Large colonic lesions may demonstrate ulceration of the overlying mucosa and thus may be difficult to distinguish from adenocarcinoma endoscopically.

Appendiceal carcinoids are most frequently found incidentally on pathologic study and are usually <2 cm. The literature demonstrates that all patients with appendiceal carcinoids <1 cm in greatest diameter do well with an appendectomy alone, with no reported incidence of recurrence. Lesions larger than 2 cm have a significantly greater incidence of spread into the draining regional lymph nodes and, therefore, require that the patient undergo a more radical resection in the form of a right hemicolectomy. Lesions between 1 and 2 cm seem to be best treated with an appendectomy. However, if any carcinoid tumor <2 cm demonstrates evidence of spread into the mesoappendix or lymphatic invasion, or if the tumor is situated at the base of the appendix (near the surgical resection margin), a return to the operating room for a formal right hemicolectomy should seriously be considered. In such situations, the age of the patient may influence the decision to return to the operating room, given the relatively benign nature of these malignancies. Thus a younger patient would likely benefit from a more radical procedure, whereas an older patient may best be served by an appendectomy alone. The surgeon must keep in mind the reported incidence of metastases for smaller appendiceal carcinoids: 0% for tumors <1 cm; 0 to 11% for lesions between 1 and 2 cm. At the time of diagnosis, 30 to 60% of patients with lesions > 2 cm have synchronous lymphatic metastases. Fortunately, the overwhelming majority of appendiceal carcinoids are <2 cm in size, and 5-year survival is 90 to 100%.

Only about 5% of all carcinoid tumors are located in the colon. These lesions most frequently arise in the cecum and ascending colon (60%). Data from the literature support limited local excision for tumors <2 cm and standard colon resection for tumors >2 cm. The 5-year survival for all patients with primary colonic carcinoid tumors is 30 to 40%.

Carcinoids of the rectum are more common than carcinoids of the colon and most are <1 cm in size and asymptomatic. They tend to be found on endoscopy being performed for evaluation of complaints unrelated to the carcinoid. Rectal carcinoids often produce prostatic acid phosphatase (80%) and many (25%) produce carcinoembryonic antigen (CEA). Thus rectal carcinoid should be included along with cancer of the prostate and adenocarcinoma of the rectum in the differential diagnosis of a patient with a rectal mass and such elevated tumor markers. Furthermore, as mentioned previously, synchronous adenocarcinoma and carcinoid coexist in approximately 7% of carcinoid patients. Rectal tumors <1 cm are adequately treated with local excision, usually accomplished via transanal excision. Lesions >2 cm are much more likely to have spread into the regional lymphatics, and thus a radical resection (anterior, low anterior, or abdominoperineal resection) is required. Rectal lesions between 1 and 2 cm can usually be adequately treated with a local excision, because lymphatic involvement is rare. But if the pathology returns suggesting a larger tumor size or evidence of lymphatic invasion, radical surgery should be considered.

When metastatic lesions cause symptoms (usually liver metastases), medical treatment with somatostatin analogues can be very helpful. Daily doses of 300 to 600 μg have been used to manage such patients. Palliative chemotherapy is otherwise not very effective. 5-FU and streptozotocin have been used with varying amounts of success. Treatment of symptomatic metastatic lesions with 131-I MIBG has been reported to be of benefit for some patients. Surgical debulking of metastatic disease may in many patients help alleviate symptoms and, despite the inability to cure the patient, should be seriously considered.

MALIGNANT MELANOMA

Primary malignant melanoma of the gastrointestinal tract is rare, and the most common site is the anus. Anal melanoma accounts for 0.25 to 1.1% of all primary tumors of the anal canal. Melanoma arises from the melanocytes in the anal canal and tends to spread both proximally into the rectum and distally out onto the anal margin. Anal melanoma is more common in females.

The tumor initially presents as a small, dark lesion, which is usually undetected or ignored by the patient and sometimes by the doctor, frequently being misdiagnosed as a hemorrhoid. By the time patients present to a surgeon, the lesions are larger, ulcerated, and frequently associated with bleeding. Sometimes the lesions are not pigmented, lowering suspicion until the diagnosis is made on biopsy. Malignant melanoma is highly invasive and spreads locally. Lymphatic spread to the inguinal, perirectal, and internal iliac lymph nodes is common at initial presentation. Hematogenous spread to the liver, lungs, brain, and bones is sometimes present at the time of diagnosis.

Melanoma of the anus is usually a lethal disease, as patients most often present in an advanced state. Prognosis is related to the size of the tumor, the depth of tumor penetration into the skin and subcutaneous tissue, and to the overall stage of the disease. The 5-year survival is dismal, ranging from 0 to 12%. Tumor thickness is measured using the Breslow and Clark classification. Workup includes CT scan of the abdomen, looking for liver metastasis as well as intra-abdominal and inguinal lymph nodes, colonoscopy, and chest X-ray. Bone scans may be indicated, depending on symptoms.

Tumor size dictates the procedure of choice in terms of patient management. Therapy is mostly surgical, supplemented by chemotherapy and/or immunotherapy. Small lesions, <2 cm and Breslow stage I, can be treated with a wide local excision. Breslow stage II lesions may be similarly treated, depending on the presence of surrounding adenopathy. Lesions thicker than this have a poor prognosis, and many authors have recommended aggressive therapy with abdominoperineal resection. Whether such a radical surgical approach improves survival is unclear. Some authors claim that wide local resection produces the same survival rate as a major resection while reducing morbidity and mortality. Abdominoperineal resection may have to performed for palliation if the tumor is large, fungating, and produces severe fecal incontinence owing to involvement of the majority of the sphincter mechanism.

Adjuvant chemotherapy has been used with or without radiation, but the results have generally been disappointing. Immunotherapy with interferon α2b has shown improved survival in node-positive cutaneous melanoma patients and may offer promise in patients suffering from anal melanoma.

SQUAMOUS CELL CARCINOMA

Squamous cell carcinoma of the colon and rectum is an extremely rare tumor, with < 100 cases reported in the literature. This large bowel lesion should be differentiated from the much more common lesion that develops in the anus. The most frequent origin of this uncommon tumor is the rectosigmoid junction. Theories regarding the cancer's origin vary from suggestions that it arises from squamous cell remnants within the colonic mucosa to postulations that it represents a metaplastic change of the columnar epithelium into a squamous variety. The tumor is extremely aggressive, and at the time of diagnosis the tumor is usually advanced. Therapy is with radical resection, but the prognosis is poor.

LYMPHOID TUMORS

LYMPHOMA

Lymphoma of the large bowel accounts for $<1\%$ of all colorectal malignancies and for 10 to 20% of primary gastrointestinal lymphomas. The right side of the colon is the most frequent site of origin, followed by the rectum. Primary colorectal lymphomas are commonly of the non-Hodgkin variety. Hodgkin lymphoma of the colorectum is rare. Association of colorectal lymphoma with long-standing ulcerative colitis and as a complication of radiation therapy, immunosuppressive therapy, and ureterosigmoidostomy has been reported by numerous authors. Lymphoma of the rectum has been increasingly reported in homosexual males, and the incidence of lymphoma is increased with concomitant presence of HIV. In general, lymphoma of the colon is more common in males.

Although lymphoma of the large bowel can be seen as part of a systemic lymphoma process, in our practice we have more commonly seen these lesions as isolated, primary large intestinal lymphomas. (This may be owing to patient referral bias, because the majority of systemic lymphomas are managed by medical specialists, and the colonic management in such cases is generally part of the overall patient management.) Lesions tend to be multicentric when they are part of a systemic manifestation.

Primary large bowel lymphomas are usually bulky, right-sided, and associated with bleeding and crampy abdominal pain. Weight loss and a change in bowel habits may also be associated symptoms. Colonic lymphomas may present in a variety of forms: mass lesions with extensive mucosal destruction, large lobulated masses with minimal destruction, mucosal nodularity resembling pseudopolyposis of inflammatory bowel disease, infiltrative forms appearing as rigid bowel segments or an annular strictures, and bulky extracolonic masses.

Lymphomas develop within the submucosal layer of the colon and spread into the mucosa and the lumen and/or deeper into the muscularis propria and the extracolonic space. Lesions usually originate as monocentric, although polycentric origin cannot be ruled out. Small tumors require differentiation from lymphatic hyperplasia, easily proven by histopathology, which reveals the polyclonal nature of hyperplasia versus the monoclonal nature of lymphoma.

Surgery is the main therapeutic approach for primary colorectal lymphoma. We have removed lesions of the right colon that have on pathologic examination turned out to be Burkitts lymphomas. When these slow-growing lymphomas have been isolated to the colon with no evidence of lymph node involvement, we have chosen only to observe these patients postoperatively. For these same tumors, some authors recommend adjuvant chemotherapy with or without local irradiation. The CHOP regimen is frequently the chemotherapy chosen. Aggressive lymphomas have been treated postoperatively with *m*-BACOD (methotrexate, bleomycin, doxorubicin, cyclophosphamide, vincristine, and dexamethasone), although there are no reports that clearly demonstrate that this regimen is superior to the CHOP regimen. When the disease is systemic or has progressed beyond the colorectum, initial treatment with chemotherapy and radiation may be helpful before surgical intervention. The risk of perforation during such medical management is always present, because the malignant cells die and necrose, and emergent surgical intervention is required on occasion.

EXTRAMEDULLARY PLASMACYTOMA

Extramedullary plasmacytoma, a malignancy of plasma cell origin, is rarely found as a primary condition of the colon and rectum. More often the colon is secondarily involved as part of disseminated multiple myeloma, and even more rarely the rectum is directly invaded by a sacral plasmacytoma. When a colonic plasmacytoma is suspected, workup for multiple myeloma, including bone marrow biopsy, should be performed before assuming a primary large bowel origin. Local excision or resection for primary lesions should suffice. When the tumors are large and bulky, radiotherapy may shrink the tumor and can be helpful preoperatively. Chemotherapy is restricted to cases of disseminated disease.

MESENCHYMAL TUMORS

FIBROMA AND FIBROSARCOMA

Benign fibromas of the colon and rectum are rare spindle cell tumors and are frequently referred to in the literature as fibromyomas. They may be asymptomatic or produce symptoms of obstruction, constipation, pain, tenesmus, and bleeding. For colonic lesions, bowel resection is appropriate. Rectal lesions diagnosed on biopsy may be treated with local excision.

The malignant counterpart, fibrosarcomas, are equally as uncommon and are usually found in the rectum. Fibrosarcoma of the colon is extremely rare. Fibrosarcoma of the rectum presents as a mass lesion that can also be asymptomatic or can produce difficulty in defecation and a sense of incomplete evacuation. Pain and bleeding may also be associated with a rectal fibrosarcoma. On endoscopy, the lesion appears similar to an adenocarcinoma, and differentiation often requires histologic examination, wherein spindle cells predominate within the biopsy specimen. Treatment is surgical and follows the same surgical guidelines as for rectal adenocarcinoma. Unfortunately, fibrosarcomas rarely respond to chemotherapy or irradiation.

MALIGNANT FIBROUS HISTIOCYTOMA

Malignant fibrous histiocytoma (MFH) is a variant of fibrosarcoma and is also rarely seen as a primary colorectal tumor. The presence of histiocyte-like cells differentiate this tumor from fibrosarcoma. Both the slow growing nature of this tumor and its propensity for recurrence are demonstrated in one of our patients in whom this cancer presented as a metastatic lesion to the colon 2 years after the excision of an MFH from the lower extremity combined with a wedge resection of a pulmonary metastasis.

LEIOMYOMA AND LEIOMYOSARCOMA

Benign smooth muscle lesions of the colon and rectum are uncommon. Usually these growths are found incidentally. Reports of leiomyomas presenting as lead points in large bowel intussusception have been published but are few. These tumors can grow as intraluminal masses or be completely extracolonic. Dumbbell tumors that grow both into the lumen and in an extracolonic fashion are more common. Leiomyomas tend to develop in the left colon. Differentiation from a malignant lesion is based on the number of mitoses on histologic examination. Gross tumor size is also important, and lesions >2.5 cm are usually malignant in nature.

Leiomyosarcomas of the colon are also very uncommon. These are usually low-grade malignant neoplasms, but they carry a poor prognosis because of the late stage in which they commonly are diagnosed. The lower the frequency of mitoses on histologic examination, the better the prognosis. Leiomyosarcomas can grow so large that complete curative resection is not possible. Debulking of such giant lesions slows the progress of the disease, and repeated operations as these lesions grow back are frequently necessary and appropriate. Metastatic spread to the liver via the portal system carries a very poor prognosis. Leiomyosarcomas are not usually radiosensitive. Chemotherapy with adriamycin-based regimens may be of some limited benefit.

Rectal leiomyosarcomas arise from the smooth muscle of the rectum and the internal sphincter. Extensive spread into the perirectal tissues is usually present. Tumors tend to recur even after what initially appears to be a curative abdominoperineal resection.

LIPOMA AND LIPOSARCOMA

Lipomas are second only to polyps as the most common benign tumors of the colon and rectum. They are most frequently detected as incidental findings at autopsy. Lipomas are well differentiated, benign fatty tumors arising from the adipose connective tissue within the wall of the large bowel. Most lipomas are submucosal (90%), and the remainder are subserosal (10%). Most colonic lipomas are asymptomatic. When tumor size exceeds 2 cm, however, they can produce symptoms including constipation, abdominal pain, diarrhea, bleeding, and intestinal obstruction. When a mass is palpable, it is more likely to be bowel obstruction with fecal impaction and/or intussusception than the actual tumor itself. However, subserosal lipoma, which usually arise from the appendices epiploicae, may be felt as abdominal masses on palpation.

Lipomas of the large bowel are found (in order of decreasing frequency) in the cecum, ascending colon, sigmoid colon, and rectum. Lipomatosis of the ileocecal valve may be visualized on colonoscopy and frequently acts as a lead point in an adult intussusception. On endoscopy, the cushion or pillow sign, when the lesion indents on pressure with biopsy forceps and remains indented after removal of the instrument, and the naked fat sign, in which a tuft of yellow tissue from the lipoma exudes into the lumen after mucosal biopsy, are telltale diagnostic signs. Asymptomatic lesions do not require treatment. When colorectal lipomas cause pain, bleeding, or obstruction, local resection or limited resection of the bowel will suffice.

Liposarcoma of the large intestine are exceedingly rare and should be evaluated and treated in a manner similar to that for leiomyosarcoma. If malignant transformation of benign colorectal lipomasis occurs at all, it is incredibly uncommon.

VASCULAR TUMORS

KAPOSI SARCOMA

Classic Kaposi sarcoma is a cutaneous disorder afflicting Italian and Jewish men of central European descent. In this form, the disease usually does not involve the rectum. However, Kaposi sarcoma has become increasingly common since the 1980s and has paralleled the rise of AIDS in the general population. This epidemic variety of Kaposi sarcoma frequently does involve the gastrointestinal tract. Kaposi sarcoma involving the bowel is also associated with immunosuppressed transplant patients.

Diarrhea, rectal bleeding, and pain are common symptoms of Kaposi sarcoma. The tumor should always be considered in the differential diagnosis of homosexual males who present with persisting diarrhea. On endoscopy, the lesions can be in the rectum and/or the colon and appear as purple, spongy growths with an irregular shape. They are usually submucosal and firm when pressed with an endoscopic instrument. Most endoscopists are appropriately reluctant to biopsy what appear to be vascular lesions; fortunately, both the patient's other medical illnesses and the endoscopic appearance of the tumors allow for a presumptive diagnosis without risking tissue sampling. When palliative treatment is required, local or limited excision may be adequate. Usually treatment of colorectal Kaposi sarcoma takes a back seat to treatment of the generalized disease (usually AIDS) and of the prevalent opportunistic infections. If palliation is required and the patient believed to be too poor a surgical candidate, radiation therapy can be helpful for localized disease. Systemic Kaposi is treated with combination chemotherapy, including adriamycin, bleomycin, vinblastine, vincristin, and etoposide.

NEURAL TISSUE TUMORS

GANGLIONEUROMA

Ganglioneuromas are neuroectodermal tumors rarely found in the colon. Neurogenic tumors more commonly develop in the rectum and within the presacral space. Even in these pelvic locations, ganglioneuromas are extremely rare. The tumors are composed of ganglion cells, Schwann cells, and nerve fibers. Treatment of rectal lesions is usually by local excision. Presacral lesions may need resection via a trans-sacral or parasacral approach.

ENDOMETRIOMA

Endometriomas are tumor-like lesions composed of ectopic endometrial tissue. When present within the mucosa of the colon and rectum (owing to full-thickness penetration from their implant site on the large bowel serosa), endometriomas usually resemble routine adenocarcinomas on endoscopy. However, most endometriomas remain on and within the large bowel wall without penetration into the lumen. There, the masses usually produce obstructive symptoms. Bleeding can also occur either from complete bowel wall penetration into the lumen or from necrosis of mucosa overlying an intramural endometrioma. Excision of the colonic or rectal segment involved by this benign growth is usually sufficient treatment. Postoperative complications, including fistula formation, are not uncommon after surgical resection of these frequently frustrating lesions. Extensive endometrial disease not amenable to surgical extirpation requires hormonal management, occasionally including bilateral oophorectomy. Medroxy progesterone acetate aids in controlling any residual tumor left behind after surgical excision.

INDEX